Ernst Schering Research Foundation Workshop 18
The Endometrium as a Target for Contraception

Springer-Verlag Berlin Heidelberg GmbH

Ernst Schering Research Foundation
Workshop 18

The Endometrium as a
Target for Contraception

H.M. Beier, M.J.K. Harper, K. Chwalisz
Editors

With 68 Figures and 14 Tables

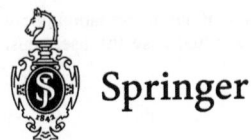 Springer

Series Editors: G. Stock and U.-F. Habenicht

Die Deutsche Bibliothek – CIP-Einheitsaufnahme
Schering-Forschungsgesellschaft <Berlin>:
Ernst Schering Research Foundation Workshop. – Berlin; Heidelberg; New York; Barcelona; Budapest; Hong Kong; London; Milan; Paris; Santa Clara; Singapore; Tokyo: Springer.
ISSN 0947-6075
NE: HST
18. The endometrium as a target for contraception. – 1997
The endometrium as a target for contraception ; with 14 tables / H.M. Beier ... ed. – Berlin; Heidelberg; New York; Barcelona; Budapest; Hong Kong; London; Milan; Paris; Santa Clara; Singapore; Tokyo: Springer, 1997
(Ernst Schering Research Foundation Workshop; 18)
ISBN 978-3-662-10325-8   ISBN 978-3-662-10323-4 (eBook)
DOI 10.1007/978-3-662-10323-4

NE: Beier, H.M. [Hrsg.]

CIP data applied for

The use of general descriptive names, registered names, trademarks, etc. in this publication does not imply, even in the absence of a specific statement, that such names are exempt from the relevant protective laws and regulations and therefore free for general use.

Product liability: The publishers cannot guarantee the accuracy of any information about dosage and application contained in this book. In every individual case the user must check such information by consulting the relevant literature.

Typesetting: Data conversion by Springer-Verlag
21/3135–5 4 3 2 1 0 – Printed on acid-free paper

Preface

Progesterone, the hormone "pro gestationem", plays a pivotal role in mammalian reproduction during almost all phases of the menstrual cycle and all stages of pregnancy. It is involved in the control of ovulation, prepares the endometrium for implantation, and, in later stages of pregnancy, is responsible for its maintenance by suppressing uterine contractility. The sudden withdrawal of progesterone action at the end of the nonfertile cycle leads to the constriction of spiral arteries and, in turn, to menstruation in human beings and nonhuman primates. The decrease in serum progesterone concentrations or its functional withdrawal in the myometrium and decidua are the most important events during parturition in various mammals.

In the uterus, progesterone controls the growth and differentiation of endometrial and myometrial cells and regulates a variety of cell functions directly by either stimulating or inhibiting structural and functional proteins, but also indirectly by functionally opposing estradiol action. In the nonpregnant uterus, there are different progesterone effects on uterine cell proliferation which vary among species. In the fertile cycle, progesterone regulates in synergism with estradiol the transport of the fertilized eggs and the cleavage stage embryos through the oviduct and induces the secretory changes in the endometrium required for implantation. During the period between ovulation and implantation, remarkable morphological and biochemical changes in the lumenal and glandular epithelial cells take place under the influence of rising progesterone levels in the human and primate endometrium. These changes include the accumulation of glycogen deposits in the basal cytoplasm, an increasing Golgi apparatus in the apical cytoplasm,

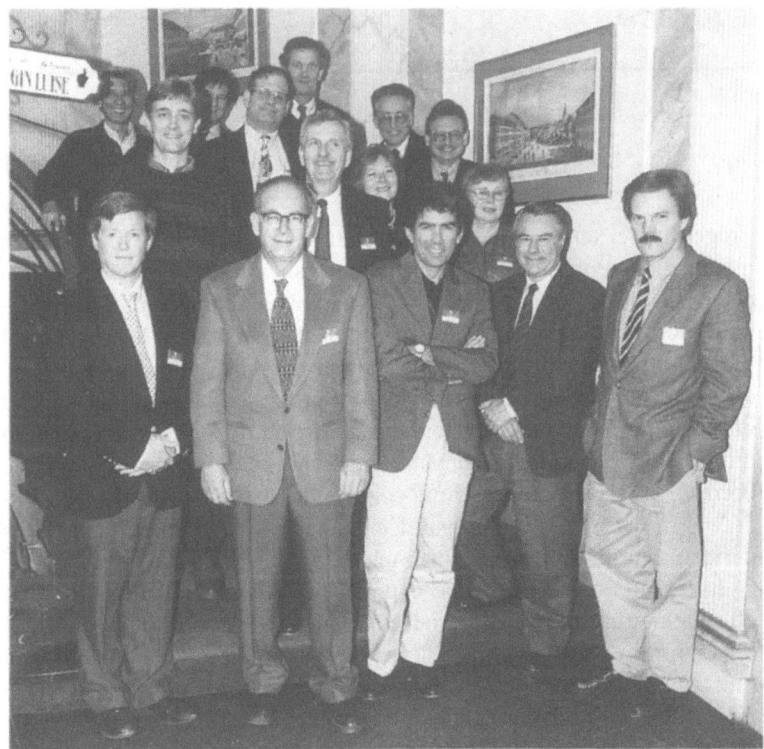

The participants of the workshop

and a continuous increase in secretory vesicles. The maximum secretory capacity of the glandular epithelium is reached a few days after the luteinizing hormone peak and remains high for several days. The secretory proteins, produced by the endometrial glands, and the cell surface proteins as well as the expression of growth factors and cytokines most likely determine the endometrial patterns of receptivity, which appear when the endometrium permits blastocyst attachment and implantation.

These changes are all dependent on progesterone action, mainly after estrogen priming. Consequently, the luteal phase endometrium, actually during the peri-implantation period, may be a very sensitive target for contraception, in particular with all components acting in competition with progesterone. During the last decade several possibilities for using progesterone antagonists in fertility regulation have been suggested, based either on the inhibition of ovulation or on the prevention of implantation after postcoital or early luteal phase treatment. However, only postcoital treatment with progesterone antagonists or their early luteal phase administration on the second day after the luteinizing hormone peak have as yet been proven to be effective in women. The contraceptive effects of progesterone antagonists in these initial clinical approaches are most likely due to their effects on the endometrium.

This volume contains the contributions of the 18th Ernst Schering Research Foundation Workshop, held in Berlin from 29 November to 1 December 1995, which was devoted to the topic of endometrial contraception, a new approach to contraception which does not rely on ovulation inhibition. Since the exact molecular mechanism of action of progesterone antagonists on endometrial receptivity and on the implantation process is still unclear, basic and clinical studies are required to demonstrate which mechanism interferes with those essential steps of the various stages of preimplantation physiology that finally lead to the establishment of implantation and pregnancy.

These fascinating possibilities of applying progesterone antagonists in reproductive medicine for the purpose of contraception brought together molecular biologists, pharmacologists, gynecologists, and endocrinologists. The various topics under discussion proved to be of considerable mutual interest, and their novelty held the attention of the delegates during all sessions of this workshop. The achievements of basic and clinical research on progesterone and its antagonists are reflected in the content of the present book. The views expressed in this volume remain the responsibility of the respective authors.

We are aware of numerous ethical and political controversies in using progesterone antagonists in reproductive medicine. However, it is our fervent hope that research in this area will continue well into the future. The ultimate aim is to improve the quality of human reproductive health. To this end we are confident that the present collection of scientific and clinical research contributions will serve as a basis for further exciting achievements in the development of new means of contraception.

We gratefully acknowledge the generous support for the production of this book and the assistance provided by the Ernst Schering Research Foundation, in particular by Dr. U.-F. Habenicht and Mrs. U. Wanke.

Henning M. Beier
Michael J.K. Harper
Kristof Chwalisz

Table of Contents

List of Editors and Contributors

Editors

H.M. Beier
Department of Anatomy and Reproductive Biology, University of Aachen,
Wendlingweg 2, 52076 Aachen, Germany

K. Chwalisz
Fertility Control and Hormone Therapy Research, Schering AG,
Müllerstraße 178, 13342 Berlin, Germany

M.J.K. Harper
CONRAD Program, 1611 North Kent Street, Suite 806,
Arlington, VA 22209, USA

Contributors

J.D. Aplin
Department of Obstetrics and Gynecology and School of Biological Sciences,
University of Manchester, Research Floor, St. Mary's Hospital,
Manchester M13 0JH, UK

H.M. Beier
Department of Anatomy and Reproductive Biology, University of Aachen,
Wendlingweg 2, 52076 Aachen, Germany

P. Bischof
Department of Obstetrics and Gynecology, University of Geneva, Maternité,
1211 Geneva 14, Switzerland

R.M. Brenner
Division of Reproductive Sciences, Oregon Regional Primate Research
Center, Beaverton, OR 97006, USA

A.J. Castelbaum
UNC-Chapel Hill, Department of Obstetrics and Gynecology,
CB#7570 Old Clinic Building, Chapel Hill, NC 27599-7570, USA

M. Chedid
Laboratory of Cellular and Molecular Biology, N.C.I.,
Bethesda, MD 20892, USA

K. Chwalisz
Fertility Control and Hormone Therapy Research, Schering AG,
Müllerstraße 178, 13342 Berlin, Germany

C. Coutifaris
University of Pennsylvania Center for Research on Reproduction
and Women's Health, Department of Obstetrics and Gynecology,
Room 778 - Clinical Research Building, 415 Curie Boulevard,
Philadelphia, PA 19104-6142, USA

H.B. Croxatto
Istituto Chileno de Medicina Reproductiva, José Ramón Gutiérrez 295,
Depto. 3, Correo 22, Casilla 96, Santiago, Chile

K.G. Csaky
Laboratory of Cellular and Molecular Biology, N.C.I.,
Bethesda, MD 20892, USA

J.E. Fortune
Department and Division of Physiology, University of Cornell,
Ithaca, NY 14853, USA

B. Fuentealba
Istituto Chileno de Medicina Reproductiva, José Ramón Gutiérrez 295,
Depto. 3, Correo 22, Casilla 96, Santiago, Chile

E.E. Furth
University of Pennsylvania Center for Research on Reproduction
and Women's Health, Department of Obstetrics and Gynecology,
Room 778 - Clinical Research Building, 415 Curie Boulevard,
Philadelphia, PA 19104-6142, USA

I. Gemperlein †
formerly: Fertility Control and Hormone Therapy Research, Schering AG,
Müllerstraße 178, 13342 Berlin, Germany

M.J.K. Harper
CONRAD Program, 1611 North Kent Street, Suite 806,
Arlington, VA 22209, USA

K.B. Horwitz
University of Colorado Health Sciences Center, 4200 East Ninth Avenue,
Campus Box B151, Denver, CO 80262, USA

S. Izumi
Department of Anatomy III, Nagasaki University School of Medicine,
1-12-4 Sakamoto, Nagasaki 852, Japan

A. King
Research Group in Human Reproductive Immunobiology,
Department of Pathology, University of Cambridge, Tennis Court Road,
Cambridge CB2 1QP, UK

R. Knauthe
Fertility Control and Hormone Therapy Research, Schering AG,
Müllerstraße 178, 13342 Berlin, Germany

T. Koji
Department of Anatomy III, Nagasaki University School of Medicine,
1-12-4 Sakamoto, Nagasaki 852, Japan

B.A. Lessey
UNC-Chapel Hill, Department of Obstetrics and Gynecology,
CB#7570 Old Clinic Building, Chapel Hill, NC 27599-7570, USA

Y.W. Loke
Research Group in Human Reproductive Immunobiology,
Department of Pathology, University of Cambridge, Tennis Court Road,
Cambridge CB2 1QP, UK

C.D. MacCalman
University of Pennsylvania Center for Research on Reproduction
and Women's Health, Department of Obstetrics and Gynecology,
Room 778 - Clinical Research Building, 415 Curie Boulevard,
Philadelphia, PA 19104-6142, USA

R. Massai
Istituto Chileno de Medicina Reproductiva, José Ramón Gutiérrez 295,
Depto. 3, Correo 22, Casilla 96, Santiago, Chile

A. Omigbodun
University of Pennsylvania Center for Research on Reproduction
and Women's Health, Department of Obstetrics and Gynecology,
Room 778 - Clinical Research Building, 415 Curie Boulevard,
Philadelphia, PA 19104-6142, USA

C.P. Puri
Institute for Research in Reproduction (ICMR), Parel Bombay, India

J.S. Rubin
Laboratory of Cellular and Molecular Biology, N.C.I.,
Bethesda, MD 20892, USA

A.M. Salvatierra
Istituto Chileno de Medicina Reproductiva, José Ramón Gutiérrez 295,
Depto. 3, Correo 22, Casilla 96, Santiago, Chile

S. Shao-Qing
National Research Institute for Family Planning, Beijing, China

O.D. Slayden
Division of Reproductive Sciences, Oregon Regional Primate Research
Center, Beaverton, OR 97006, USA

S.G. Somkuti
UNC-Chapel Hill, Department of Obstetrics and Gynecology,   .
CB#7570 Old Clinic Building, Chapel Hill, NC 27599-7570, USA

J.F. Strauss III
University of Pennsylvania Center for Research on Reproduction
and Women's Health, Department of Obstetrics and Gynecology,
Room 778 - Clinical Research Building, 415 Curie Boulevard,
Philadelphia, PA 19104-6142, USA

G.S. Takimoto
University of Colorado Health Sciences Center, 4200 East Ninth Avenue,
Campus Box B151, Denver, CO 80262, USA

X.C. Tian
Department and Division of Physiology, Cornell University,
Ithaca, NY 14853, USA

L. Tung
University of Colorado Health Sciences Center, 4200 East Ninth Avenue,
Campus Box B151, Denver, CO 80262, USA

L. Yuan
UNC-Chapel Hill, Department of Obstetrics and Gynecology,
CB#7570 Old Clinic Building, Chapel Hill, NC 27599-7570, USA

D. de Ziegler
Columbia Laboratories France, 19, rue du Général Foy, 75008 Paris, France

1 The Molecular Biology of Progesterone Receptors: Why Are There Two Isoforms?

K.B. Horwitz, L. Tung, and G.S. Takimoto

1.1 Introduction

Progesterone is the reproductive and pregnancy hormone. Females without it are infertile. The major target tissues for progesterone are the ovary, uterus, mammary gland, and brain. Synthetic progestational agents are used for contraception and hormone replacement therapy and antiprogestins are in clinical trials for contraception and for the treatment of cancers and uterine disorders. The agonists and antagonists act at their target tissues by binding to progesterone receptors (PR) which consist of two isoforms: human B receptors (hPR$_B$) are 933 amino acids in length, while human A receptors (hPR$_A$) lack the N-terminal 164 amino acids, but are otherwise identical to B receptors. When A and B isoforms are present in equimolar amounts, they dimerize and bind DNA as three species: A/A and B/B homodimers, and A/B heterodimers. This heterogeneity has complicated the study of antiprogestins since each isoform and dimeric species has a unique ligand response profile that varies with the gene and cell in question (Horwitz 1992, and references therein). This chapter reviews recent work from our laboratory dealing with the two isoforms of human PR, focusing on antiprogestin actions in breast cancer cells. These studies have allowed us to pose, but not yet answer, the question in the title of this chapter.

The structure of PR and other members of the steroid receptor family of proteins has been extensively reviewed (Horwitz 1992; Truss and Beato 1993, and references therein). Briefly, these receptors are intranuclear transcription factors whose DNA binding capacity is activated by ligand occupancy. Receptors bind as dimers to specific transcriptional enhancers called hormone response elements (HRE) and regulate gene expression. DNA binding is effected through a DNA binding domain

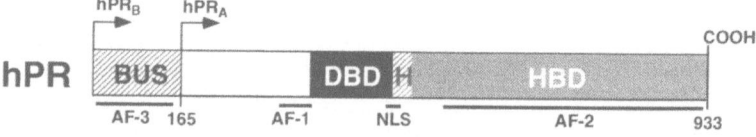

Fig. 1. Model of human progesterone receptors (*hPR*), showing origin of B receptors (*hPR$_B$*) and A receptors (*hPR$_A$*). *BUS*, B-upstream segment; *DBD*, DNA binding domain; *H*, hinge region; *HBD*, hormone binding domain; *NLS*, nuclear localization signal; *AF*, activation function

(DBD) composed of two zinc fingers. The DBD also has weak dimerization functions and may be involved in other protein–protein interactions. Upstream of the DBD is an N-terminal region that usually contains at least one activation function (AF1). However, the 164 amino acid hPR B-receptor upstream segment (BUS) in the far N-terminus contains another activation function (AF3). Downstream of the DBD is a nuclear localization sequence (NLS), followed by a C-terminal region that contains the hormone binding domain (HBD), a strong dimerization domain, a second transcriptional activation function (AF2), and other regions involved in protein–protein interactions (Fig. 1).

1.2 Conventional Inhibitory Actions of Antiprogestins

Two fundamentally different mechanisms underly the actions of antagonist–hPR complexes. The first of these is the classical effect of antagonists; namely, their ability to directly inhibit agonist actions (Horwitz 1992). In this scenario, agonist-occupied hPR regulate transcription by binding as dimers to PREs present on the promoter of the regulated gene. Antagonist-occupied hPR complexes also bind to PREs but are transcriptionally inert. Thus, by this mechanism, antagonist inhibition involves competition between the two ligands, agonist vs. antagonist, for hPR occupancy, followed by competition between the two ligand hPR classes for binding to PREs. With agonists, DNA binding leads to a specific transcriptional response, while with antagonists, the DNA binding is nonproductive (Fig. 2a). It follows that the nonproductive or inhibitory potency of an antagonist is controlled by numerous factors, which include its affinity for the receptors, the affinity of antagonist-occupied hPR complexes for PREs, the number of PREs on a promoter, and probably other factors. As will be discussed below, the two hPR isoforms often have unequal inhibitory potency. In general we find that at equimolar concentrations, antagonist-occupied A receptors are stronger transcriptional and proliferation inhibitors than B receptors.

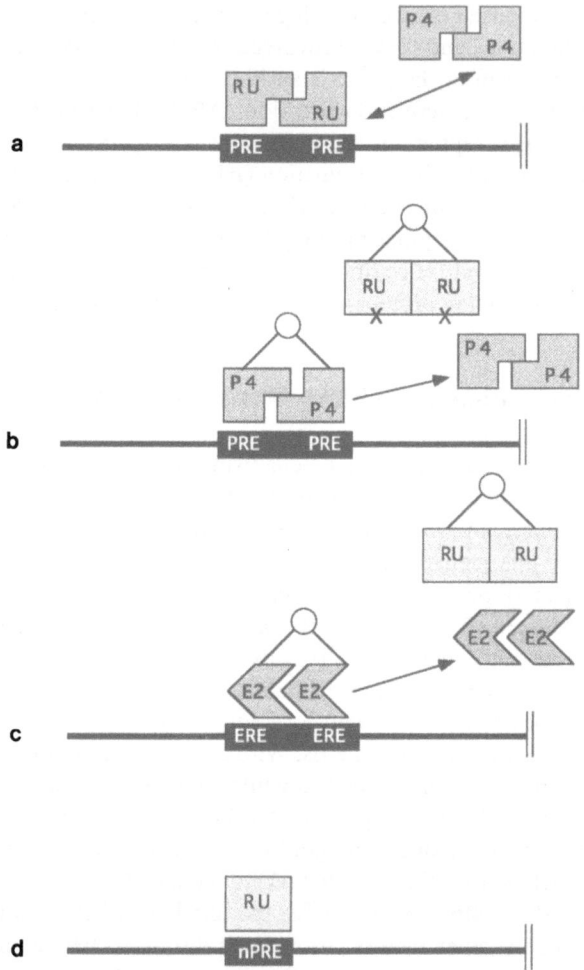

Fig. 2a–d. Antiprogestin inhibition as described in the text. **a** Conventional mechanism: progesterone response element (*PRE*)+ A≥B. **b** Progesterone receptor (PR)-specific accessory factors: PRE+ A>B. **c** Squelching of general factor: PRE–, A-only. **d** Negative PRE: PRE–, A-only. A receptors are depicted as *squares*; B receptors are *L-shaped. RU*, RU486; *P4*; progesterone; *E2*, estradiol bound to estrogen receptors; *ERE*, estrogen response element; *nPRE*, negative PRE

1.3 Nonconventional Inhibitory Actions of Antiprogestins

In addition to their inhibitory effects through direct competition at PREs, new evidence suggests that antiprogestin-occupied hPR can be inhibitory without DNA binding at PREs. Truss et al. (1994) used in vivo footprinting of the mouse mammary tumor virus (MMTV) promoter to show that under conditions in which antiprogestin–hPR complexes inhibit transcription by PRE-bound agonist complexes, the antagonist–hPR complexes are not bound to the PREs. We have shown in unpublished studies that antiprogestin-occupied hPR mutants whose DNA binding specificity has been switched from a PRE to an estrogen response element (ERE) can nevertheless still inhibit transcription by a constitutively active PRE-bound hPR. The mechanisms underlying this inhibition by a receptor that cannot bind a PRE are unknown but could, in theory, be due to squelching of a specific accessory factor required by the PRE-bound receptors (Fig. 2b). Again, in our hands, A receptors are more potent inhibitors than B receptors through this pathway.

Additionally, it is now becoming evident that antagonist-occupied A receptors, but not B receptors, have more general inhibitory properties than previously thought. As discussed further below, antagonist-occupied A receptors can inhibit transactivation by ER from ERE–reporter construct – inhibition that again, does not require receptor binding to PREs. The mechanisms are unknown, but squelching of one or more general factors common to the function of several steroid receptors can be envisioned (Fig. 2c).

Finally, another mechanism for inhibition – once more restricted to A receptors – is through noncanonical DNA binding sites (nPREs) analogous to the negative glucocorticoid response elements (nGREs). One such nPRE has been described in the bovine prolactin promoter (Cairns et al. 1993). Our unpublished studies show that antiprogestin-occupied A receptors, but not B receptors, inhibit constitutive transactivation through this promoter (Fig. 2d).

1.4 Novel Stimulatory Actions
of Antagonist-Occupied hPR$_B$

In addition to novel mechanisms by which antagonist-occupied hPR can be inhibitory, we have been exploring conditions under which antiprogestins can have agonist-like effects. We find that regardless of the model system in which such agonist-like effects can be elicited, it is a property restricted to B receptors (Fig. 3). Again, we find that antago-

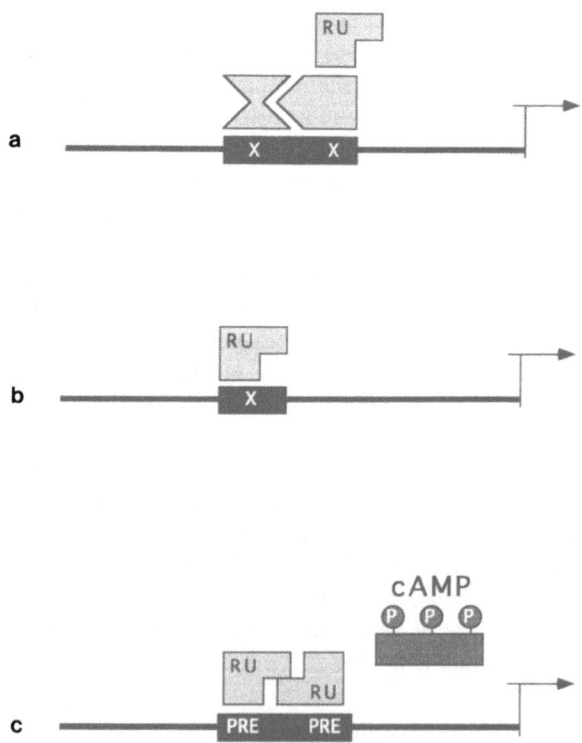

Fig. 3a–c. Activation by antiprogestins – human progesterone receptor B only. **a** Progesterone response element (*PRE*) independent tethering: PRE⁻. **b** Novel DNA binding site: PRE⁻. **c** Phosphorylated coactivator: PRE⁺. *RU*, RU486; *P*, phosphate; *X*, DNA binding site for unknown proteins

nist-occupied hPR_B have inadvertent stimulatory actions through DNA-binding sites or DNA-binding proteins that do not involve the canonical PREs. These novel agonist-like effects could, in theory, affect not only genes that contain PREs, but even genes that were never meant to be regulated by hPR and upon which agonists have no effects. Such mechanisms could explain how an antiprogestin can inadvertently regulate genes that are not normally progesterone targets. There are several experimental models which demonstrate these unusual mechanisms.

1.5 PRE-Independent Transactivation of the Thymidine Kinase Promoter

We have studied the transcription by antagonist-occupied hPR using a chloramphenicol acetyltransferase (CAT) reporter driven by a PRE cloned upstream of the thymidine kinase (*tk*) promoter (Tung et al. 1993). Transient transfection of HeLa cervicocarcinoma cells with an hPR_A expression vector and treatment with the agonist R5020 leads to a 20-fold increase in CAT transcription compared to basal levels. As expected, none of three antiprogestins, RU486, ZK112993, or ZK98299, stimulate transcription. Instead, the antiprogestins typically suppress basal levels. However, in cells expressing hPR_B, not only the agonist, but all three antagonists strongly stimulate CAT transcription. We were surprised that ZK98299 was an activator because, in our hands, receptors occupied by this antagonist do not bind to DNA in vitro or in vivo. This suggested that the activation was independent of PRE binding. We therefore removed the PRE from the *tk* promoter–reporter to test this theory. As expected, agonist-dependent transcription was abolished when the PRE was removed, but, in support of our hypothesis, the anomalous antagonist-dependent activation was retained. Similar results were observed with a B receptor mutant whose DNA-binding specificity was altered so that it would no longer recognize a PRE. When occupied by antiprogestins, these mutant B receptors still activated transcription of the PRE-containing reporter.

Recent data show that other members of the steroid receptor superfamily can have effects independent of the canonical HREs. Potential mechanisms fall into two broad categories. Either the receptors bind to novel DNA sites that differ substantially from the consensus

HREs, or the receptors do not bind DNA at all, but are tethered by other DNA-binding proteins instead (Oro et al. 1988; Sakai et al. 1988; Diamond et al. 1990; Yang-Yen et al. 1990; Jonat et al. 1990; Schüle et al. 1990; Miner and Yamamoto 1991; Kutoh e tla. 1992). By the latter mechanism, two factors establish protein–protein contacts on the DNA, but only one of the two actually binds DNA. However, both the DNA-bound protein and its tethered partner contain a DBD. This model is of particular significance for antagonist-occupied, hPR$_B$-mediated transcription, because we also find a requirement for an intact DBD. Thus, an hPR$_B$ mutant lacking an ordered first zinc finger fails to stimulate transcription when occupied by RU486. In addition to its DNA-binding function, the DBD of steroid receptors is implicated in mediating protein–protein interactions (Diamond et al. 1990; Yang-Yen et al. 1990; Schüle et al. 1990), perhaps through conserved surfaces that face away from the DNA. Indeed, several recent studies show that glucocorticoid receptors (GR) and c-Jun repress one another's activity by protein–protein binding mechanisms that are independent of DNA binding. Nevertheless, to produce repression, an intact GR DBD is required. Additionally, a dimerization function has been assigned to the second zinc finger (Härd et al. 1990), providing further evidence that the DBD mediates protein interactions. We speculate that induction of transcription by antagonist-occupied hPR$_B$ can proceed through a mechanism in which the receptors are tethered to a DNA-bound protein partner, but do not bind DNA themselves (Fig. 3a). Thus, hPR$_B$ could function by linking an activator protein bound to the *tk* promoter to the basal transcriptional machinery. Alternatively, antagonist-occupied hPR$_B$ may bind to novel, as yet undefined, DNA elements (Fig. 3b). In either scenario, the transactivation would be PRE independent.

1.6 Antagonist-Occupied Human hPR$_B$ Are Switched to Agonists by cAMP

By contrast, we have described an entirely different antagonist-mediated activation scenario, in which hPR do have to be bound to DNA (Sartorius et al. 1993). Because we have a specific interest in the actions of steroid antagonists in breast cancer, we studied antiprogestins in a derivative of T47D human breast cancer cells which express high endogenous levels of both PR isoforms and which are stably transfected with the MMTV promoter cloned upstream of the CAT gene. Treatment of these cells with R5020 produces high levels of CAT. When tested alone, the three antiprogestins RU486, ZK98299, and ZK112993 are unable to stimulate transcription, and all three inhibit R5020-mediated transcription. Thus, in this model, all three antiprogestins are good antagonists, presumably through the conventional pathway shown in Fig. 3a.

However, when cellular cAMP levels are raised, two of the antagonists demonstrate a surprisingly strong agonist activity: when present alone, RU486 and ZK112993 are antagonists, but in the presence of 8-Br-cAMP, they become agonists. In contrast, despite elevated cAMP levels, ZK98299 remains an antagonist. Recall that ZK98299-occupied hPR either do not bind to DNA at PREs or have anomalous DNA-binding properties. From this and other controls we deduce that in order for antiprogestins to switch to agonists under cAMP control, the receptors have to be bound to DNA, presumably at PREs.

The amplification effects of cAMP are not limited to PR. While PR levels are overexpressed in T47D cells, the levels of GR, androgen receptors (AR), and estrogen receptors (ER) are extremely low. In addition to PR, the PREs of the MMTV promoter can be regulated by AR and GR (Cato et al. 1987). However, the MMTV promoter lacks an ERE and is not regulated by ER. In T47D cells expressing the MMTV-CAT reporter, neither dexamethasone nor dihydrotestosterone stimulate CAT transcription, suggesting that GR and AR levels are too low in these cells to activate this promoter in the absence of other influences. However, when cAMP levels are raised, the cells acquire sensitivity to the steroid hormones, resulting in strong transcription. Thus, 8-Br-cAMP sensitizes the MMTV promoter to the actions of glucocorticoids and androgens. In contrast, no transcriptional amplification is seen with estradiol, consistent with the inability of ER to bind the MMTV promoter. Since the MMTV promoter lacks an ERE, this again suggests that the cooperativity between 8-Br-cAMP and PR, AR, and GR requires that the receptors be DNA bound. In fact, when tamoxifen–ER complexes are tested on an ERE-containing promoter-reporter, they become strong transactivators if cAMP levels are raised. Thus, cAMP-induced amplification of transcription is a general property of antagonist-occupied steroid receptors (Sartorius et al. 1993).

Signal transduction pathways ultimately converge at the level of transcription to produce patterns of gene regulation that are specific to the gene and cell in question. Composite promoters may be regulated by multiple independent and interacting factors. In extreme cases, a transcription factor can yield opposite regulatory effects from one DNA-binding site due to modulation by a second factor. A case in point are GR, which regulate proliferin gene transcription either positively or negatively. The direction of transcription by glucocorticoids is selected by DNA-bound Jun and Fos, which are postulated to interact with GR at PREs. cAMP-responsive signal transduction pathways are often involved in such cooperative interactions. These models suggest that on complex promoters, nonreceptor factors, among which are cAMP-regulated proteins, can interact with steroid receptors to select the direction of transcription (Diamond et al. 1990; Gruol et al. 1986).

Our studies demonstrate that cAMP can amplify the transcriptional signals of agonist-occupied steroid receptors and can switch the activity of some antiprogestins to render them potent agonists, an effect that can have unintended clinical consequences. We believe that this switching requires that hPR bind to DNA, but that it is not due to ligand-independent phosphorylation of the receptor or direct activation of the receptors by protein kinase A-dependent pathways. We find that elevated cAMP levels do not enhance phosphorylation of hPR in breast cancer cells nor do they modulate the hormone-dependent phosphorylation induced by progestins, and therefore conclude that cAMP does not directly influence hPR activity by phosphorylating the receptors (Sartorius et al. 1993). Instead, our data are consistent with a model in which the direction of transcription by DNA-bound hPR is indirectly regulated by "coactivator" proteins whose activity is perhaps controlled by cAMP-dependent phosphorylation (Fig. 3c). This cooperativity between two signal transduction pathways, one involving steroid receptors, another involving cAMP-regulated proteins, requires that the steroid receptors bind to DNA. It therefore does not occur on the MMTV promoter with ER or when hPR are occupied by ZK98299. However, it does occur with many steroid receptors when they are bound to their cognate HREs, suggesting that the "coactivator" is a general mediator of steroid hormone-induced transcription. As we show again below, PR A receptors do *not* activate transcription by this route, suggesting that there are fundamental differences between the mechanisms of action of the two PR isoforms.

1.7 New T47D Breast Cancer Cell Lines for the Independent Study of Progesterone B and A Receptors: Only Antiprogestin-Occupied B Receptors Are Switched to Agonists by cAMP

The studies with wild-type T47D cells described above do not permit analysis of the relative contributions of B or A receptors to the synergism observed with cAMP, since these cells contain mixtures of both receptors. However, their constitutive high level production of PR have made T47D cells the major model in which to study the actions of progesterone in human breast cancer cells, unencumbered by the need for estradiol priming. Because of several special phenotypic properties of T47D cells and because factors other than receptors may be missing in persistently receptor-negative cells, we thought it prudent to retain the T47D cellular milieu in developing new models to study the independent actions of the two PR isoforms (Sartorius et al. 1994a). First we needed a PR-negative T47D subline. We developed a monoclonal PR-negative cell line, called T47D-Y, by selecting a PR-negative subpopulation from a parental T47D line that contained mixed PR-positive/PR-negative cells identified by flow cytometry. T47D-Y cells are PR-negative immunologically and by ligand binding assays, by growth resistance to progestins, by failure of a cell extract to bind a PRE in vitro, and by failure to transactivate PRE-regulated promoters.

T47D-Y cells were then stably transfected with expression vectors encoding one or the other hPR isoform, and two monoclonal cell lines were selected that express only B receptors (called T47D-YB), or only A receptors (called T47D-YA). The ectopically expressed receptors are at approximately wild-type levels, are properly phosphorylated, and, like endogenously expressed receptors, they undergo ligand-dependent downregulation. The expected B/B or A/A homodimers are present in cell extracts from each cell line, but A/B heterodimers are missing in both (Sartorius et al. 1994a).

To study isoform-specific transcriptional effects of agonists and antagonists when cAMP levels are raised, YA or YB cells were transiently transfected with the MMTV-CAT reporter and treated with R5020 or the three antiprogestins in the presence or absence of 8-Br-cAMP. 8-Br-cAMP alone does not stimulate CAT synthesis in either cell line. In YA cells, R5020-occupied A receptors are relatively weak transactivators, but their activity is strongly enhanced by cAMP. The three antipro-gestins RU486, ZK98299, or ZK112993 have no intrinsic agonist-like activity alone, and 8-Br-cAMP does not alter this.

In the B receptor-containing YB cells, R5020-regulated transcription is very strong, with little further cAMP amplification. However, 8-Br-cAMP strongly enhances the transcription by two of the antagonists, RU486 and ZK112993. These antiprogestins are inactive alone, but become strong agonists when 8-Br-cAMP is added. The antagonist ZK98299 is entirely different since it has no intrinsic agonist activity alone, and no enhancement is produced by 8-Br-cAMP.

These studies using our new stable cell lines show that the two PR isoforms behave dissimilarly in their cooperativity with cAMP. With regard to the agonist R5020, the synergism between cAMP and agonist-occupied receptors is most pronounced in YA cells. We speculate that in YA cells, cAMP sensitizes the MMTV promoter to the weak signal transmitted by R5020-occupied A receptors. This is similar to the man-ner in which cAMP amplifies the weak signals transmitted by hormone-occupied GR and AR in wild-type T47D cells. Since in YB cells agonist-occupied B receptors are already strong transactivators, cAMP has only modest further effects on this isoform.

With regard to progesterone antagonists, the isoform specificity of the cAMP effect is even more interesting. We find absolutely no effect of cAMP in YA cells, perhaps due to the fact that the antagonists (specifically RU486 and ZK112993) exhibit no agonist-like activity on A receptors. Is there no minimal signal for cAMP to amplify? In con-trast, the two antagonists appear to have some weak agonist-like activity in YB cells; hence, cAMP strongly amplifies this signal, converting the antagonist-occupied B receptors to potent agonists. Therefore, it is significant that B receptors occupied by the antiprogestin ZK98299 are not subject to this functional switching by cAMP. We speculate that ZK98299-occupied PR are physically removed from cAMP control by their failure to bind DNA. This again implies that cooperativity between PRE-bound PR and a cAMP-regulated coactivator accounts for the transcriptional synergism as depicted in Fig. 3c.

In studies, the details of which will be reported elsewhere, we find that cell growth regulation by progestins is also modulated by cellular cAMP levels. In the first 48 h of treatment, R5020 stimulates prolifera-tion, and the antiprogestins inhibit the agonist. However, when cAMP levels are raised the antiprogestin RU486 has agonist-like proliferative effects – but only in YB cells. We believe that the ratio of B to A receptors in tumors, and perhaps also in normal progesterone target tissues, controls the response to progestational agents. In the future not only the tumor PR status, but also the PR isoform distribution will have to be defined. Additionally, the PR isoform distribution in normal tissues may dictate their responses to progestational agents.

1.8 A Receptors Are Transdominant Repressors of B Receptors Without Binding a PRE

If B and A receptors are so different, what happens when the two are mixed? To determine the effects of A receptors on antagonist-stimulated transcription by B receptors, expression vectors encoding hPR_B and increasing levels of hPR_A were cotransfected into HeLa cells together with the PRE-tk-CAT reporter, and the cells were treated with either R5020 or RU486. hPR_B alone stimulate CAT transcription in this model whether or not the receptors are occupied by agonist or antagonist, while hPR_A alone are stimulatory only when they are agonist occupied. In fact, when RU486 is bound to hPR_A, transcription is always suppressed below basal levels. When the two receptor isoforms are coexpressed, strong transcription is maintained in the presence of the agonist, regardless of the hPR_B to hPR_A ratio. However, in the presence of the antagonist and at approximately equimolar amounts of the two receptors, the transcriptional phenotype of hPR_A predominates, so that hPR_B-stimulated transcription is almost entirely extinguished (Tung et al. 1993).

When hPR_A and hPR_B are equimolar, a 1:2:1 ratio of A/A, A/B, and B/B dimers is expected. The extensive inhibition by A receptors suggested that A/B heterodimers have the same inhibitory activity as A/A homodimers and that only B/B homodimers are stimulatory. However, presence of the two competing homodimers complicates functional analysis of the heterodimers, and B/B homodimers probably account for the incomplete suppression of transcription seen when A and B receptors are mixed. Therefore, we decided to construct receptors containing only heterodimers. For this we used the special properties of c-Jun and c-Fos.

When they are mixed, c-Jun and c-Fos preferentially form heterodimers over homodimers by at least 1000-fold (O'Shea et al. 1989). Therefore, to force heterodimerization of hPR, the leucine zippers of c-Fos or c-Jun were fused to the C-terminus of hPR_A or hPR_B (Mohamed et al. 1994). These chimeric hPR retain agonist and antagonist binding capacity, and agonist or antagonist-occupied hPR_A-Jun and hPR_B-Fos, when each is expressed alone, have the same transcriptional phenotype as the wild-type receptors. However, when the two are cotransfected, the weak residual transcription seen with wild-type RU486-occupied B/A receptor mixtures is entirely eliminated. Thus, CAT levels are reproducibly below control values with B-Fos/A-Jun heterodimers. These data confirm the A-dominance hypothesis and show that antagonist-occupied pure A/B heterodimers exhibit exclusively the inhibitory transcriptional phenotype of antagonist-occupied A/A homodimers.

The dominance of A receptors is observed even when the antagonist used is ZK98299. Because ZK98299-occupied A receptors do not bind to a PRE, these data imply that their inhibitory effects, like the stimulatory effects of antagonist-occupied B receptors, are mediated by novel non-PRE-dependent mechanisms. This was confirmed by experiments in which the antagonist-occupied A receptor DBD specificity mutant, which cannot bind a PRE, was used as the competing receptor species. On PRE-*tk*-CAT, activation of CAT transcription by RU486-occupied wild-type hPR_B was completely inhibited by the antagonist-occupied hPR_A-DBD specificity mutant.

Our studies demonstrate that A receptors can inhibit the activity of B receptors (Sartorius et al. 1993). In related studies it has been shown that A receptors also inhibit the activities of other members of the steroid receptor family, including ER (Vegeto et al. 1993; McDonnell and Goldman 1994). Thus, the dominant inhibitory effects of A receptors are extensive and may explain some of the "antiestrogenic" actions reported for antiprogestins. The mechanisms underlying these "trans" inhibitory effects are unknown. Meyer et al. (1989) demonstrated several years ago that transcription by PR is inhibited by coexpressed ER and that both PR and GR inhibit activation by ER. They suggested that steroid receptors compete for limiting transcription factors that they all use in common. Since ER and PR bind to different DNA response elements, their mutual inhibition appears to occur without direct DNA binding of the interfering receptor. Thus, when PR interferes with ER action, the gene being suppressed need not contain a PRE or be otherwise progestin regulated, as modeled in Fig. 3c.

1.9 A Third Transactivation Function of Human Progesterone Receptors Located in the Unique N-Terminal Segment of the hPR$_B$ – the BUS

Why do B receptors differ from A receptors? We postulated that the unique 164 amino acid BUS is in part responsible for the functional differences between the two isoforms and constructed a series of hPR expression vectors encoding BUS fused to individual downstream functional domains of the receptors (Sartorius et al. 1994b). These include the two transactivation domains, AF1 located in a 90 amino acid segment just upstream of the DBD and NLS and AF2 located in the HBD. BUS is a highly phosphorylated domain and contains the serine residues responsible for the hPR$_B$ triplet protein structure. The construct containing BUS-DBD-NLS binds tightly to DNA when aided by accessory nuclear factors. In HeLa cells, BUS-DBD-NLS strongly and constitutively activates CAT transcription from a promoter containing two progesterone response elements (PRE$_2$-TATA$_{tk}$-CAT) to levels comparable to those of hormone-activated, full-length B receptors. Thus, we conclude that this construct contains an autonomous third transactivation function, AF3.

In HeLa cells, transcription levels with BUS-DBD-NLS are equivalent to those seen with full-length hPR$_B$ and are higher than those seen with hPR$_A$. Additional studies show that BUS specifically requires an intact hPR DBD in order to be transcriptionally active. DBD mutants that cannot bind DNA, or whose DNA binding specificity have been altered, cannot cooperate in BUS transcriptional activity. This suggests that the autonomous AF3 activity resides in a discontinuous domain formed from BUS and the hPR DBD. We also find that the autonomous function of BUS-DBD-NLS is promoter- and cell-specific. BUS-DBD-NLS does not transactivate MMTV-CAT in HeLa cells and poorly transactivates PRE$_2$-TATA$_{tk}$-CAT in the PR-negative T47D-Y breast cancer cells. In the latter, however, transcription can be restored either by elevating cellular levels of cAMP or by linking BUS to AF1 or AF2, each of which alone is also inactive in T47D-Y cells. Thus, while in T47D-Y cells each AF alone is inactive, when AF3 is linked to either of the other two AFs (AF3 + AF1 or AF3 + AF2), strong transcription is regenerated, which is approximately equal to that obtained with B receptors. These data suggest that in the appropriate cell or promoter context, BUS can supply an important transactivation function in two different ways: either by autonomously activating transcription in the absence of the other two AFs, as it does in HeLa cells on PRE_2-TATA$_{tk}$-CAT; or by synergizing with the other AFs as it does in T47D-Y cells on PRE_2-TATA-CAT (Sartorius et al. 1994b). Is it the autonomous function of BUS that produces agonist-like effects from antagonist-occupied B receptors?

1.10 Summary

This year represents the twentieth anniversary of our first demonstration that human breast cancers contain PR, and are markers of hormone dependence (Horwitz et al. 1975). These receptors are now routinely measured in tumors not only as markers of hormone dependence, but also of disease prognosis. Theoretically, their central function in breast cancers should not be as markers, however, but as effectors of the proliferative signals of endogenous progesterone in premenopausal women and as targets for the therapeutic effects of progestins and antiprogestins. At present, PR are rarely measured for these functional purposes. As the aforegoing shows, the actions of PR are complex, and responsiveness to progestin agonists or antagonists will depend on the gene whose activity is being measured, the peculiarities of the cell and tissue under study, and, most importantly, the PR isoform that predominates in a tissue or tumor. Thus, while this chapter has focused on progesterone actions in the breast and breast cancer, the principles described here will undoubtedly also apply to other progesterone target tissues, including the female reproductive tract, the ovaries, the brain, and bone. We believe the differential expression of PR isoforms, perhaps under developmental and hormonal control, serves to fine-tune responsiveness to this important reproductive hormone. It follows that knowledge, not just of the PR content of a tissue, but of the expression of B vs. A receptors in that tissue, will be vital to understanding the effects of progestins therein.

Additionally, recent studies with PR have forced us to revise the standard model of steroid receptor action. The conventional model, which depicts receptors as ligand-activated proteins that bind to specific DNA sequences at "consensus" HREs and activate transcription, is not incorrect. It is, however, oversimplified, as studies with PR demonstrate. This should not have been surprising given the complex regulatory demands on these receptors. These demands include requirements for both positive and negative transcriptional regulation; for tissue specificity of action; and for regulation of composite and simple gene promoters. It should also not have been surprising, given the complex structural organization of these proteins. This includes multiple covalent modifications by phosphorylation and multiple functional domains that control intramolecular contacts, intermolecular protein–protein interactions, and DNA binding. Finally, given the fact that steroid antagonists are synthetic rather than natural hormones, it is perhaps not surprising that their binding produces structural alterations in the receptors that unveil additional novel interactive capabilities.

Thus, while antiprogestins can indeed competitively inhibit agonists by forming nonproductive receptor–DNA complexes, this is not their sole mechanism of action. Depending on the promoter and cell regulated, antiprogestin effects may also be mediated by receptor interactions with coactivators whose function is in turn controlled by nonsteroidal signals. Therefore, when two different signaling pathways are simultaneously activated, they can cooperate to produce unintended effects. Additionally, it seems clear from several studies that antagonist-occupied receptors can act without binding to canonical PREs, or without binding to DNA at all, relying perhaps on tethering proteins. This may be a consequence of the unusual allosteric structure imparted on the receptors by synthetic ligands. For some of these unusual actions, the receptors may even be monomeric rather than dimeric. Because of these, and undoubtedly other mechanisms yet to be discovered, the most serious mistake that investigators can make when studying antiprogestins is to assume that a specific mechanism is operating.

It is our contention that these novel actions begin to explain two properties of steroid antagonists that have puzzled investigators. One is the common observation that antagonists are agonists in some normal tissues. The other, which is an extension of the first, is that in malignant cells, antagonists can acquire agonist-like properties as tumors progress, leading to treatment failure. Although such tumors are called "resistant," they may in fact be responding quite well to the antagonist!

With respect to receptor protein structure, we are only beginning to appreciate its complexity. For example, it appeared at first blush that the structural independence of functional domains permitted the analysis of receptor fragments by fusing them to heterologous proteins. However, we now know that important functional domains can overlap, that other functional domains may be discontinuous, and that one domain can modulate the activity of another. This means that analysis of receptor fragments in chimeras is an incomplete test of domain function and that we need innovative experimental strategies to understand this intra-molecular cross-talk. Finally, what could be more unexpected than finding that one receptor isoform can inhibit not just its partner, but even distantly related receptor cousins! Be prepared for more surprises from this fascinating protein family.

Acknowledgments. The studies described herein were generously supported by the NIH through CA26869, CA55595, and DK48238, by the National Foundation for Cancer Research, by the U.S. Army, and by the Johnson and Johnson Focused Giving Program. Versions of this chapter have been published elsewhere.

References

Cairns C, Cairns W, Okret S (1993) Inhibition of gene expression by steroid hormone receptors via a negative glucocorticoid response element. DNA Cell Biol 12:695–702

Cato ACB, Henderson D, Ponta H (1987) The hormone response element of the mouse mammary tumor virus DNA mediates the progestin and androgen induction of transcription in the proviral long terminal repeat region. EMBO J 6:363–368

Diamond MI, Miner JN, Yoshinaga SK, Yamamoto KR (1990) Transcription factor interactions: selectors of positive or negative regulation from a single DNA element. Science 249:1266–1272

Gruol DJ, Campbell NF, Bourgeois S (1986) Cyclic AMP-dependent protein kinase promotes glucocorticoid receptor function. J Biol Chem 261:4909–4914

Härd T, Kellenbach E, Boelens R et al (1990) Solution structure of the gluco-corticoid receptor DNA-binding domain. Science 249:157–160

Horwitz KB (1992) The molecular biology of RU486. Is there a role for an-tiprogestins in the treatment of breast cancer? Endocr Rev 13:146–163

Horwitz KB, McGuire WL, Pearson OH, Segaloff A (1975) Predicting re-sponse to endocrine therapy: a hypothesis. Science 189:726–727

Jonat C, Rahmsdorf HJ, Park K-K, Cato AC, Gebel S, Ponta H, Herrlich P (1990) Antitumor promotion and antiinflammation: down-modulation of AP-1 (fos/jun) activity by glucocorticoid hormone. Cell 62:1189–1204

Kutoh E, Stromstedt P-E, Poellinger L (1992) Functional interference between the ubiquitous and constitutive octamer transcription factor 1 (OTF-1) and the glucocorticoid receptor by direct protein-protein interaction involving the homeo subdomain of OTF-1. Mol Cell Biol 12:4960–4969

McDonnell DP, Goldman ME (1994) RU486 exerts antiestrogenic activities through a novel progesterone receptor A form-mediated mechanism. J Biol Chem 269:11945–11949

Meyer ME, Gronemeyer H, Turcotte B, Bocquel M-T, Tasset D, Chambon P (1989) Steroid hormone receptors compete for factors that mediate their en-hancer function. Cell 57:433–442

Miner JN, Yamamoto KR (1991) Regulatory cross-talk at composite response elements. Trends Biol Sci 16:423–426

Mohamed KM, Tung L, Takimoto GS, Horwitz KB (1994) The leucine zippers of c-Fos and c-Jun for progesterone receptors dimerization: mechanisms of A-dominance in the A/B heterodimer. J Steroid Biochem Mol Biol 51:241–250

Oro AE, Hollenberg SM, Evans RM (1988) Transcriptional inhibition by a glucocorticoid receptor-β-galactosidase fusion protein. Cell 55:1109–1114

O'Shea EK, Rutkowski R, Stafford WF III, Kim PS (1989) Preferential het-erodimer formation by isolated leucine zippers from Fos and Jun. Science 245:646–648

Sakai DD, Helms S, Carlstedt-Duke J, Gustafsson JÅ, Rottman FM, Yamamoto KR (1988) Hormone-mediated repression of transcription: a negative glucocorticoid response element from the bovine prolactin gene. Genes Dev 2:1144–1154

Sartorius CA, Tung L, Takimoto GS, Horwitz KB (1993) Antagonist-occupied human progesterone receptors bound to DNA are functionally switched to transcriptional agonists by cAMP. J Biol Chem 5:9262–9266

Sartorius CA, Groshong SD, Miller LA, Powell RL, Tung L, Takimoto GS, Horwitz KB (1994a) New T47D breast cancer cell lines for the independent study of progesterone B- and A receptors: only antiprogestin-occupied B-receptors are switched to transcriptional agonists by cAMP. Cancer Res 54:3868–3877

Sartorius CA, Melville MY, Hovland AR, Tung L, Takimoto GS, Horwitz KB
(1994b) A third transactivation function (AF3) human progesterone receptors located in the unique, N-terminal segment of the B-isoform. Mol Endocrinol 8:1347–1360

Schüle R, Rangarajan P, Kliewer S, Ransone LJ, Bolado J, Yang N, Verma IM,
Evans RM (1990) Functional antagonism between oncoprotein c-Jun and
the glucocorticoid receptor. Cell 62:1217–1226

Truss M, Beato M (1993) Steroid hormone receptors: interaction with deoxyribonucleic acid and transcription factors. Endocr Rev 14:459–479

Truss M, Bartsch J, Beato M (1994) Antiprogestins prevent progesterone receptor binding to hormone responsive elements in vivo. Proc Natl Acad Sci
USA 91:11333–11337

Tung L, Mohamed KM, Hoeffler JP, Takimoto GS, Horwitz KB (1993) Antagonist occupied human progesterone B-receptors activate transcription
without binding to progesterone response elements, and are dominantly inhibited by A-receptors. Mol Endocrinol 7:1256–1265

Vegeto E, Shahbaz MM, Wen DX, Goldman ME, O'Malley BW, McDonnell
DP (1993) Human progesterone receptor A form is a cell- and promoter-
specific repressor of human progesterone receptor B function. Mol Endocrinol 7:1244–1255

Yang-Yen H-F, Chambard J-C, Sun Y-L, Smeal T, Schmidt TJ, Drouin J, Karin
M (1990) Transcriptional interference between c-Jun and the glucocorticoid
receptor: mutual inhibition of DNA binding due to direct protein-protein interaction. Cell 62:1205–1215

2 Hormonal Regulation of the Paracrine Growth Factors HGF and KGF in the Endometrium of the Rhesus Macaque

R.M. Brenner, O.D. Slayden, T. Koji, S. Izumi, M. Chedid,
K.G. Csaky, and J.S. Rubin

2.1 Introduction

The endometrium, as with many mucosal tissues, consists of glandular, stromal, and vascular components. Recent research in various species has shown that the stromal component secretes mediators that affect various epithelial functions. More and more evidence is accumulating which suggests that specific soluble mediators secreted by stromal cells under steroid hormone influence participate in the mitogenic and differentiative responses of endometrial epithelia during normal adult reproductive life (Cunha et al. 1985, 1987; Bigsby and Cunha 1986; Brenner and Slayden 1994; Brenner et al. 1990).

Until recently the nature of these particular mediators was unknown. However, two polypeptide growth factors that fit the requirements for such hormonally modulated, secreted, stromal-epithelial mediators have recently been described. These are keratinocyte growth factor (KGF; also known as FGF-7) and hepatocyte growth factor (HGF; also known as scatter factor). Both are mesenchymally derived, secreted epithelial mitogens whose receptors are epithelial cell specific tyrosine kinases (Rubin et al. 1993; Finch et al. 1989). Both can be regulated by several factors, including steroid hormones. Our laboratory has reported that progesterone (P) upregulates KGF in the primate endometrium, and we now have evidence that HGF is upregulated by estradiol (E_2) in this tissue. In this chapter we summarize our findings and offer the view that in the endometrium HGF is an estromedin, that is, a paracrine mediator of estrogen effects, and KGF a progestomedin, a paracrine mediator of progestin action. These growth factors and their receptors may be important new targets for the development of endometrial-based contraceptives. Although numerous other growth factors of various families are present in the endometrium that also may serve as such targets, we limit this review to KGF and HGF, as little has been published concerning these mitogens in the endometrium.

Keratinocyte Growth Factor. Early work showed that KGF mRNA is present in four different fibroblast cell lines and in the dermis of mouse skin, but absent from seven different epithelial cell lines and mouse epidermis (Finch et al. 1989). The KGF peptide is mitogenic, as measured by an in vitro proliferation assay, in three epithelial cell lines but has no effect on two fibroblast lines or on an endothelial cell line (Rubin et al. 1989). The recent literature on KGF, which has been extensively reviewed (Rubin et al. 1995), supports the hypothesis that KGF acts primarily as a one-way paracrine factor, from fibroblasts to epithelial cells.

A high-affinity receptor for KGF (KGFR) was isolated by expression cloning (Miki et al. 1991). Specific binding was effectively displaced by low concentrations of KGF and acidic fibroblast growth factor (aFGF, or FGF-1), but substantially higher concentrations of basic fibroblast growth factor (bFGF, or FGF-2) were required for a similar effect (Bottaro et al. 1990). Structural analysis of amino acid sequences predicted from the cDNAs for mouse KGFR and human KGFR revealed that KGFR is a variant of fibroblast growth factor receptor-2 (FGFR-2) and contains a unique 49 amino acid region near the *trans*-membrane domain. Subsequent binding analysis confirmed that the 49 amino acid sequence is responsible for the greater binding affinity of KGF for KGFR. Other studies have shown that the KGFR mRNA is expressed only in certain epithelial cells and is absent from all fibroblasts tested (Miki et al. 1992, 1991; Bottaro et al. 1993).

Several reports document the effects of KGF in animals. For example, both intratracheal and systemic administration of a single dose of KGF (5 mg/kg) in rats induced extensive proliferation of type II pneumocytes in the lung (Ulich et al. 1994b). KGF administered by either intravenous, intraperitoneal, or subcutaneous routes induced ductal hyperplasia in the mammary glands of both male and female rats (Ulich et al. 1994a). All effects of KGF were reversible by discontinuing KGF administration (Rubin et al. 1995). These data clearly suggest a physiological role for KGF in a number of mammalian epithelial cell types, although there are as yet no reports on its effects in the endometrium.

We have reported that KGF mRNA in rhesus monkey endometrium is dramatically increased during the luteal phase to levels 50- to 100-fold higher than in the follicular phase, and that this increase can be similarly induced by P action in estrogen-primed ovariectomized rhesus monkeys (Koji et al. 1994). A review of our findings is presented below.

Hepatocyte Growth Factor. HGF was originally described as a mitogen for hepatocytes during liver regeneration (Lindroos et al. 1991). In vivo administration of HGF to mice facilitated regenerative repair in the kidney after renal injuries (Kawaida et al. 1994) and stimulated liver regeneration after partial hepatectomy (Ishiki et al. 1992). HGF also has been called a "motogen" as it can stimulate movement (scattering) of epithelial cells (Stoker et al. 1987), a "morphogen" as it can stimulate tubule formation in canine kidney cells in culture (Montesano et al. 1991), and an "angiogen," as it can induce angiogenesis in the rabbit cornea and proliferation/migration of endothelial cells in culture (Grant et al. 1993; Bussolino et al. 1992). The promoter region of the HGF gene has been sequenced and a number of regulatory elements identified (Liu et al. 1994). These include (among others) two estrogen response elements.

HGF is secreted into the extracellular environment, where it is proteolytically cleaved into an active conformation by various HGF convertases, including plasminogen activator and other serine proteases (Miyazawa et al. 1992; Naldini et al. 1992; Boccaccio et al. 1994). Tissue-type plasminogen activator (PA) is upregulated by E_2 in the human endometrium (Berthois et al. 1991), and urokinase-type PA is also present. Both could activate HGF in the endometrium during menses.

The receptor for HGF is encoded by the c-Met proto-oncogene. This is a heterodimeric tyrosine kinase, a glycoprotein with an extracellular, and a transmembrane subunit found primarily in epithelial cells, especially in the proliferative compartment (Di Renzo et al. 1991) but also detected in endothelial cells, melanocytes, and microglial cells (Boccaccio et al. 1994). The c-Met promoter has been sequenced and various response elements detected, including several Sp1 sites, two AP2 sites and a consensus site for PEA3, a site responsive to growth factors and tissue-type PA (Gambarotta et al. 1994). Studies of an endometrial carcinoma cell line showed that the c-Met promoter has interleukin (IL)-1 and IL-6 responsive sites, and that IL-1, IL-6, tumor necrosis factor (TNF)-α, and E_2 can all upregulate c-Met mRNA (Moghul et al. 1994). This report also confirmed that HGF can also enhance the expression of its own receptor and increase expression of the urokinase-type PA mRNA, an enzyme responsible for cleaving pro-HGF to an active form (Boccaccio et al. 1994; Pepper et al. 1992). Thus HGF may be capable of autoamplifying its own effects through upregulating both its own receptor and an enzyme responsible for its activation in the extracellular matrix.

Clearly HGF has many of the properties one would expect in a factor that would facilitate cyclic endometrial regeneration and participate in estrogen-dependent endometrial growth. Consequently it shares with KGF the potential for being a target of endometrial-based contraception. In the following we review our data on these peptides and their receptors in the rhesus monkey endometrium.

2.2 Materials and Methods

2.2.1 Animals, Tissues, and Cell Lines

Uteri were obtained from ovariectomized as well as cycling rhesus monkeys (*Macaca mulatta*). Cycling monkeys were sampled during the midfollicular and midluteal phases as determined by assessment of serum E_2 and P levels (Brenner et al. 1983). Artificial cycles were initiated by treating the spayed monkeys with a 3-cm Silastic capsule (Dow Corning, Midland, Mich., USA) packed with crystalline E_2 for 14 days to stimulate an artificial proliferative phase. Subsequently a 6-cm silastic capsule of P was inserted for an additional 14 days to produce an artificial luteal phase. Tissues were removed for analysis at the end of either the artificial follicular or luteal phases. In some cases the E_2 and P implants remained in place for 4 additional weeks of E_2+P treatment before sampling. In some cases animals were treated continuously with E_2 for 28 days and sampled. In other cases the P implant was removed at the end of the artificial luteal phase, with the E_2 implant left in place, and uteri were collected by laparotomy on days 1, 6, and 14 after P withdrawal. Some animals were treated with E_2 for 14 days and subsequently with E_2 plus P plus RU-486 for 14 days. RU-486 (1 mg/kg) was injected daily i.m. in ethanol (Slayden et al. 1993). Finally, some animals were treated for 14 days with E_2, after which time the E_2 implant was removed, a P implant inserted for 14 days, and then tissue removed.

After removal each uterus was quartered, and the endometrium of one quarter was cut into thin slices, embedded in Tissue Tek OCT compound (Miles, Elkhart, Ind., USA), frozen in liquid propane, and then stored over liquid nitrogen (Koji and Brenner 1993) for analysis by in situ hybridization and immunocytochemistry. The remaining uterine tissue was dissected into endometrial and myometrial segments and frozen in liquid nitrogen for RNA preparation. Various other rhesus monkey tissues (lung, liver) were collected from healthy, naturally cycling monkeys that were being euthanized for other studies at our institution. Decidual tissues were obtained by cesarean section at 45 days of gestation from a rhesus macaque. In all cases these tissues were frozen and stored as described above. In some cases tissues for immunocytochemistry were microwaved before freezing as previously described (Slayden et al. 1995a)

M426 human embryonic lung fibroblasts were used as positive controls for KGF (Rubin et al. 1989; Finch et al. 1989) and HGF (Rubin et al. 1991) and negative controls for KGFR (Miki et al. 1992) and c-Met (Slayden et al. 1995b). MCF-7 cells and B5/589 human mammary epithelial cells (Stampfer and Bartley 1985; a gift of M. Stampfer, University of California, Berkeley, Calif., USA) were used as positive controls for KGFR. After harvesting all cells were frozen in liquid nitrogen and stored at −80°C for RNA preparation.

2.2.2 RNA Preparation, Northern Blotting, and Probes

Frozen materials were homogenized in 4 M guanidine thiocyanate, homogenized, and centrifuged. The RNA was isolated by cesium chloride centrifugation (Ausubel et al.1994), electrophoresed, transferred by capillary action onto Nytran membranes, and hybridized overnight at 42°C with random primed [^{32}P]cytidine triphosphate (dCTP) labeled cDNA probes. After hybridization filters were washed and exposed to X-ray film. After exposure blots were stripped by washing at 80°C and rehybridized with additional probes.

Mouse glial fibrillary acidic protein (GFAP) cDNA (1.2 kbp; Lewis et al. 1984) and the 1.1-kb EcoR1/HindIII fragment of the rat ribosomal cDNA (Low et al. 1990; Rothblum et al. 1982) were provided courtesy of Michael Melner, Department of Obstetrics and Gynecology, Vanderbilt University (Nashville, Tenn., USA). The human glyceraldehyde 3-phosphate dehydrogenase (GAPDH) cDNA [PstI-XbaI fragment of cDNA was obtained from ATCC (nr. 57090; Tso et al. 1985)]. Human KGF cDNA (0.68 kbp; Koji et al. 1994) coded for the 5' untranslated region and the first exon (Kelley et al. 1992; Finch et al. 1989). Human

KGFR cDNA (0.15 kbp) was provided courtesy of Paul Finch, Mt. Sinai Hospital (New York, N.Y., USA). Human HGF cDNA (2.2 kbp) consisted of the entire coding sequence (Rubin et al. 1991).

A rhesus monkey specific c-Met cDNA was prepared based on the human c-Met sequence (GenBank no. J02958). Rhesus monkey lung total RNA was reverse transcribed and polymerase chain reaction (PCR) was carried out with appropriate primers. The PCR products (5 µl) were electrophoresed on 1.5% agarose gels, and a single 400-bp band was identified, subcloned, and sequenced. The DNA sequence of the monkey c-Met cDNA fragment was 96% homologous to nucleotides 458–836 of the human sequence (GeneBank no. J02958).

Probes for northern and Southern hybridization were labeled with [^{32}P]dCTP by random priming with an oligo-labeling kit. Probes for in situ hybridization were labeled with digoxigenin dUTP by random priming with a labeling kit.

Sense and antisense strands corresponding to nucleotides 539–583 of the human KGF cDNA sequence (Finch et al. 1989) were synthesized. These 45 mer oligodeoxynucleotides (oligo-DNAs) were labeled at the 3' end with [^{32}P-α]ATP (Henderson et al. 1991) by terminal deoxynucleotidyl transferase (Boehringer Mannheim, Germany). The specific activities of these oligo-DNAs were 0.6–1.4×10^9 cpm/µg DNA.

2.2.3 KGFR Detection by Reverse Transcriptase PCR

KGFR mRNA in the endometrium was detected by the reverse transciptase (RT) PCR technique (Izumi et al. 1996; Slayden et al. 1994). Control RNAs, including RNA from M426 cells (a negative control) and RNA from B5/859 cells (a positive control), were also analyzed. The PCR products were electrophoresed and transferred to Nytran. The specific bands were identified by Southern hybridization with random primed [^{32}P]dCTP-labeled KGFR cDNA probes prepared from the KGFR-specific exon (Miki et al. 1992) of the human KGFR cDNA.

2.2.4 In Situ Hybridization and Histological Techniques

The procedures for preparing frozen sections (5 μm), attaching them to gelatin-coated slides, fixation, pretreatments, and hybridization of the sections were all as previously described (Koji and Brenner 1993). Some sections were hybridized with labeled KGF cDNA probes in the presence of an excess amount of unlabeled KGF cDNA (17-fold) to validate the sequence specificity of the signal. The Ki-67 proliferation marker was identified by immunocytochemistry as previously described (Slayden et al. 1993) to identify proliferating cells. Glycolmethacrylate sections of monkey uterus were prepared and stained with hematoxylin as described previously (Slayden et al. 1993).

A unique chimeric molecule consisting of KGF fused to the hinge region and Fc portion of mouse IgG (KGF-HFc) has been shown to be effective as a probe to detect KGF binding activity (presumptive KGFR) in tissue sections (LaRochelle et al. 1995). (This reagent was supplied courtesy of Dr. William LaRochelle, NIH, Bethesda, Md., USA.) After an overnight incubation at 4°C with the fusion molecule, standard immunocytochemical procedures were used to reveal KGF-binding sites.

2.3 Results

2.3.1 Progesterone Upregulates KGF mRNA in Rhesus Endometrium

Endometrial and myometrial RNAs were extracted from uteri after different hormonal treatments. Figure 1 shows that the 2.4-kb KGF transcript was barely detectable in endometrium of spayed (lane 1) or E_2-treated (lane 3) monkeys but was abundant in the endometrium after treatment with E_2+P (lane 5). KGF mRNA was detectable at low level in myometrium of spayed animals (lane 2), but its level of expression was essentially unchanged by E_2 or E_2+P treatment (lanes 4, 6). In the same northern blot a typical 2.4-kb band of KGF mRNA was detected in total RNA from M426 human fibroblasts, a KGF-positive cell line (lane 7), but not from B5/589 cells, a KGF-negative cell line (lane 8).

Figure 2 shows that in animals treated for 14 days with combined E_2+P the degree of endometrial KGF mRNA expression was very high

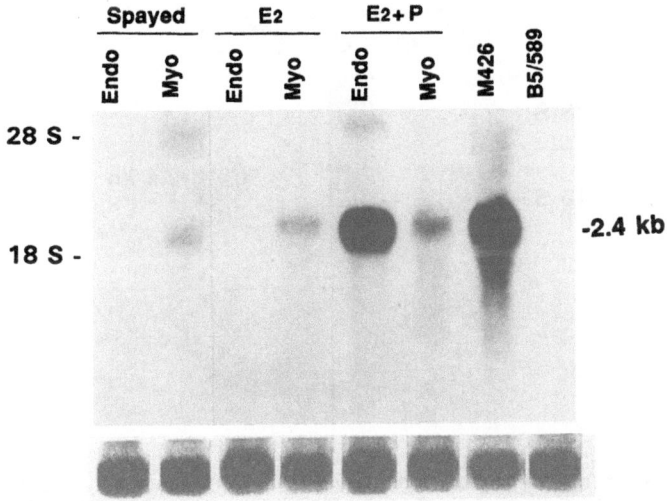

Fig. 1. Northern blot of total uterine RNA from hormonally treated animals hybridized with ^{32}P-labeled KGF cDNA. Lanes 1, 2, spayed animals; lane 1, endometrium; lane 2, myometrium; lanes 3, 4, E$_2$-treated animals; lane 3, endometrium; lane 4, myometrium; lanes 5, 6, E$_2$+P treated animals; lane 5, endometrium; lane 6, myometrium; lane 7, KGF-positive M426 cell line; lane 8, KGF-negative B5/589 cell line. 2.4 kb marks KGF mRNA, which was greatly enhanced by E$_2$+P treatment in endometrium and was present but essentially invariant in myometrium under all hormonal conditions. Below, the signal after reprobing with a cDNA probe against GAPDH, confirming that equivalent amounts of RNA were loaded and transferred in all lanes. (Koji et al. 1994; reproduced from The Journal of Cell Biology, 1994, vol 125, pp. 393-401, by copyright permission of The Rockefeller University Press)

(E$_2$+P; lane 1), and that this effect was blocked by the P antagonist RU-486 (lane 2). E$_2$ was not required during P action because KGF mRNA was elevated by P in animals treated first with E$_2$ for 14 days and then for 14 days with P alone (E$_2$, P; lane 3). Also, endometrial KGF mRNA expression was minimal during the follicular phase (lane 4) and highly abundant in the luteal phase (lane 5) of the natural cycle. Together these data support a role for P but not E$_2$ in stimulating large increases in expression of endometrial KGF mRNA.

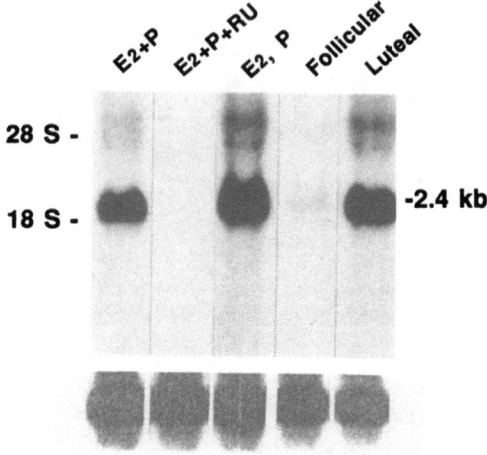

Fig. 2. Northern blot of total endometrial RNA from hormonally treated and naturally cycling macaques hybridized with ^{32}P-labeled KGF cDNA. *Lane 1*, E$_2$, then E$_2$+P; *lane 2*, E$_2$, then E$_2$+P+RU-486; *lane 3*, E$_2$, followed by P alone (E$_2$, P); *lane 4*, follicular phase of the menstrual cycle; *lane 5*, luteal phase of the menstrual cycle. *2.4 kb* marks KGF mRNA, which was elevated in P-dominated tissues whether E$_2$ was present or absent. The effect of P was antagonized by RU-486. *Below*, the signal on these blots after reprobing with a cDNA probe against GAPDH. (Koji et al. 1994; reproduced from *The Journal of Cell Biology*, 1994, vol 125, pp. 393–401, by copyright permission of The Rockefeller University Press)

2.3.2 Endometrial KGF mRNA Expression Is Increased by Long-Term P Treatment

We also examined KGF mRNA expression in animals treated first for 14 days with E$_2$ then with E$_2$+P for either 1, 3, 7, 14, or 42 days (6 weeks). KGF mRNA expression was upregulated within 1 day of P treatment and continued to increase many fold over the subsequent 6-week treatment period (Fig. 3).

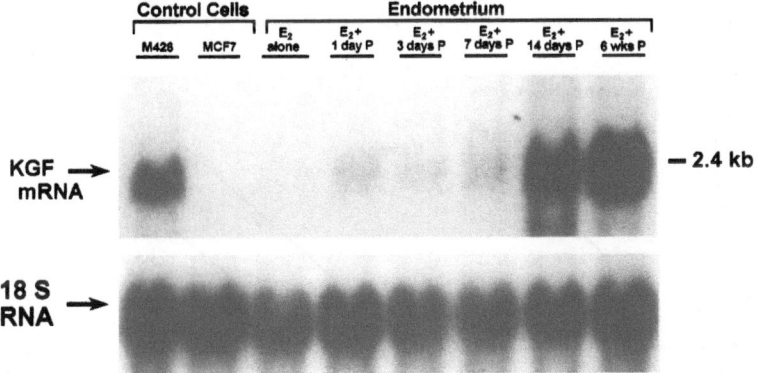

Fig. 3. Northern blot of total RNA from control cells and endometria from various hormonal treatments hybridized with ^{32}P-labeled KGF cDNA. *Lane 1,* M426 cells, KGF positive control; *lane 2,* MCF7 cells, KGF negative control; *lane 3,* E_2 alone (14 days); *lane 4,* E_2+1 day P; *lane 5,* E_2+3 days P; *lane 6,* E_2+7 days P; *lane 7,* E_2+14 days P; *lane 8,* E_2+6 weeks P. *2.4 kb* marks KGF mRNA, which is slightly upregulated by 1 day of P treatment, increases substantially by 14 days, and appears to increase even further after 6 weeks of P treatment. *Below,* the signal after reprobing with a cDNA probe against 18S RNA confirming that equivalent amounts of RNA were present in all lanes

2.3.3 Progesterone Increases KGF Protein Levels in Endometrium

We also measured KGF protein under different hormonal conditions with a sensitive two-site enzyme-linked immunosorbent assay as previously described (Koji et al. 1994). In this assay recombinant KGF was detectable at subnanogram amounts (Fig. 4), and endometrial tissue extracts showed readily detectable KGF-immunoreactive material. Figure 4 and Table 1 show that KGF protein was substantially higher in endometrium from animals in the luteal phase or treated with E_2+P than in endometria from the follicular phase or from animals treated only with E_2. These data indicate that KGF protein was present in the endometrium and was elevated in P-dominated tissue.

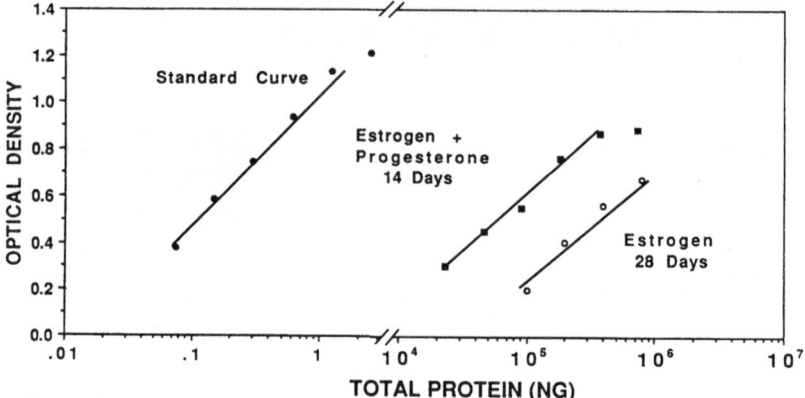

Fig. 4. Enzyme-linked immunosorbent assay of KGF protein in homogenates of rhesus monkey endometrium. Protein was extracted from the endometrium of animals subjected to different hormonal treatments, and serial dilutions of each sample were assayed along with dilutions of a recombinant human KGF standard as described in Sect. 2.2. Each data point was the mean value of duplicate measurements. (Koji et al. 1994; reproduced from *The Journal of Cell Biology*, 1994, vol 125, pp. 393–401, by copyright permission of The Rockefeller University Press)

Table 1. KGF concentration in rhesus monkey endometrium

Animal number	Hormonal state	KGF concentration (ng/mg tissue protein)
11762	E_2+P 14 days	4.0
14958	E_2+P 14 days	3.5
11989	E_2+P 14 days	2.1
14581	Luteal phase	1.1
9360	Follicular phase	0.26
11671[a]	Follicular phase+E_2	0.12

Hormonal state, phase of menstrual cycle or hormone treatment: 14 days E_2+P, treated for 14 days with an E_2 implant and then for 14 days with implants of E_2 and progesterone.

[a] Rhesus monkey 11671 (follicular phase+E_2) was an animal injected with 42 μg/kg E_2 28 h before surgery during late follicular phase of the menstrual cycle to produce highly elevated levels of E_2 to mimic the natural preovulatory E_2 surge.

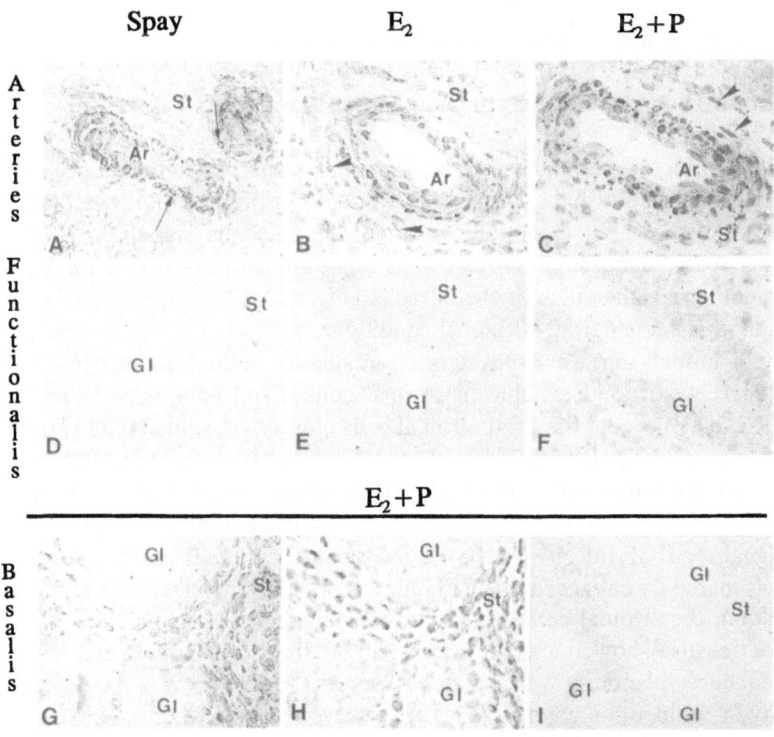

Fig. 5A–I. In situ hybridization of KGF mRNA with digoxigenin-labeled cDNA. **A** Artery, spayed. A distinct signal is evident in the cytoplasm of the smooth muscle cells that constitute the tunica media of the artery (*Ar*). Stromal (*St*) cells lack any significant signal. **B** Artery, E₂ treated. The signal evident in the cytoplasm of the smooth muscle cells of the artery wall is about the same strength as in the spayed animals. A few perivascular stromal cells (*arrowheads*) show a distinct signal. **C** Artery, P treated. The signal in the cytoplasm of the smooth muscle cells of the artery wall is about the same as in the E₂ treated animals. Some perivascular stromal cells show an increased signal. **D** Functionalis, spayed. The glands (*Gl*) and the periglandular stromal regions are negative for KGF mRNA. **E** Functionalis, E₂ treated. The glands and the periglandular stroma are negative as in the spayed animals. **F** Functionalis, P treated. The glands and the periglandular stroma are negative as in the E₂-treated animals. **G** Basalis, P treated. The glands are negative, but the stroma shows a substantially increased, distinct signal for KGF mRNA. **H** Basalis, P treated. This is a phase micrograph of the identical section as in **G**. The signal in the stroma is enhanced while the glands remain negative. **I** Basalis, P treated, competition control. Competition with excess unlabeled probe greatly suppresses the stromal signal. ×400

2.3.4 KGF mRNA Is Expressed Most Intensely
in the Stromal Cells of the Basalis Region
and the Perivascular Stroma and Musculature of Spiral Arteries

To examine the cellular localization of KGF transcript in the uterus we performed in situ hybridization. During all hormonal conditions there was a distinct but essentially invariant, cytoplasmic signal for KGF mRNA in the muscular-stromal walls of the spiral arteries (Fig. 5A–C). Endometrial glandular epithelial cells (Fig. 5D–F) were negative for KGF mRNA under all hormonal conditions.

In animals that were spayed or E_2-treated (or in the follicular phase) signals were nondetectable in stromal cells of all endometrial zones (Fig. 5D,E) except for a few stromal cells closely associated with spiral arteries (Fig. 5A,B). In P-treated (or luteal phase) animals the stromal cells in the *functionalis* zone had nondetectable signals (Fig. 5F); however, the stromal cells of the *basalis* zone showed a definite cytoplasmic signal for KGF mRNA (Fig. 5H). The stromal cell KGF mRNA signal was markedly enhanced by phase microscopy (Fig. 5I). During P-domination, the stromal cells in the perivascular regions around the spiral arteries also showed a small increase in the level of staining (Fig. 5C). Sequence specificity was shown by the great reduction of signal intensity in competition controls (Fig. 5I). Excess stringency controls, GFAP probe controls, and RNase pretreated controls were all negative (data not shown; see Koji et al. 1994).

2.3.5 Progesterone Stimulates Proliferation
in the Basalis and the Spiral Arteries

In E_2-treated and follicular phase animals there was a substantial number of Ki-67 positive cells in the glands of the functionalis (Fig. 6A) and only a minimal number in the glands of the basalis (Fig. 6C). In contrast, in E_2 plus P-treated and luteal-phase animals glandular proliferation was not observed in the functionalis (Fig. 6B) but was stimulated in the basalis (Fig. 6D). In addition, the spiral arteries proliferated under P influence. During the follicular phase (Fig. 6A) there were few Ki-67 cells in the walls of the spiral arteries, while in P-dominated

E₂   E₂+P

F
u
n
c
t
i
o
n
a
l
i
s

B
a
s
a
l
i
s

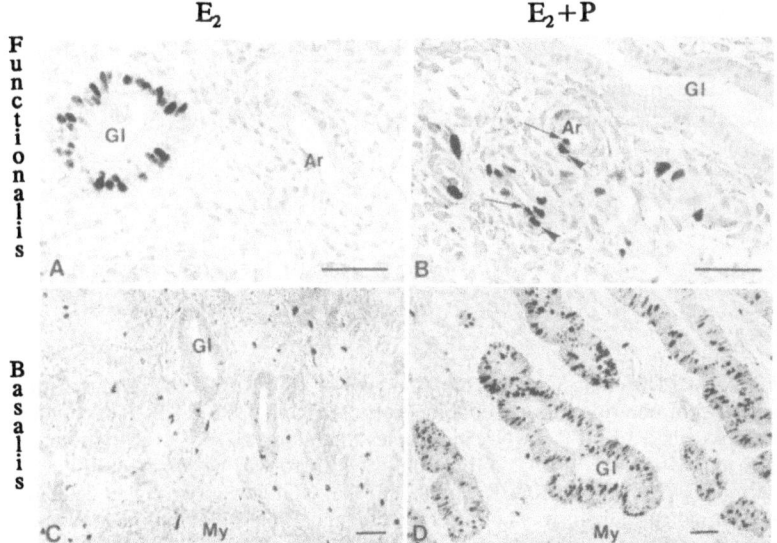

Fig. 6A–D. Proliferating cells as indicated by Ki-67 staining. **A,C** Micrographs from an E₂ treated animal. **B,D** Micrographs from an animal sampled on day 21 of the natural luteal phase (P-dominated). **A** Functionalis, E₂ treated. Ki-67 staining is evident in many glandular epithelial cells but is absent from the walls of the adjacent artery. Functionalis, P dominated. Ki-67 staining is absent from the glandular epithelial cells but is evident in many of the endothelial (*arrows*) and smooth muscle cells (*arrowheads*) of the spiral arteries. **C** Basalis, E₂ treated. A region of the basalis near the myometrial (*My*) border. Ki-67 staining is evident in some stromal cells but is minimal in the glandular epithelium. **D** Basalis, P dominated. A region of the basalis near the myometrial border. Ki-67 staining is now greatly increased in the glandular epithelium and minimal in the stroma. **A,B** ×400; **C,D** ×160. (Koji et al. 1994; reproduced from *The Journal of Cell Biology*, 1994, vol 125, pp. 393–401, by copyright permission of The Rockefeller University Press)

animals (Fig. 6B) there were numerous Ki-67 positive vascular smooth muscle, perivascular stromal, and endothelial cells in the spiral arteries.

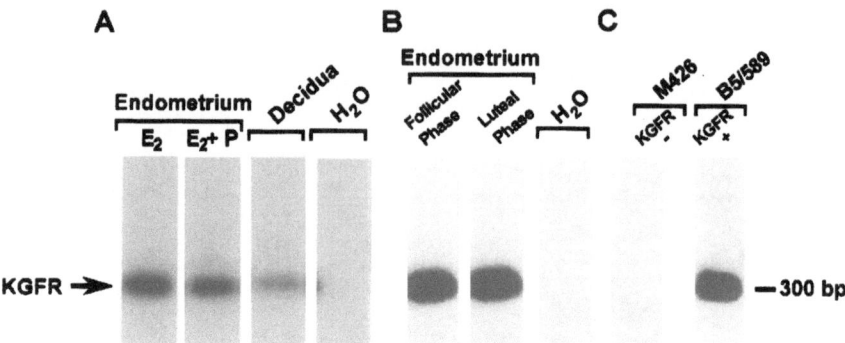

Fig. 7A–C. Different Southern blot analyses of KGFR RT-PCR products prepared from control cell and endometrial total RNA. The RT-PCR technique clearly detected KGFR mRNA in samples of endometrial RNA from hormonally treated animals (**A,B**). **A** Blot indicates there was no apparent effect of hormonal treatment on KGFR signal, and that KGFR was present in decidua. **B** Blot indicates there was no difference in signal intensity amplified between samples collected during the follicular and luteal phases of the natural menstrual cycle. KGFR mRNA was readily detectable in RNA prepared from human B5/589 cells (positive control), and no signal was amplified from total RNA from human M426 cells (negative control). In each PCR reaction one sample contained no RNA (H_2O) as a negative methological control

2.3.6 The KGF Receptor

Although we found that expression of KGFR mRNA was below the sensitivity of northern analysis, we obtained useful information on KGFR expression in endometrium through the use of RT-PCR technology and ligand histochemistry with KGF-HFc.

Southern hybridization of PCR products from endometrium were obtained after various hormonal treatments; a decidual sample from a 45-day pregnant rhesus monkey and KGFR-positive and negative cell lines are shown in Fig. 7. In endometrium, including the decidual tissue, KGFR mRNA was detected under all hormonal conditions, and there was little evidence of quantitative change in expression.

However, ligand histochemistry with the KGF-HFc reagent did reveal specific hormonal effects on KGFR expression. For example, in estrogenized animals binding activity was present on the basolateral

$$E_2 \qquad\qquad E_2+P$$

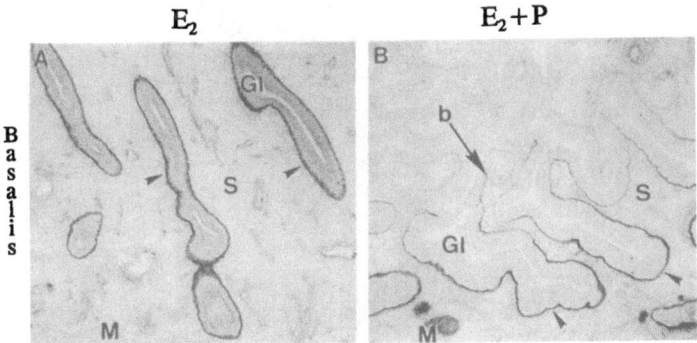

Fig. 8A,B. KGF binding activity in endometrium as indicated by ligand histochemistry with the KGF-HFc fusion molecule. The micrographs are of the basalis region near the myometrial (*M*) border. *Gl,* gland; *S,* stroma. **A** 14-day E_2 treatment. There is an intense signal in the basement membrane region (*arrowheads*) of the glands. ×100 **B** 14 days of E_2 then 14 days of E_2+P treatment. The deepest basalis glands retained their binding capacity, but there was a marked P-induced fall-off in signal (*large arrow*) where the lower basalis blends into the functionalis. ×250

membrane region of the luminal and glandular epithelial cells in both the functionalis and basalis zones (Fig. 8A). However, after subsequent E_2+P treatment, binding activity disappeared from the functionalis and was retained only in the deepest regions of the basalis (Fig. 8B) and the spiral arteries. When sections were incubated with a control fusion molecule that lacked the KGF ligand (HFc alone), no binding activity was detected (data not shown).

2.3.7 HGF mRNA Is Upregulated by Estradiol and Suppressed by P

Figure 9 shows that HGF mRNA was readily detectable in endometria from rhesus monkeys treated with E_2 alone for 28 days, but was only barely detectable in endometria from monkeys treated first for 14 days with E_2 then for 14 additional days with E_2+P. Additional evidence suggesting E_2-dependent HGF mRNA upregulation was found in tis-

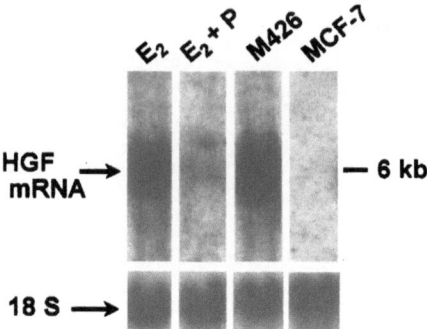

Fig. 9. Northern blot analysis of HGF mRNA expresion in the endometrium of spayed-hormone treated monkeys. Levels of HGF mRNA were increased by E_2 treatment for 14 days, and suppressed by sequential E_2+P treatment for 14 days. A strong signal was detected in M426 cell RNA (positive control), and no signal was detected in MCF-7 cell RNA (negative control)

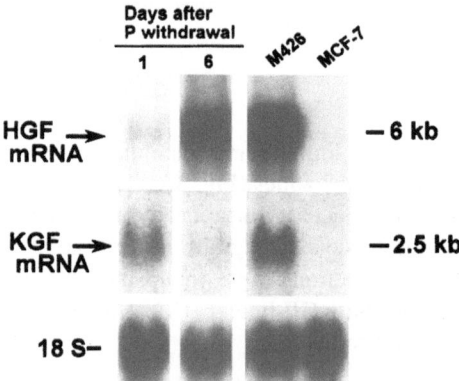

Fig. 10. Northern blot analysis of HGFmRNA, KGF mRNA, and 18S RNA in the endometrium on days 1and 6 after P withdrawal, during LFT. Endometrial total RNA was hybridized with a ^{32}P-labeled cDNA for HGF, and the blots were then stripped and reprobed for KGF mRNA and 18S RNA. Withdrawal of P and continuation of E_2 treatment resulted in an increase in HGF transcript and a decrease in KGF transcript. 18S RNA was equivalently expressed in all lanes

sues removed subsequent to P withdrawal in the presence of E_2 during the induced luteal-follicular transition (LFT). Figure 10 is a representative northern blot which shows that expression was very low on day 1 but was substantially elevated by day 6. We stripped this blot and reprobed it for KGF mRNA and 18S RNA. KGF mRNA was elevated on day 1 and then diminished considerably by day 6, as would be expected for a P-dependent message. The 18S mRNA signal did not vary significantly between days 1 and 6 after P withdrawal. These data on upregulation of HGF by E_2 have been confirmed in additional animals, and they suggest that HGF mRNA expression is suppressed by P and elevated by E_2. The increase in HGF mRNA after P withdrawal in the presence of E_2 is consistent with a role for HGF in the E_2-dependent endometrial proliferation that begins around day 4.5 of the LFT (McClellan et al. 1990).

2.3.8 The HGF Receptor c-Met Is Present Under All Hormonal Conditions in Rhesus Endometrium

We designed a monkey-specific c-Met probe and evaluated expression of c-Met mRNA in endometria obtained under various hormonal conditions. The data in Fig. 11 suggest there is little change in the expression of this gene under different hormonal conditions.

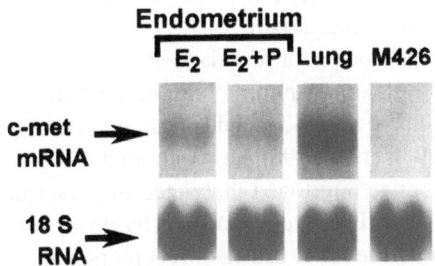

Fig. 11. Northern blot analysis of c-Met mRNA in the endometrium of rhesus monkeys. *Lane 1*, Endometrium treated 14 days with E_2; *lane 2*, endometrium treated with 14 days E_2 then 14 days E_2+P; *lane 3*, rhesus monkey lung (positive control); *lane 4*, M426 cells (negative control). The data suggest that there were no clear effects of hormones on c-Met mRNA expression

2.4 Discussion

The above data indicate that KGF, HGF, and their respective receptors KGFR and c-Met are present in the rhesus macaque endometrium. Both growth factors appear to be dramatically affected by hormones. During the cycle HGF expression increases under E_2 influence and decreases when P levels rise, even though E_2 levels remain elevated. This is the typical pattern of an E_2-dependent, P-antagonized molecule. KGF expression increases when P rises even when E_2 is absent and decreases when P falls even though E_2 is present; this pattern is characteristic of a P-dependent molecule.

There also appear to be cyclic changes in the distribution of KGFR, as KGF binding activity was found on all the glands, from the luminal surface to the myometrial border under E_2 influence, but was restricted to the basalis glands and the spiral arteries during $E_{2+}P$ treatment. The HGF receptor, c-Met, appeared to be constitutively expressed.

What physiological roles might these potent mitogens play? Three different waves of epithelial proliferation occur in the macaque endometrium during the menstrual cycle. The first is the repair phase, immediately after menstruation, when the ragged surface of the endometrium heals. This surface healing is highly analogous to reepithelialization during wound healing and is known to be estrogen independent (Ferenczy et al. 1979). Because KGF falls during this phase, it probably plays little role in such healing. HGF mRNA transcription increases substantially during this phase and HGF could possibly play a role in endometrial surface repair.

The second wave begins a few days after menstrual surface repair. During the LFT the glandular epithelium in the functionalis, but not the basalis, proliferates in an E_2-dependent manner. In a previous report on the LFT (McClellan et al. 1990) we speculated that estrogen stimulated the stroma to produce a mitogen that acted in paracrine fashion on the glandular epithelium. That suggestion was based on our observation that during days 4–5 of the LFT: estrogen receptors were detectable in the stroma but not the epithelium of the proliferating glands. An indirect effect of estrogen on epithelial proliferation, mediated by the stroma, thus seemed plausible. Because HGF, a stromally derived epithelial mitogen, increases after P falls and remains elevated under E_2 treatment, this molecule is a likely candidate for the proposed estrogen-dependent stromal mitogen.

The third wave of mitosis occurs during the luteal phase, when the basalis glands and the spiral arteries proliferate in a P-dependent manner, while the glands of the functionalis cease to proliferate. The P dependence of this burst of proliferation in the basalis of the macaque endometrium during the luteal phase has been well documented (Okulicz et al. 1993; Padykula et al. 1989; Bensley 1951; Bartelmez 1951), although little evidence for similar basalis gland proliferation has been found in women (Tabibzadeh and Sun 1992). However, extensive P-dependent growth of the spiral arteries is common to both women and macaques. As reviewed above, in situ hybridization showed that during P treatment KGF mRNA expression is strongest in the stromal cells located around and between the glands of the basalis. Our histochemical studies with the KGF-HFc fusion molecule indicated those glands are the only ones to retain KGF binding activity in the luteal phase. The temporal and spatial correlation between P-dependent KGF mRNA expression, KGF binding activity, and P-dependent basalis gland epithelial proliferation are all consistent with a role for KGF as a stromally derived endometrial progestomedin.

In situ hybridization also revealed KGF transcripts in the perivascular stroma and the smooth muscle cells of the spiral arteries, and ligand histochemistry with the KGF-HFc fusion molecule indicated that KGF binding activity was evident in these vessels. However, the precise localization of the signal was not clear. Electron microscopy is needed to delineate more precisely the KGF binding sites in these arteries. Although KGF has not previously been considered a mitogen for vascular muscle or endothelium (Rubin et al. 1989), the possibility exists that these particular arteries have a unique dependence on the KGF/KGFR system.

There are several other growth factors that may interact with KGF in the endometrium. Together, KGF and insulin-like growth factor (IGF)-I (or insulin at pharmacological doses) stimulated proliferation of BALB/MK mouse epidermal keratinocytes in a chemically defined medium more effectively than KGF alone (Rubin et al. 1989). P has been shown to increase the levels of several IGF binding proteins (Giudice et al. 1991b) and IGF-II mRNA was detected in secretory phase human endometrium (Giudice et al. 1991a). Thus, during P domination in-

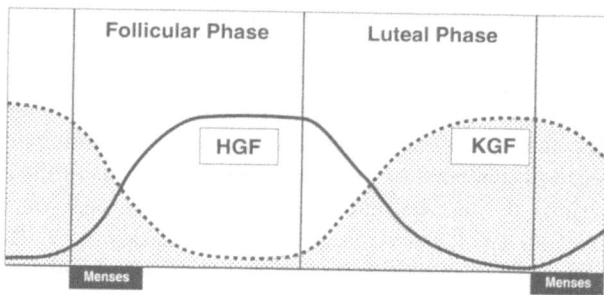

Fig. 12. A summary diagram that depicts the "yin-yang" relationship between HGF and KGF during the menstrual cycle in the rhesus macaque. The cyclic shifts in expression of HGF and KGF correlates with the cyclic shifts in proliferative activity from the functionalis to the basalis and the spiral arteries

creased levels of IGF-binding proteins, IGF-II, and KGF may act in concert, together with other growth factors, to mediate P action in the primate endometrium.

Finally, KGF produced by cells in and around the spiral arteries could directly enhance the proliferation and/or migration of the embryonic trophoblast, which invades and canalizes the spiral arteries during the early stages of implantation (Enders and King 1991). We recently reported that the trophoblastic epithelium of the villi of 30-day-old macaque placentas express KGFR mRNA and can bind ^{125}I-labeled KGF (Izumi et al. 1996). Whether the invading trophoblast also expresses KGFR during the earliest stages of implantation remains to be established.

KGF might also play a role in the proliferation of the surface epithelium that results in the temporary epithelial plaque which forms during implantation in rhesus macaques (Enders and Hendrickx 1988). Research in Sengupta's laboratory has shown that this response is P dependent, as RU-486 significantly inhibits plaque formation during experimental decidualization (Ghosh et al. 1992; Ghosh and Sengupta 1989). Because the surface epithelium lacks progesterone receptors during the luteal phase (Brenner et al. 1991; Okulicz et al. 1990; Hild-Petito et al. 1992), it is likely that the P-dependent proliferation of these cells is mediated indirectly by the P receptor-positive stromal elements. Whether the KGF/KGFR system is involved in this or other aspects of implantation is currently unknown. KGF and its receptor are present in human endometrium (Pekonen et al. 1993), but little is known about its regulation or precise cellular distribution in women.

In summary, our search for hormonally regulated, stromally derived growth factors in the endometrium has been rewarding. A "yin-yang" relationship appears to exist during the cycle as HGF rises when KGF falls and vice versa (Fig. 12). There are of course many other cell-cell signaling molecules that participate in a complex intercellular network that mediates endometrial function, but an analysis of these multiple elements is beyond the scope of this brief review.

Targeted inhibition of KGF and/or HGF action at the endometrial level may provide a new form of endometrial contraception. Inhibition of HGF action might inhibit regeneration of the endometrium during the LFT and lead to an atrophied endometrium, unable to develop a full progestational response or to support implantation. Inhibition of KGF might prevent spiral artery development and full glandular differentiation, again resulting in tissues unable to support or sustain implantation. If such inhibitors were to be effective, specialized means of local delivery would have to be developed, as these two growth factors play important roles in other organ systems, including the lungs and integument. Whether KGF and/or HGF can be targeted to create a new form of endometrial contraception remains to be determined. Whatever the outcome of such efforts, studies of these two hormonally regulated mitogens should greatly increase our understanding of the factors that mediate the actions of E_2 and P in the primate endometrium.

Acknowledgments. We gratefully acknowledge assistance with immunocytochemistry and in situ hybridization procedures by Kunie Mah, molecular procedures by Geraldine Murray, and word processing assistance from Angela Adler. This study was supported by NIH grants HD 07675 (O.D.S.), HD19182, HD18185, and HDRR00163 (R.M.B.). This is publication no. 2000 of the Oregon Regional Primate Research Center. The Morphology, Hormone Assay, Cell Culture and Molecular Biology Core laboratories provided by Population Center grant P30 HD18185 were invaluable to these studies.

References

Ausubel FM, Brent R, Kingston RE et al (eds) (1994) Current protocols in molecular biology. Greene, Wiley

Bartelmez GW (1951) Cyclic changes in the endometrium of the rhesus monkey (Macaca mulatta). Contrib Embryol 34:99–144

Bartelmez GW (1951) Cyclic changes in the endometrium of the rhesus monkey (*Macaca mulatta*). Contrib Embryol 34:99-144.

Bensley CM (1951) Cyclic fluctuations in the rate of epithelial mitosis in the endometrium of the rhesus monkey. Contrib Embryol 34:87–98

Berthois Y, Salat-Baroux J, Cornet D, De Brux J, Kopp F, Martin PM (1991) A multiparametric analysis of endometrial estrogen and progesterone receptors after the postovulatory administration of mifepristone. Fertil Steril 55:547–554

Bigsby RM, Cunha GR (1986) Estrogen stimulation of deoxyribonucleic acid synthesis in uterine epithelial cells which lack estrogen receptors. Endocrinology 119:390–396

Boccaccio C, Gaudino G, Gambarotta G, Galimi F, Comoglio PM (1994) Hepatocyte growth factor (HGF) receptor expression is inducible and is part of the delayed-early response to HGF. J Biol Chem 269:12846–12851

Bottaro DP, Rubin JS, Ron D, Finch PW, Florio C, Aaronson SA (1990) Characterization of the receptor for keratinocyte growth factor. Evidence for multiple fibroblast growth factor receptors. J Biol Chem 265:12767–12770

Bottaro DP, Fortney E, Rubin JS, Aaronson SA (1993) A keratinocyte growth factor receptor-derived peptide antagonist identifies part of the ligand binding site. J Biol Chem 268:9180–9183

Brenner RM, Slayden OD (1994) Cyclic changes in the primate oviduct and endometrium. In: Knobil E, Neill JD (eds) The physiology of reproduction. Raven, New York, p 541

Brenner RM, Carlisle KS, Hess DL, Sandow BA, West NB (1983) Morphology of the oviducts and endometria of cynomolgus macaques during the menstrual cycle. Biol Reprod 29:1289–1302

Brenner RM, West NB, McClellan MC (1990) Estrogen and progestin receptors in the reproductive tract of male and female primates. Biol Reprod 42:11–19

Brenner RM, McClellan MC, West NB, Novy MJ, Haluska GJ, Sternfeld MD (1991) Estrogen and progestin receptors in the macaque endometrium. In: Bulletti C, Gurpide E (eds) The primate endometrium. New York Academy of Sciences, New York, p 149

Bussolino F, Di Renzo MF, Ziche M, Bocchietto E, Olivero M, Naldini L, Gaudino G, Tamagnone L, Coffer A, Comoglio PM (1992) Hepatocyte growth factor is a potent angiogenic factor which stimulates endothelial cell motility and growth. J Cell Biol 119:629–641

Cunha GR, Bigsby RM, Cooke PS, Sugimura Y (1985) Stromal-epithelial interactions in adult organs. Cell Differ 17:137–148

Cunha GR, Bigsby RM, Donjacour AA, Cooke PS (1987) Hormonal regulation of epithelial morphogenesis, growth and cytodifferentiation in fetal and adult urogenital tracts: roles of mesenchymal-epithelial interactions. In: Wolff JR, Sievers J, Bräutigam W (eds) Mesenchymal-epithelial interactions in neural development. Springer, Berlin Heidelberg New York, p 223

Di Renzo MF, Narsimhan RP, Olivero M, Bretti S, Giordano S, Medico E, Gaglia P, Zara P, Comoglio PM (1991) Expression of the Met/HGF receptor in normal and neoplastic human tissues. Oncogene 6:1997–2003

Enders AC, Hendrickx AG (1988) Implantation and early embryonic development in primates. In: Brans YW, Kuehl TJ (eds) Nonhuman primates in perinatal research. Wiley, New York, p 139

Enders AC, King BF (1991) Early stages of trophoblastic invasion of the maternal vascular system during implantation in the macaque and baboon. Am J Anat 192:329–346

Ferenczy A, Bertrand G, Gelfand MM (1979) Studies on the cytodynamics of human endometrial regeneration III. In vitro short-term incubation historadioautography. Am J Obstet Gynecol 134:297–304

Finch PW, Rubin JS, Miki T, Ron D, Aaronson SA (1989) Human KGF is FGF-related with properties of a paracrine effector of epithelial cell growth. Science 245:752–755

Gambarotta G, Pistoi S, Giordano S, Comoglio PM, Santoro C (1994) Structure and inducible regulation of the human MET promoter. J Biol Chem 269:12852–12857

Ghosh D, Sengupta J (1989) Endometrial responses to a deciduogenic stimulus in ovariectomized rhesus monkeys treated with oestrogen and progesterone. J Endocrinol 120:51–58

Ghosh D, De P, Sengupta J (1992) Effect of RU 486 on the endometrial response to deciduogenic stumulus in ovariectomized rhesus monkeys treated with oestrogen and progesterone. Hum Reprod 7:1048–1060

Giudice LC, Lamson G, Rosenfeld RG, Irwin JC (1991a) Insulin-like growth factor-II (IGF-II) and IGF binding proteins in human endometrium. Ann NY Acad Sci 626:295–307

Giudice LC, Milkowski DA, Lamson G, Rosenfeld RG, Irwin JC (1991b) Insulin-like growth factor binding proteins in human endometrium: steroid-dependent mesenger ribonucleic acid expression and protein synthesis. J Clin Endocrinol Metab 72:779–787

Grant DS, Kleinman HK, Goldberg ID, Bhargava M, Nickoloff BJ, Polverini P, Rosen EM (1993) Scatter factor induces blood vessel formation in vivo. Proc Natl Acad Sci USA 90:1937–1941

Henderson GS, Conary JT, Davidson JM, Stewart SJ, House FS, McCurley TL (1991) A reliable method for Northern blot analysis using synthetic oligonucleotide probes. Biotechniques 10:190–197

Hild-Petito S, Verhage HG, Fazleabas AT (1992) Immunocytochemical localization of estrogen and progestin receptors in the baboon (Papio anubis) uterus during implantation and pregnancy. Endocrinology 130:2343–2353

Ishiki Y, Ohnishi H, Muto Y, Matsumoto K, Nakamura T (1992) Direct evidence that hepatocyte growth factor is a hepatotrophic factor for liver regeneration and has a potent antihepatitis effect vivo. Hepatology 16:1227–1235

Izumi S, Slayden OD, Rubin JS, Brenner RM (1996) Keratinocyte growth factor and its receptor in the rhesus macaque placenta during the course of gestation. Placenta 17:123–135

Kawaida K, Matsumoto K, Shimazu H, Nakamura T (1994) Hepatocyte growth factor prevents acute renal failure and accelerates renal regeneration in mice. Proc Natl Acad Sci USA 91:4357–4361

Kelley MJ, Pech M, Seuanez HN, Rubin JS, O'Brien SJ, Aaronson SA (1992) Emergence of the keratinocyte growth factor multigene family during the great ape radiation. Proc Natl Acad Sci USA 89:9287–9291

Koji T, Brenner RM (1993) Localization of estrogen receptor messenger ribonucleic acid in rhesus monkey uterus by nonradioactive in situ hybridization with digoxigenin-labeled oligodeoxynucleotides. Endocrinology 132:382–392

Koji T, Chedid M, Rubin JS, Slayden OD, Csaky KG, Aaronson SA, Brenner RM (1994) Progesterone-dependent expression of keratinocyte growth factor mRNA in stromal cells of the primate endometrium: keratinocyte growth factor as a progestomedin. J Cell Biol 125:393–401

LaRochelle WJ, Dirsch OR, Finch PW, Cheon H-G, May M, Marchese C, Pierce JH, Aaronson SA (1995) Specific receptor detection by a functional keratinocyte growth factor-immunoglobulin chimera. J Cell Biol 129:357–366

Lewis SA, Balcarek JM, Krek V, Shelanski M, Cowan NJ (1984) Sequence of a cDNA clone encoding mouse glial fibrillary acidic protein: structural conservation of intermediate filaments. Proc Natl Acad Sci USA 81:2743–2746

Lindroos PM, Zarnegar R, Michalopoulos GK (1991) Hepatocyte growth factor (hepatopoietin A) rapidly increases in plasma before DNA synthesis and liver regeneration stimulated by partial hepatectomy and carbon tetrachloride administration. Hepatology 13:743–749

Liu Y, Michalopoulos GK, Zarnegar R (1994) Structural and functional characterization of the mouse hepatocyte growth factor gene promoter. J Biol Chem 269:4152–4160

Low KG, Allen RG, Melner MH (1990) Association of proenkephalin transcripts with polyribosomes in the heart. Mol Endocrinol 4:1408–1415

McClellan MC, Rankin S, West NB, Brenner RM (1990) Estrogen receptors, progestin receptors and DNA synthesis in the macaque endometrium during the luteal–follicular transition. J Steroid Biochem Molec Biol 37:631–641

Miki T, Fleming TP, Bottaro DP, Rubin JS, Ron D, Aaronson SA (1991) Expression cDNA cloning of the KGF receptor by creation of a transforming autocrine loop. Science 251:72–75

Miki T, Bottaro DP, Fleming TP, Smith CL, Burgess WH, Chan AM, Aaronson SA (1992) Determination of ligand–binding specificity by alternative splicing: two distinct growth factor receptors encoded by a single gene. Proc Natl Acad Sci USA 89:246–250

Miyazawa K, Shimomura T, Kitamura A, Kondo J, Morimoto Y, Kitamura N (1992) Molecular cloning and sequence analysis of the cDNA for a human serine protease responsible for activation of hepatocyte growth factor: structural similarity of the protease precursor to blood coagulation factor XII. J Biol Chem 267:20493–20496

Moghul A, Lin L, Beedle A, Kanbour-Shakir A, DeFrances MC, Liu Y, Zarnegar R (1994) Modulation of c-Met proto-oncogene (HGF receptor) mRNA abundance by cytokines and hormones: evidence for rapid decay of the 8 kb c-MET transcript. Oncogene 9:2045–2052

Montesano R, Matsumoto K, Nakamura T, Orci L (1991) Identification of a fibroblast-derived epithelial morphogen as hepatocyte growth factor. Cell 67:901–908

Naldini L, Tamagnone L, Vigna E, Sachs M, Hartmann G, Birchmeier W, Daikuhara Y, Tsubouchi H, Blasi F, Comoglio PM (1992) Extracellular proteolytic cleavage by urokinase is required for activation of hepatocyte growth factor/scatter factor. EMBO J 11:4825–4833

Okulicz WC, Savasta AM, Hoberg LM, Longcope C (1990) Biochemical and immunohistochemical analyses of estrogen and progesterone receptors in the rhesus monkey uterus during the proliferative and secretory phases of artificial menstrual cycles. Fertil Steril 53:913–920

Okulicz WC, Balsamo M, Tast J (1993) Progesterone regulation of endometrial estrogen receptor and cell proliferation during the late proliferative and secretory phase in artificial menstrual cycles in the rhesus monkey. Biol Reprod 49:24–32

Padykula HA, Coles LG, Okulicz WC, Rapaport SI, McCracken JA, King NW Jr, Longcope C, Kaiserman-Abramof IR (1989) The basalis of the primate endometrium: A bifunctional germinal compartment. Biol Reprod 40:681–690

Pekonen F, Nyman T, Rutanen E (1993) Differential expression of keratinocyte growth factor and its receptor in the human uterus. Mol Cell Endocrinol 95:43–49

Pepper MS, Matsumoto K, Nakamura T, Orci L, Montesano R (1992) Hepatocyte growth factor increases urokinase-type plasminogen activator (u-PA) and u-PA receptor expression in Madin-Darby canine kidney epithelial cells. J Biol Chem 267:20493–20496

Rothblum LI, Parker DL, Cassidy B (1982) Isolation and characterization of rat ribosomal DNA clones. Gene 17:75–77

Rubin JS, Osada H, Finch PW, Taylor WG, Rudikoff S, Aaronson SA (1989) Purification and characterization of a newly identified growth factor specific for epithelial cells. Proc Natl Acad Sci USA 86:802–806

Rubin JS, Chan AM, Bottaro DP, Burgess WH, Taylor WG, Cech AC, Hirschfield DW, Wong J, Miki T, Finch PW et al (1991) A broad-spectrum human lung fibroblast-derived mitogen is a variant of hepatocyte growth factor. Proc Natl Acad Sci USA 88:415–419

Rubin JS, Bottaro DP, Aaronson SA (1993) Hepatocyte growth factor/scatter factor and its receptor, the c-met proto-oncogene product. Biochimica et Biophysica Acta 1155:357–371

Rubin JS, Bottaro DP, Chedid M, Miki T, Ron D, Cunha GR, Finch PW (1995) Keratinocyte growth factor as a cytokine that mediates mesenchymal-epithelial interaction. In: Goldberg I, Rosen E (eds) Epithelial mesenchymal interactions in cancer. Birkhäuser, Basel

Slayden OD, Hirst JJ, Brenner RM (1993) Estrogen action in the reproductive tract during antiprogestin treatment. Endocrinology 132:1845–1856

Slayden OD, Izumi S, Wilson I, Vijayaraghavan S, Rubin JS, Finch P, Brenner RM (1994) Keratinocyte growth factor (KGF) and KGF receptor (KGFR) mRNAs in the cervix, placenta, and decidua of rhesus macaques. In: Abstracts of SSR annual meeting (held in Ann Arbor, MI, 24-27 July 1994), p 121, no 267

Slayden OD, Koji T, Brenner RM (1995a) Microwave stabilization enhances immunocytochemical detection of estrogen receptor in frozen sections of macaque oviduct. Endocrinology 136:4012–4021

Slayden OD, Murray G, Izumi S-I, Rubin JS, Chedid M, Brenner RM (1995b) Steroids regulate hepatocyte growth factor (HGF) mRNA in the reproductive tract of rhesus macaques. In: Program and abstracts of the 28th annual meeting of SSR (held at University of California, Davis, 9-12 July) 161, no 419

Stampfer MR, Bartley JC (1985) Induction of transformation and continuous cell line from normal human mammary epithelial cells after exposure to benzo(a)pyrene. Proc Natl Acad Sci USA 82:2394–2398

Stoker M, Gherardi E, Perryman M, Gray J (1987) Scatter factor is a fibroblast-derived modulator of epithelial cell mobility. Nature 327:239–242

Tabibzadeh S, Sun XZ (1992) Cytokine expression in human endometrium throughout the menstrual cycle. Hum Reprod 7:1214–1221

Tso JY, Sun X-H, Kao T, Reece KS, Wu R (1985) Isolation and characterization of rat and human glyceraldehyde-3-phosphate dehydrogenase cDNAs: genomic complexity and molecular evolution of the gene. Nucleic Acids Res 13:2485–2502

Ulich TR, Yi ES, Cardiff R, Yin S, Bikhazi N, Biltz R, Morris CF, Pierce GF (1994a) Keratinocyte growth factor is a growth factor for mammary epithelium in vivo. Am J Pathol 144:862–868

Ulich TR, Yi ES, Longmuir K, Yin S, Biltz R, Morris CF, Housley RM, Pierce GF (1994b) Keratinocyte growth factor is a growth factor for type II pneumocytes in vivo. J Clin Invest 93:1298–1306

3 Cell Biological Aspects of the Implantation Window

H.M. Beier

3.1 Introduction

"Implantation window" is a widely used and remarkably well understood term in reproductive biology and medicine. This term emerged
from suggestions by Psychoyos (1963), McLaren (1973), and Finn and
Martin (1974) when they asked whether estrogens in mice and rats may
control the physiological status of a "sensitive" or "nonsensitive," of a
"receptive" or "nonreceptive" endometrium to achieve implantation of

Table 1. Time frames of the implantation window

Time frames (days of the cycle)	Markers	Methods	Reference
15–24	Uterine secretion protein patterns	Electrophoretical separation and laser densitometry of uterine secretion samples of endocrinologically normal patients (in vitro fertilization because of androgenic factor)	Beier-Hellwig et al. (1989)
19–21	Pinopodes (apical protrusions of epithelial cells)	Scanning electron microscopy of endometrial biopsy samples	Nikas et al. (1995)
20–24	Embryonic signals (hCG of trophoblast cells)	Embryo transfer in patients of an IVF/ET-program in cycles without stimulation, hCG chemiluminescence assay in maternal serum	Bergh and Navot (1992)
20–24	Integrins $\alpha_v\beta_3$, $\alpha_1\beta_1$, $\alpha_4\beta_1$	Histochemistry of endometrial biopsy samples	Lessey et al. (1995)

the blastocyst. However, the term has mainly been applied to the concept of an "endometrial" window. Biologically this term could be extended to cover all of the physiological changes associated with implantation, by the endometrium, the corpus luteum, and the blastocyst. Consequently one could consider an "implantation window" as well at the "luteal" or at the "embryonic" level and call it "luteal" or "embryonic" window. Each of the main aspects of this term "implantation window" requires precise description and definition for scientific understanding. It is equally important, however, that we focus our attention on the adequate level of methodological approach, when we scientifically use the terms "receptivity" or "implantation window." Since the level of methodological resolution may be either at the organ, tissue, cellular, or molecular level, the status of receptivity entails various patterns of complexity.

To date there are no widely accepted criteria for evaluating endometrial receptivity in reproductive medicine. Novel methodological approaches include classical means such as light and electron microscopy, cell and tissue culture, and biochemical and physicochemical analyses. However, the most promising means are available by molecular biology and gene technology, which will resolve cell physiology up to switching-on and-off specific genes. Final confirmation of receptivity will be taught to the investigator rather by the blastocyst itself than by any polymerase chain reaction readings. It is this crucial phenomenon of receptivity which will be the decisive question for any clinical investigation on the newly envisaged "endometrial contraception" which is based on the strategic concept of inhibition or prevention of a receptive stage of the endometrium. This in turn should prevent the early establishment of pregnancy and act as a locally restricted contraceptive mechanism.

Nevertheless, the terms "receptivity" and "implantation window" are currently used synonymously to describe the physiological and structural stage of the endometrium during the luteal phase of the cycle in which attachment and implantation of the blastocyst can be achieved. The time frame of the implantation window is set differently by various investigators according to different cell biological markers and levels of methodological resolution (see Table 1).

3.2 The Endometrium: A Complex Organ and Not Just a Simple Tissue

The endometrium represents the mucosa, lining the uterine cavity. The common description that this mucosa consists of two principal cell populations, namely "epithelial" and "stromal" cells, is a simplification which is no longer justified. The epithelial cell population is comprised of the surface epithelium and of the various glandular epithelium cells, which are found in the tubular glands of the stratum functionale and stratum basale (Fig. 1). The "stroma" is found to contain the reticular connective tissue of the mucosa, filled abundantly with lymphocytes and granulocytes during the luteal phase of the menstrual cycle. This reticular connective tissue is comprised of a very special population of fibroblasts which can be rapidly transformed into decidualized cells if an embryo has started to attach and to implant. These specialized cells are found in any menstrual cycle as predecidualized cells, which are located preferentially within the perivascular compartments of the stratum functionale. The abundantly proliferating blood vessels seem to

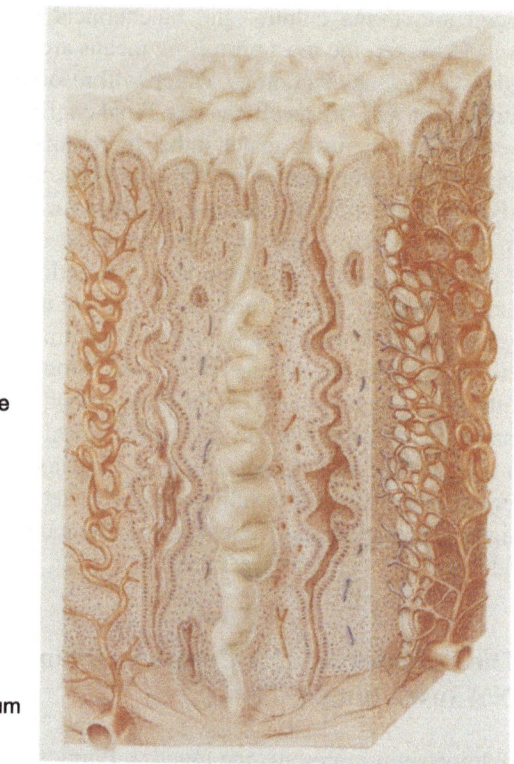

Stratum
functionale

Stratum
basale

Myometrium

Fig. 1. Histological diagram of human endometrium during the luteal phase of the cycle. The epithelial cells are distributed at the endometrial surface and lining all glands. The "stroma" is filled with fibroblasts, predecidual cells, and numerous blood vessels. This picture is a common textbook version; however, it does not take into account our new insights into the differentiated cell populations of the "stroma," particularly the immunocompetent cells (see Fig. 2). (With kind permission from Breckwoldt et al. 1994, Medical Service Munich)

play an extremely important role within the mucosa. Basal anastomosing arteries branch into the terminal "spiral" arteries, which sprout into capillaries that drain the periglandular and subepithelial compartments into venous sinuses. It is from the blood vessels, where an enormous number of lymphocytes, granulocytes, and macrophages immigrate into

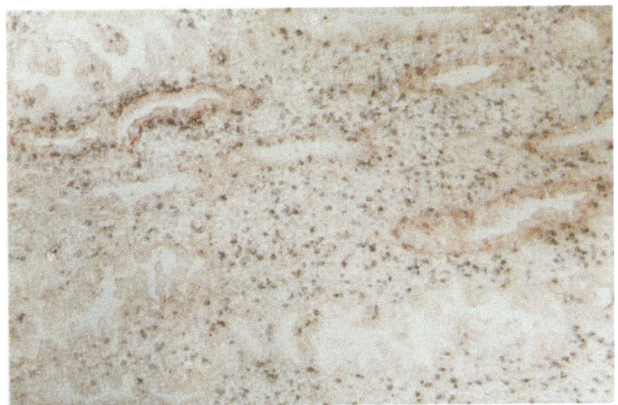

Fig. 2. Endometrial section from the late luteal phase, day 28 of the cycle, showing the abundant appearance of immunocompetent cells (*blue staining*). There is a large number of CD56^{bright} cells, evenly distributed, some appearing in closer contact to the glands. Counterstaining (*red*) of the epithelial gland cells by BTC 41 antibodies (Takara) against β3-integrins. Cryosection, ×125

the compartment of the "stroma" (Fig. 2), and where all endocrine signals for endometrial proliferation and transformation originate.

3.3 Steroid Hormone Receptors

Estrogens and progesterone are the key hormones which regulate the endometrial cycle. Estradiol also controls the synthesis of estrogen and progesterone receptors. These steroid receptors have been used as cellular marker molecules to identify various stages of differentiation of endometrial cells because their expression can be followed easily by immunohistochemical staining (Fig. 3). However, the timing of steroid receptor expression did not prove a useful marker system for assessing endometrial receptivity. At the beginning of the luteal-phase downregulation of epithelial estradiol and progesterone receptors was found to be a phase-specific and consistent phenomenon. However, no further correlation was found with cellular transformations, which in turn could

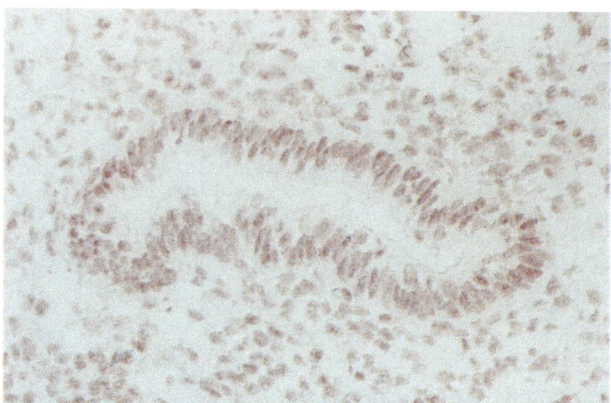

Fig. 3. Endometrial section from the late proliferative phase, day 14 of the cycle, showing positive immunoreaction for the progesterone receptors within the nuclei of epithelial and stromal cells. Both cell types express the progesterone receptor strongly. Cryosection, ×500

define the frame of an implantation window (Classen-Linke et al. 1995a).

3.4 Adhesion Molecules

Other molecules have been proposed in recent years to be significant markers. These are thought to be expressed in relation to the endometrial transformation into the stage of receptivity, by such expression signaling a particular surface condition or epithelial stage, which may facilitate adhesion or initiation of implantation. Adhesion molecules seem to play an important role in the interactions between the blastocyst and the endometrial surface, when physiologically attachment and cellular contacts are established, and also when invasion of the trophoblast cells occurs, and complex control of the invading cells takes place. Adhesion molecules, such as integrins, are deeply involved in control or guidance of the trophoblast during these delicately balanced stop-and-go activities (Bronson and Fusi 1996).

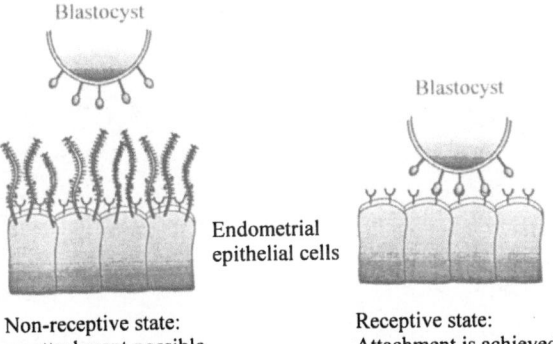

Fig. 4. Model of mouse blastocyst attachment to endometrial epithelium. The diagram shows an attachment-competent mouse embryo binding to the apical surface of endometrial epithelial cells after these cells have converted from the nonreceptive to the receptive state. Removal of mucin glyoproteins (*bottle-brush-like structures*) is requisite to making the apical surface accessible to the embryo. Upon removal of the mucins, HSPG binding proteins (*short structures*) of the endometrial cell surface become accessible to HSPGs (*drumstick-like structures*) displayed on the blastocyst surface, permitting attachment. (Modified from Carson et al. 1995)

However, there are some other intriguing candidate molecules including large carbohydrates, mucin glycoproteins, and heparan sulfate proteoglycans, which have been suggested for facilitation of embryo attachment (Aplin, this volume; Hey et al. 1994; Carson et al. 1995). Conversion of the blastocyst's and the endometrial epithelium's surfaces from a nonadhesive to an adhesive state obviously involves several alterations in the expression of adhesive molecules. Shortly after hatching from the zona pellucida the mouse blastocyst becomes competent for attachment (Fig. 4). The acquisition of this competence is associated with the increased expression of heparan sulfate proteoglycans (HSPG) on the external surface of the trophoblast (trophectoderm). Mucin glycoproteins are believed to provide a barrier at many mucosal surfaces. In particular, the mucin MUC-1 is expressed abundantly at the apical surface of mouse endometrial epithelial cells. MUC-1 is hormonally regulated and drastically reduced prior to uterine receptivity in the mouse. As a result, smaller molecules displayed at the apical surface

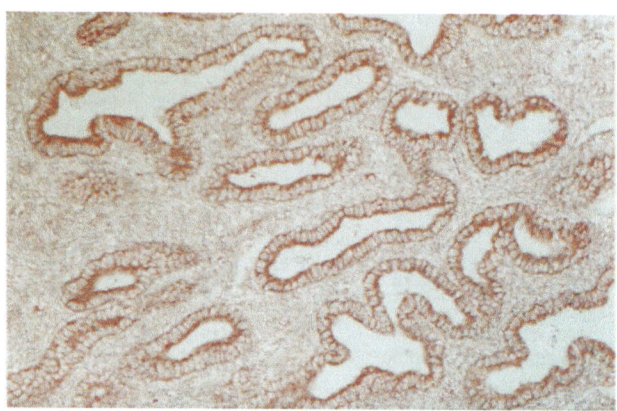

Fig. 5. Endometrial section from the luteal phase, day 23 of the cycle, showing the strong expression of β3-integrins (*red staining*). The immunostaining was performed by BTC 41 antibodies (Takara) and is localized all over the cytoplasm of the epithelial cells of most of the glands. Paraffin section, ×500

may become more accessible as functional receptors for HSPGs and for the support of embryo attachment (Carson et al. 1995).

Integrins are cell adhesion molecules interacting with macromolecules of the extracellular matrix. They are composed of α- and β-chains, and their differential expression of 14 different α-subunits and 8 different β-subunits confers their immense variability. The differential combination of α- and β-subunits results in a series of molecules of unique properties, some of which may be suitable for sustaining successive interactions between trophectoderm/trophoblast cells and endometrial cell populations to achieve implantation and early placentation. It has been a challenging idea that integrins are adhesion forces which get the free-floating blastocyst to a "touch down" at the endometrial surface, where initiation of implantation can start readily.

Highly specific antibodies have been useful to localize expressed integrin subunits in endometrial tissue sections, particularly in sections of biopsies (Fig. 5). While some integrin chains are constitutively expressed, a few subunits show phasic epithelial expression (Tabibzadeh 1992; Lessey et al. 1992, 1994, 1995; Bischof et al. 1993; Classen-Linke et al. 1995b). Lessey et al. (1994, and this volume) have described a histochemical scoring system which was determined by visual assessment and turned into an empirical pattern of integrin expression in the endometrium during the menstrual cycle. These authors suggest that the simultaneous assessment of expression of three heterodimeric molecules ($\alpha_v\beta_3$, $\alpha_1\beta_1$, $\alpha_4\beta_1$) may be used as diagnostic approach of a receptive endometrial stage (Table 1) or of various infertility types.

Even though many of the various molecules may in fact be involved in the one or the other significant step of embryonic-maternal interaction, any acceptable overall regulatory concept describing the one and only mode of implantation is still in its early infancy.

3.5 Surface Specializations: The Pinopodes

The initial step of blastocyst attachment to the endometrial surface is thought to involve extraction of fluid from the uterine lumen by specialized cellular apical protrusions (Fig. 6). These specialized bulging sur-

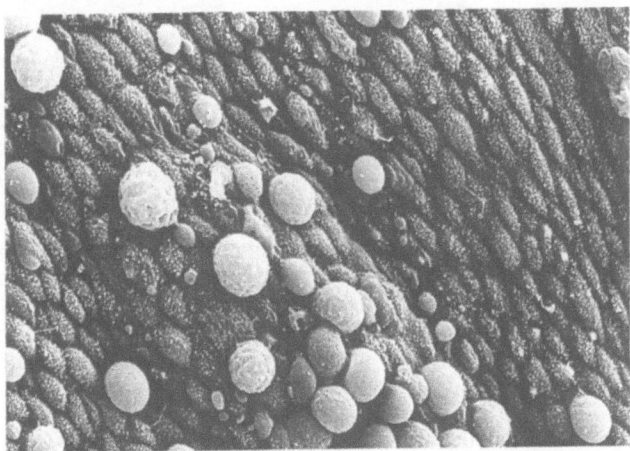

Fig. 6. Scanning electron micrograph showing the apical surface of the luminal uterine epithelium in an endometrial sample obtained from a patient at day 11 of the cycle after clomiphen treatment (100 mg each day from day 5 to day 9 of the cycle). Fully developed pinopodes appear at the edge of a funnel-shaped gland opening. SEM, ×3600

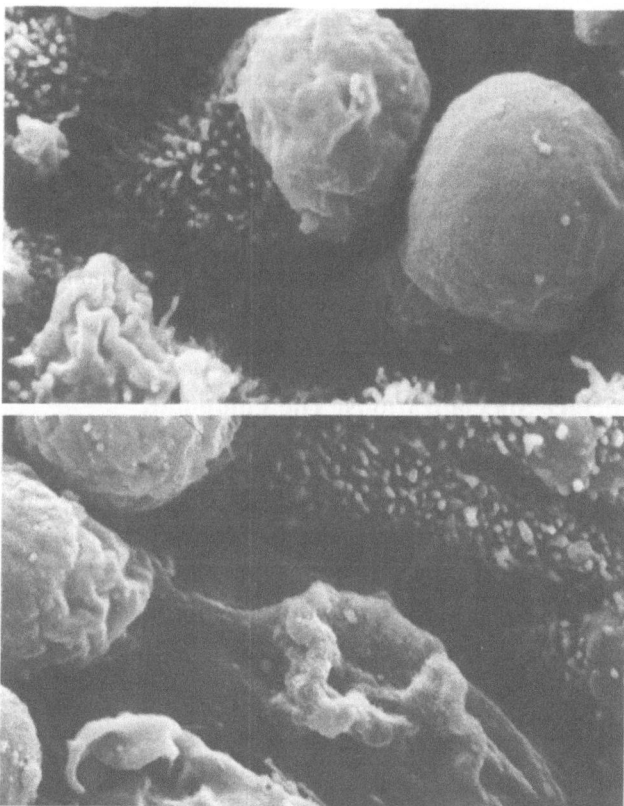

Fig. 7 *(above).* Scanning electron micrograph showing larger magnifications of pinopodes in various stages of their morphological development (same patient as Fig. 6). *Right,* a fully extended apical protrusion; *left,* a nearly completely wrinkled structure possibly in the process of shrinking. This indicates that pinopodes more frequently are shrinking than being pinched off. SEM, ×17000

Fig. 8 *(below).* Scanning electron micrograph showing pinopodes in various stages of their morphological development (same patient as Fig. 6). *Center,* the remnants of a pinched off pinopode. The others *(left)* show pinopode stages of shrinking. SEM, ×17000

face membranes have been described as "pinopodes" (Parr and Parr 1974; Psychoyos 1994; Nikas et al. 1995). These descriptions postulate that pinopodes are progesterone-dependent cellular organelles, appearing for only 2–3 days between days 19 and 21 of the normal menstrual cycle. However, there is no conclusive evidence that these structures have any clearcut predictive value as "markers" of the implantation window (Table 1). We have shown by scanning electron microscopy that these apical protrusions are preferentially seen at the funnel-shaped openings of the glands, and that they are membrane specializations supposedly for easier transmembrane carrier processes, possibly in both directions. Occasionally these pinopodes are pinched off (Figs. 7, 8), releasing probably more fluid than they may have taken up.

3.6 Paracrine Modulation of Endometrial Function

Modern cell biology has unraveled the molecules responsible for the fine tuning of endocrine regulation. Many functions of endometrial cells are regulated by potent intercellular signals, the cytokines. These molecules act as paracrine or even autocrine factors from cell to cell or from a cell via extracellular pathways back on the same cell. Cytokines were initially recognized as factors involved in immune reactions. However, recent research results clearly indicate that cytokines represent the network of polypeptide signals which cell populations of complex tissues such as the endometrium need for local and for immediate cell-cell communication. There is ample evidence that cytokines participate in the modulation of estrogen and progesterone control of endometrial differentiation, transformation, and stepwise achievement of receptivity and thus enable the embryo to implant.

Cytokines such as interleukin-1, tumor necrosis factor-α, transforming growth factor-α, epidermal growth factor, and colony-stimulating factor-1 (macrophage colony-stimulating factor) are obviously involved in establishing regional specific distribution of various cell populations and their differential proliferative activity within the endometrium. Particular microenvironmental conditions may be created by the assembly of cytokine-responsive cells which are attracted around cells that produce membrane-bound cytokines. On the other hand, cytokines may be released by certain cells and attract other responsive cells. Conse-

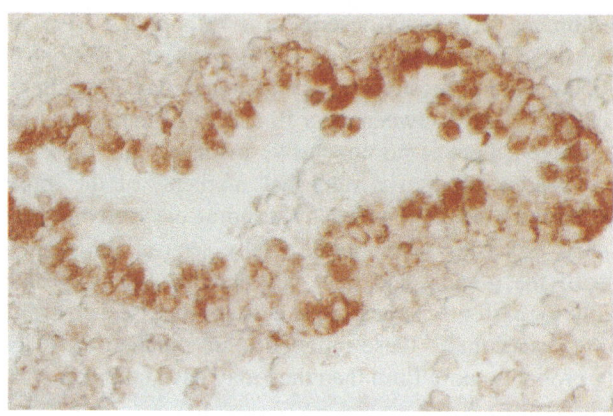

Fig. 9. Endometrial section from the luteal phase, day 24 of the cycle, showing immunoreaction of leukemia inhibitory factor (*red staining*). This section demonstrates a strong response for leukemia inhibitory factor located in the apical cytoplasm and apical protrusions of glandular epithelial cells. Paraffin section, ×500

quently, local production and paracrine effects of cytokines may be decisive modulatory events to polarize tissue compartments, such as the basalis and functionalis of the human endometrium. From these stromal compartments, particularly from lymphoid cell aggregates, major modulations of glandular and lumenal epithelium, on epithelial cell differentiation and function may be initiated by cytokines, for example, as has been shown for interferon-γ and transforming growth factor-α. Further effects on epithelial cells cycles and on the preparation of menstrual processes have been shown by interleukin-1 and by interleukin-1 mediated effects by elaboration of interleukin-6 (Tabibzadeh and Sun 1992; Simon et al. 1995).

Individual molecules of the cytokine family may be understood as characters of an alphabet or code. Therefore an information transmitted to target cells may be the product of several cytokines or the net effects of a battery of regulatory peptides rather than being made up of only one single cytokine (see Tabibzadeh 1994)

The expression of genes for cytokines and their receptors has gained particular attention in research on early mammalian development, which appears in synchrony with endometrial differentiation to achieve receptivity. Various cytokines (growth factors) such as insulin-like growth factors I and II, epidermal growth factor, transforming growth factor-α, platelet-derived growth factor-A, colony-stimulating factor-1, and leukemia inhibitory factor (Fig. 9) are expressed in temporal and spatial variables to serve a most sophisticated pattern of events which finally accomplishes embryonic and trophoblastic development. Thus, paracrine modulations may enable a molecular cross-talk between endometrial cells and blastocyst cells contributing locally to the endocrine embryo-maternal dialogue. The molecular network of cytokines being involved in cellular control of this complex tissue, however, does not represent a departure from the traditional view that steroids are the main forces in pulling the strings for endometrial function. Finally, cytokines enlarge our understanding of the intricate cellular operations which achieve receptivity and immunological tolerance of the endometrium.

3.7 Composition of Endometrial Secretion

In the uterus the fluid layer on the inner surface of the lumen contains a considerable amount of protein. These proteins are transudates of serum origin, leakage products of apoptotic and sloughed-off cells, and products of the release of local glandular secretion (Beier 1974). All components of transudate, leakage, and secretion material vary in composition and amount during the menstrual cycle depending on ovarian hormonal control. Due to steroid hormone influence, viscosity, and biochemical composition in terms of electrolyte concentration, glucosaminoglycans, glycogen, peptide, and protein contents change. Estrogens control the permeability of capillary endothelia and thus transudation; progesterone is responsible for the secretory activity and the control of apoptosis of endometrial epithelia (Terada et al. 1989; Rotello et al. 1991). Physicochemically, estrogen decreases the viscosity of uterine secretion while progesterone stimulates an increase of viscosity.

From cell kinetic studies we know that cellular proliferation of the endometrial epithelium and glands initiates synthesis and immediate protein secretion into the lumen. A significant increase in such macromolecules characterizes the preimplantation milieu in which conditioning for implantation takes place. Production and transformation of the protein composition in uterine secretion are regularly generated depending on the corresponding peripheral blood levels of ovarian hormones (Beier and Mootz 1979). However, in up to 30% of patients endometrial histology appears not to correspond with steroid hormone levels in blood serum, clinically resulting in a defective luteal phase (Crosignani 1988).

More than two decades ago we presented the first protein biochemical analyses of human uterine secretion (Beier et al. 1970; Beier and Beier-Hellwig 1973). At that time uterine fluid with an amount of protein large enough for electrophoretical resolution was obtained by gently flushing the uterine lumen after hysterectomy. Today methodological improvements in the analysis of minute fluid volumes have made it possible to intensively investigate samples of protein in small amounts such as 60–80 µg. Sodium dodecyl sulfate (SDS) treatment of proteins further permits a useful resolution of protein patterns. Systematic and comparative analysis has revealed numerous characteristic variations and alterations of protein patterns of uterine secretion in patients from infertility clinics, the definition of which has lead to more accuracy in diagnosing normality or deficiency of endometrial performance.

3.8 Biochemical Analysis of the Uterine Secretion Proteins

After SDS treatment of the protein samples there appears a considerable number of protein bands in acrylamide gel electrophoresis, particularly among the lower molecular weight fractions (Fig. 10). This area is represented by the bands between M_r 68 kDa (marker: albumin) and M_r

Fig. 10. Protein patterns of human uterine secretion at various stages of the menstrual cycle. For comparison, a protein pattern of human blood serum (*HSP*) is shown. The patterns demonstrated are from the phases of quiescence (*QUP*), early proliferation (*EPP*), complete proliferation (*CPP*), and the luteal phase (*LUP*). *Left*, molecular weight ranges. Particular families of protein bands are indicated by the areas of group A, group B, and group C. Albumin (*Alb*), histones (H2A, H2B, H3, and H4), cyclophilin (*Cyp*), transthyretin (*Tty*), haptoglobin (*Hpg*), and both chains of hemoglobin [α-globin (α-*gl*) and β-globin (β-*gl*)] are indicated. Sodium dodecyl sulfate polyacrylamide gel electrophoresis was performed in a polyacrylamide gradient of 8.3%–16.6%, Comassie blue staining

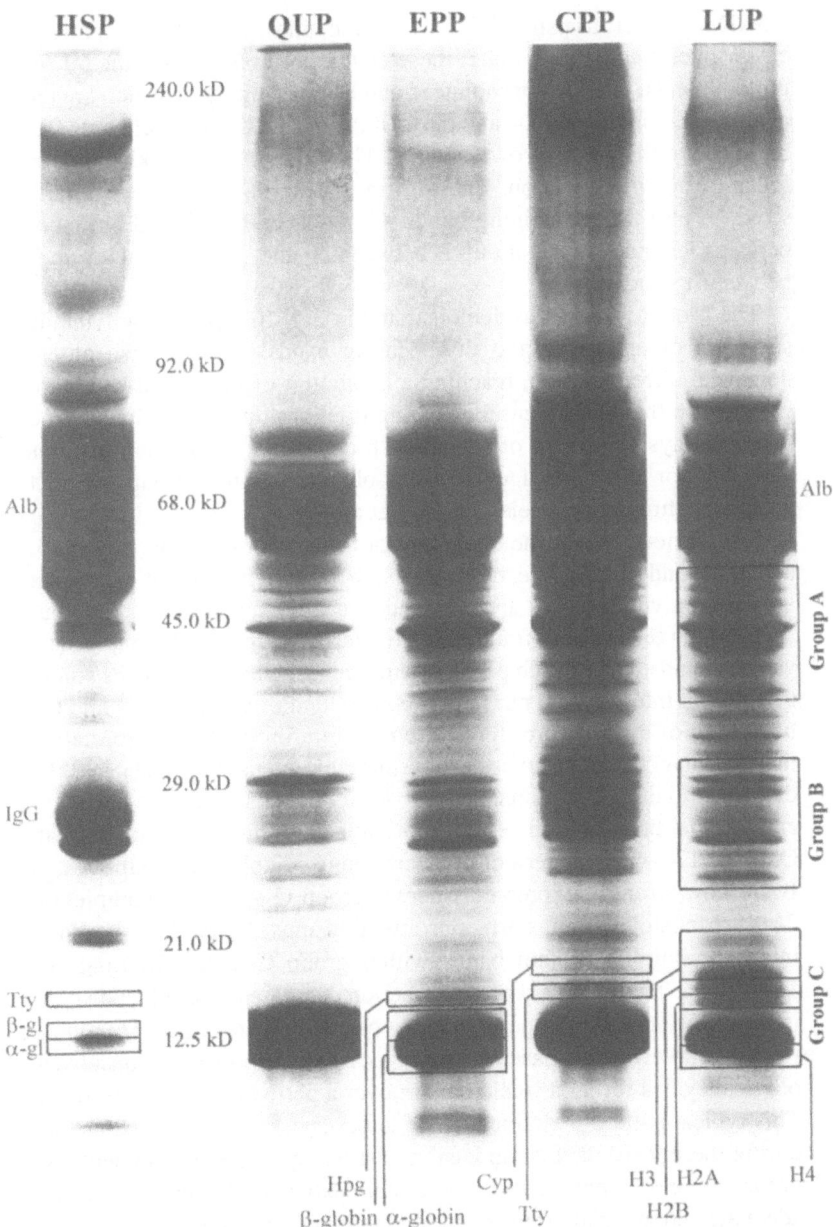

Fig. 10. Legend see p. 64

6.5 kDa (marker: trypsin inhibitor from the lung). The totally expressed electrophoretical pattern under these conditions comprises some 60–70 protein bands, the most pronounced and heavy staining of which are the albumin fraction at 68 kDa and those of the α- and β-chains of hemoglobin close to the position of 12.5 kDa. The bands below 68 kDa are the focus of our investigation. These form three groups of very similarly sized, in part faintly staining bands. Group A is represented by bands between 45 and 34 kDa, group B between 29 and 25 kDa, and group C between 18 and 12 kDa.

The protein patterns as demonstrated in Fig. 10 represent a dynamic spectrum of appearing and disappearing bands in the course of endometrial differentiation, reaching a maximum of individual bands together with the most intensely staining fractions during the time period between days 15 and 24 of the ideal 28-day cycle. All protein patterns analyzed for the normal cycle were obtained from patients without hormonal stimulation (Beier-Hellwig et al. 1988).

It is obvious that at the beginning of the menstrual cycle, days 1–5, and at the end of the cycle, days 25–28, there are a number of bands that are missing while others are only very weakly expressed, except albumin and the α-/β-globin fraction. Particularly group A and group C lack various bands during such phase of quiescence, which represents something of an intermediate phase between the end of the secretory and the beginning of the next proliferative phase, reinforcing the interpretation that for diagnostic reasons the physiological menstrual cycle may be divided into three functional states instead of two. During the period of endometrial proliferation several more intensely staining bands appear. On days 12–14 the pattern of proliferation is completed. Groups A and B are now strongly expressed whereas group C awaits its completion 24–48 h postovulation. Particular attention must be paid to the three intensely staining protein bands within group C at the M_r range of 15–18 kDa. The 12.5-kDa protein fraction decreases in width and staining intensity during the periovulatory period and stays less prominent for the whole luteal phase. As early as 24–48 h postovulation physiological cycles reveal a stable pattern over a period of up to 9–10 days. This typical pattern is defined as the luteal-phase pattern. It seems that during these 9–10 days of an ideal menstrual cycle there is no decrease or vanishing of components of the protein patterns. This pattern reflects adequate endometrial performance and may be considered a "receptive" uterine milieu, which represents on the level of protein biochemical investigation the window of implantation, which here is open from day 15 to day 24 (Beier-Hellwig et al. 1989, 1994, 1995).

3.9 Identification of Significant Protein Bands

The most obvious changes during the luteal phase are the individual protein bands in group C, with an M_r range between 12.0 and 18.0 kDa. After SDS polyacrylamide gel electrophoresis (PAGE), using 15% PAA gels, the resolved proteins were transferred to a Millipore Immobilon-P membrane using the discontinuous semidry blotting method for 45 min at 5 mA/cm^2 at 15°C. After staining with Comassie brilliant blue G250, the three bands between 14.0 and 18.0 kDa were excised and frozen at −20°C. These samples were processed for amino acid sequencing using the Applied Biosystems 477A pulsed liquid protein sequencer (Biochemisches Institut, University of Giesen, Germany). The sequence P-E-P-A-K-(X)-A-P-A-P, clearly identified histone H2B. The identity was 90% in an overlap of the ten amino acids.

Consequent investigations using comigration of histones H2A, H2B, H3, and H4 (commercially available from Boehringer, Mannheim, Germany) in SDS-PAGE revealed convincing evidence that all of these histones had corresponding protein bands in the uterine secretion samples (Hilmes et al. 1993; Beier-Hellwig et al. 1995). Finally, we were able to present definite proof of molecular identity by immunological identification using polyclonal antibodies directed specifically to histones H2A, H2B, H3, and H4. These antibodies had been produced in rabbits (Institut de Biologie Moleculaire et Cellulaire, CNRS, Strasbourg, France). There were no cross-reactions with human blood serum samples or with uterine secretion samples from the follicular phase. We have obtained clear evidence by molecular biological investigations (northern blot, in situ hybridization) that the histones H2A, H2B and H3 are controlled by ovarian steroid hormones during the menstrual cycle. By contrast, the histone H4 is not regulated by steroids but represents rather a constitutive component of uterine secretion (Hilmes et al. 1995, 1996).

Further identification of lower molecular size protein bands of uterine secretion electrophoretic (USE) patterns revealed that another interesting cell protein migrates in two isoforms of approximately 17 and 18 kDa. The isolated protein was sequenced at the first ten amino acids as V-N-P-T-V-F-F-D-I-A, which represents a 100% identity in the overlap of these ten amino acids and identifies this protein as cyclophilin A (peptidyl-prolyl-*cis-trans*-isomerase A; EC 5.2.1.8). This protein is composed of a total of 164 amino acids (Harding 1991). Cyclophilins are receiving increasing attention because they are involved in the conformation of steroid hormone receptors, bound to the nonactivated receptor molecule together with the heat shock proteins hsp70 and hsp90. These proteins belong to the important components of the receptor complex that can accomplish their specific functions only after protein folding. There is evidence that this cyclophilin is involved in estrogen receptor biochemistry on the basis of the results of Ratajczak et al. (1993) and those shown for the progesterone receptor (Lebeau and Baulieu 1994; Fischer 1994).

In another identification we have defined two serum proteins to be part of the USE pattern, the subunits of which are migrating as bands in the group C region. The sequence S-P-T-G-T-G-E-S-K, which represents an 88.9% identity in the overlap of these nine amino acids, identified the protein as transthyretin (prealbumin). This serum protein comprises 147 amino acids, of which 21 form the signal peptide. Transthyretin is a binding protein for thyroxin. The subunits of the protein are arranged as a homotetramer. Two pairs of loops from an internal molecular channel where two binding sites for thyroxine are located. Fewer than 1% of these protein molecules are normally involved in thyroxine transport. About 40% of the transthyretin circulates in a tight protein-protein complex with the plasma retinol binding protein, the specific transport protein for vitamin A. The stoichiometry and polarization data suggest four binding sites for molecular mass of 54|980; the monomeric subunit migrates in PAGE at approximately at the 15-kDa position.

The sequence V-D-S-G-N-D-V-T-D-I-A-D-D-G led to the identification of haptoglobin 1. This analysis represents a 100% identity in the overlap of these 14 amino acids. The protein has a signal peptide of 18 amino acids and a total of 347 amino acids. The peptide content of the native molecule is 84%; consequently 16% of the carbohydrates are part of the molecule. Haptoglobin normally binds free plasma hemoglobin. The hemoglobin usually binds as a dimer of an α-chain and one β-glo-

Table 2. Proteins of human endometrial secretion involved in assessments of USE by PAGE, laser densitometry, and western blotting

Protein	Molecular weight	Number of AA residues	SDS-PAGE localization	Comments on origin and/or function
α-Globin	15000	141	12.0 kDa	Hemoglobin α-chain, serum protein
Histone H4	11236	102	12.0 kDa	Cellular protein, basic nuclear protein
β-Globin	16000	146	12.5 kDa	Hemoglobin β-chain, serum protein
Histone H2A	13960	129	13.0 kDa	Cellular protein, basic nuclear protein
Histone H2B	13775	125	15.0 kDa	Cellular protein, basic nuclear protein
Transthyretin (one subunit of homotetramer)	13745	147	15.0 kDa	Syn. prealbumin, serum protein, hormone binding protein
Histone H3	15273	135	16.0 kDa	Cellular protein, basic nuclear protein
Haptoglobin 1 (α-chain dimer)	17686	166	17.0 kDa	Serum protein, hemoglobin binding protein
Cyclophilin A	17881	164	17.0 kDa	Cellular protein, protein folding enzyme (peptidyl-prolyl-cis/trans-isomerase)
Albumin	66290	585	66.0 kDa	Main serum protein, hormone binding protein

bin chain. Haptoglobin is found in extracellular compartments in all body tissues. The molecule forms a tetramer of two α_1- and two β-chains. Although the haptoglobin β-chain is clearly related to serine proteases, haptoglobin has no enzymatic activity. A common haptoglobin allele codes for a variation with different amino acid positions in the α-chain, resulting in an α_2-chain.

Further, from the USE protein pattern we identified the sequence V-L-S-P-A-D-K-T-N-V-K-A as the α-chain of hemoglobin (α-globin). There was a 100% identity in the overlap of the 12 amino acids. Our minisequence represents the first 12 amino acids from a total of 141 in this molecule. Another sequence from a USE protein band resulted in 12

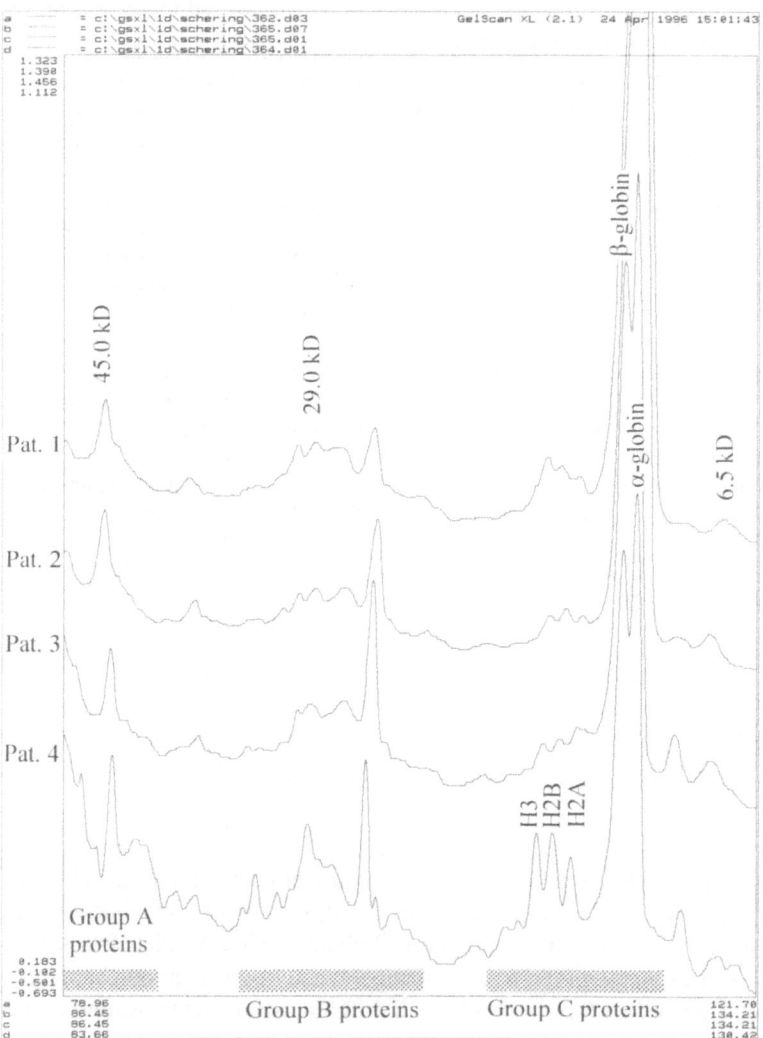

Fig. 11. Legend see p. 71

amino acids, V-H-L-T-P-E-E-K-S-A-V-T, which was clearly identified as the β-chain of hemoglobin (β-globin). There was a 100% identity in the overlap of these 12 amino acids. This molecule comprises a total of 146 amino acids. It has an approximate molecular size of 15 kDa, very similar to that of the α-globin. Both chains, α-globin and β-globin, migrate in PAGE separation close to the 12.5-kDa position.

Further efforts to identify USE pattern protein bands is currently underway in our laboratory. Table 2 presents the protein bands so far identified by isolation, sequencing, and immunological reactions.

3.10 Assessment of USE Patterns

So far the monitoring of the menstrual cycle in the clinical procedure lacks any reliable and significant assessment of the so-called "endometrial factor" that might serve as a useful predictive parameter for a receptive endometrium or the implantation window. The endometrium regularly reacts as the target tissue of the ovarian hormones. Consequently, histological dating has proven to be a sensitive indicator of ovarian function, reflecting perturbations of the physiological balances of ovarian steroids. On the other hand, however, it is not the case that normal or sufficient steroid hormone levels measured in blood plasma guarantee a normal endometrial development.

Numerous reports in the literature indicate that insufficient histological transformation of the endometrium occurs despite a normal progesterone output during the luteal phase. Rarely, even an atrophic endometrium is present, together with normal ovarian function. Jones (1949, 1976) was the first to propose a defective endometrial response to

---

◀ **Fig. 11.** Laser densitometric assessment of human uterine secretion electrophoretic (USE) samples from the early luteal phase (day 2 after luteinizing hormone peak). This figure demonstrates four USE resolutions within segments of the molecular weight ranges from 6.5 to 45.0 kDa. The samples express the typical adequate luteal-phase patterns within the cycle of conception. Each patient experienced a normal clinical pregnancy which began in this cycle. Sodium dodecyl sulfate polyacrylamide gel electrophoresis was performed in a polyacrylamide gel gradient of 8.3%–16.6%. Laser densitometry was performed by a helium-neon laser at 633 nm. Histones H2A, H2B, and H3, and α- and β-globins are indicated

hormonal stimulation as a cause of luteal inadequacy. As noted above, endometrial transformation generally depends absolutely on steroid hormone control of the ovary. The dynamic process of transformation is paralleled by a remarkable and characteristic secretory activity. Circumstantially, the endometrial reaction may be dissociated from hormonal control. Under such conditions the physiological dependency is broken down, and the endometrium turns out to be completely refractory or provides partial response only in that proliferation and/or transformation is started but not completed. Thus the endometrium loses the capacity to build up the full composition of protein patterns in uterine secretion needed as a prerequisite for support of the implantation. The physiological cycle appears as a dynamic sequence of a continuously changing protein release which in turn can be analyzed by the sequentially changing protein patterns seen in PAGE.

Furthermore, the pathological alterations of USE patterns in patients of the infertility clinic can be sensitively assessed. We have investigated, for example, protein patterns from stimulated cycles of patients who presented with tubal factor of infertility and underwent stimulation for in vitro fertilization but could not receive embryo transfer. In such examples of follicular growth stimulation we have observed different individual endometrial responses: (a) physiological luteal-phase patterns, whereendometrial preparation is adequate, (b) USE pattern diagnosis reflecting the quiescence phase of the physiological cycle, where there is no endometrial response to stimulation, (c) USE pattern diagnosis revealing a protein pattern that is pseudoproliferative, where the endometriumis capable of partial response only and appropriate transformation is not achieved, and (d) USE pattern diagnosis revealing abortive secretion only, where the endometrium is not capable of answering the steroid hormone stimulation and there is only a rudimentary response.

Intensive work is in progress in our laboratory to determine and interpret protein patterns of uterine secretion under various stimulation conditions (human menopausal gonadotropin and gonadotropin-releasing hormone analogues, GnRHa). We have evidence that densitometric tracing of the SDS-PAGE samples of USE protein patterns will serve as a promising means for clinical evaluation. This may eventually lead to new approaches for luteal-phase management. Even in a cycle of conception, an assessment of USE protein patterns is possible. Diagnostic analyses of samples obtained on day 2 after the peak in luteinizing hormone (LH) expressed patterns of "adequate" luteal phases. These samples were taken from patients in conception cycles that went on to normal clinical pregnancies (Fig. 11).

3.11 Progesterone Regulates Endometrial Receptivity and the Expression of Proteins

Progesterone antagonists were initially studied in our rabbit model using particularly uteroglobin synthesis and release (Beier et al. 1987, 1991). Based on these investigations we used the competitive receptor antagonists to progesterone for more detailed studies of progesterone effects on human endometrial proteins. Since mifepristone (RU-486) is the only registered progesterone antagonist that is permitted for clinical administration (e.g., in France, United Kingdom, and Sweden), this compound was the first to be studied for its effect on the human luteal phase. Earlier investigations at the Karolinska Hospital in Stockholm (Swahn et al. 1990, 1991) on dose finding and classical clinical parameters had demonstrated that a single dose of 200 mg mifepristone given orally on day 2 after the LH peak inhibits the establishment of pregnancy and allows undisturbed menstrual bleeding. Also, with this protocol it has been found that mifepristone is not effective in decreasing the epithelial progesterone receptor concentration in the endometrium and, in turn, retarding endometrial maturation. However, it did not alter the serum concentration of follicle-stimulating hormone, estradiol, and progesterone.

Following the same protocol, we investigated the effect of a single administration of 200 mg mifepristone on the uterine secretion protein pattern assessed by USE. Uterine secretion samples were obtained from the first four patients at day 6 after LH peak in a nontreated control cycle. The following cycle served as the treatment cycle, when 200 mg mifepristone was given at day LH+2, and again the uterine secretion sample was obtained at day LH+6. The most striking changes following mifepristone treatment occurred among the histone bands in group C of the USE pattern. Two of the patients showed significant reductions of the H2A and H3 peaks, whereas the peak in the position of H2B revealed only partial reduction compared to the control (Fig. 12). Some

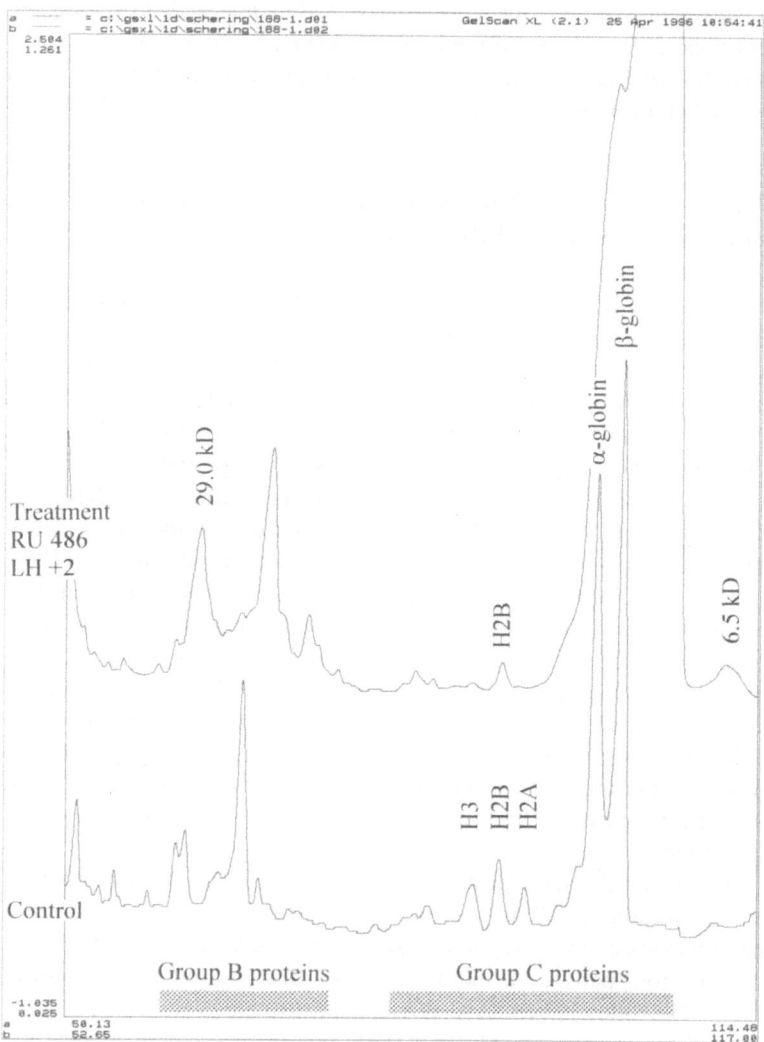

Fig. 12. Legend see p. 75

additional protein bands of group A and group B appeared markedly changed after progesterone antagonist administration. However, more detailed information will be available only after more patients have been investigated. Two of the four patients showed only a relatively weak response to mifepristone; these two displayed a significantly abnormal cycle history, beginning with an unusually extended control cycle. Consequently we need to include more individuals in this study. However, preliminary evidence shows that progesterone-dependent events in the luteal phase of the human cycle can be altered significantly by progesterone antagonists; particularly the appearance of several single endometrial proteins can be inhibited partly or totally.

Fertility-regulating approaches by progesterone antagonists have been numerous; however, only the postovulatory or early luteal-phase administration has proven effective in preventing pregnancies (Glasier et al. 1992; Gemzell-Danielsson et al. 1993). Since this treatment during the early luteal phase has been a successful contraceptive strategy, and we have observed significant changes within the uterine secretion protein patterns of these patients, we may deduce at least that the proteins under investigation can serve as markers for subtle changes in endometrial function which prevent the development of normal receptivity. An alternative approach to this postovulatory this means of contraception is the administration of progesterone antagonists during the whole cycle of the women, either daily or once a week. This strategy emerged from primate studies in which pregnancies were totally inhibited (Ishwad et al. 1993; Chwalisz et al. 1995; Katkam et al. 1995). In this context, an extremely interesting scientific aspect of the study of Katkam et al. (1995) was that low-dose onapristone treatment (2.5 mg or 5 mg every 3 days) for 4–7 consecutive cycles prevents pregnancy

◀ **Fig. 12.** Laser densitometric assessment of human uterine secretion electrophoretic (USE) samples from day 6 after luteinizing hormone (LH) peak. Treatment with the progesterone antagonist mifepristone (RU-486, 200 mg) was performed at day 2 after the LH peak. The control sample was assessed equally after collection the USE sample at day 6 after LH peak of the preceding nontreated control cycle. Significant changes appear in the histone bands H2A, H2B, and H3. Further changes can be recognized in higher molecular weight ranges. Sodium dodecyl sulfate polyacrylamide gel electrophoresis was performed in a high density gel (15% polyacrylamide). Segment of laser densitometry is shown between 6.5 kDa and 40.0 kDa

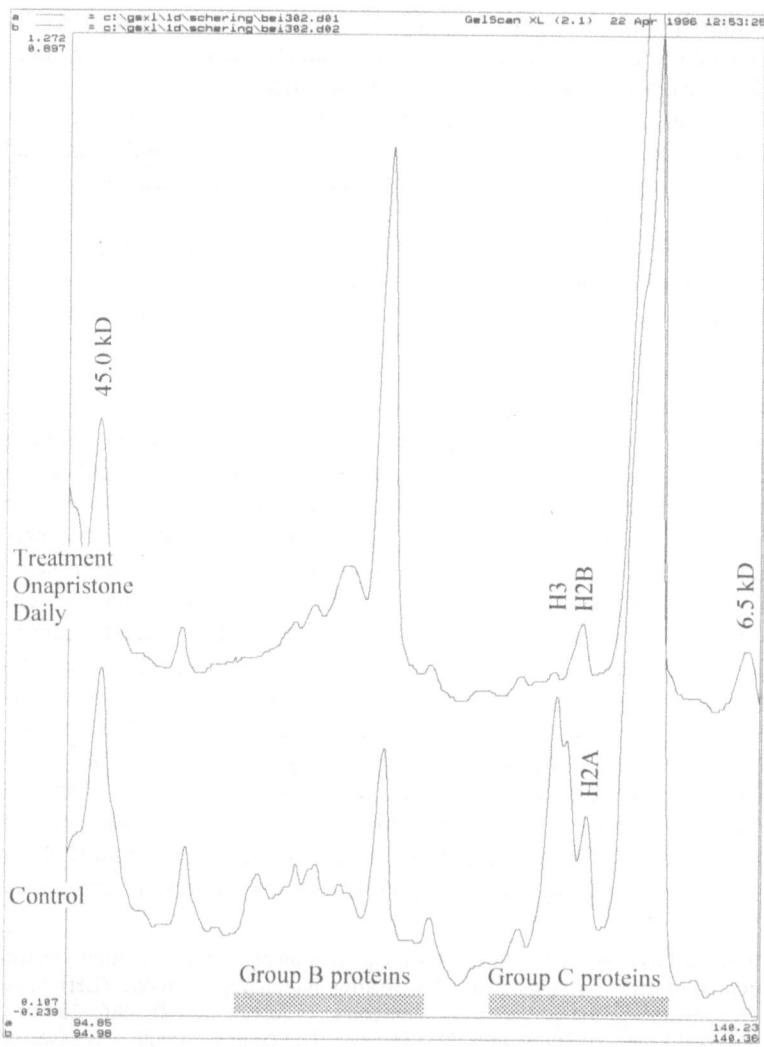

Fig. 13. Legend see p. 77

without disturbing the menstrual cycle and without inhibiting ovulation in the majoriy of cycles. However, anovulation and luteal insufficiency occurred in some animals during prolonged treatment. The contraceptive effect in the ovulatory cycles seems primarily to be related to the retardation of endometrial development, resulting in inhibition of endometrial receptivity. It appears likely that a dose or treatment regimen of onapristone that will inhibit endometrial receptivity and prevent implantation without affecting the menstrual cycle even on prolonged treatment could be identified.

Several detailed studies in animal models (Beier 1986; Hegele-Hartung and Beier 1986; Niemann et al. 1987) showed that numerous cellular and molecular steps of endometrial transformation were inhibited or delayed when progesterone was cut off from its normal triggering and regulation of luteal phase events. By inhibiting normal endometrial transformation and luteal function the basis for establishing pregnancy was prevented.

We have investigated endometrial secretory proteins in one of the first clinical studies on continuous low-dose progesterone antagonist treatment to achieve endometrial contraception. In this Schering study onapristone was administered either daily (1, 3, or 10 mg) or once a week (10, 30, or 100 mg). Onapristone and mifepristone are both selective progesterone antagonists, however, with clearly different actions at the molecular level. Unlike mifepristone, onapristone does not induce stable receptor dimers and inhibits the binding of the hormone–hormone receptor complex at the hormone responsive element of the DNA. This yields different pharmacological dynamics and a half-life of only 2–3 h for onapristone, compared to one of 24–48 h for mifepristone. As demonstrated in Figs. 13 and 14, the assessment of

---

◀ **Fig. 13.** Laser densitometric assessment of human uterine secretion electrophoretic (USE) samples from day 5 after luteinizing hormone (LH) peak. Treatment with the progesterone antagonist onapristone (ZK-98299, 10 mg daily) was performed throughout the whole cycle. The control sample was assessed equally after collecting the USE sample at day 5 after LH peak of the preceding nontreated control cycle. Significant changes appear in the histone bands H2A, H2B, and H3. Futher changes can be recognized in the higher molecular weight ranges. Sodium dodecyl sulfate polyacrylamide gel electrophoresis was performed in a polyacrylamide gel gradient of 8.3%–16.6.%. Segment of laser densitometry is shown between 6.5 kDa and 45.0 kDa

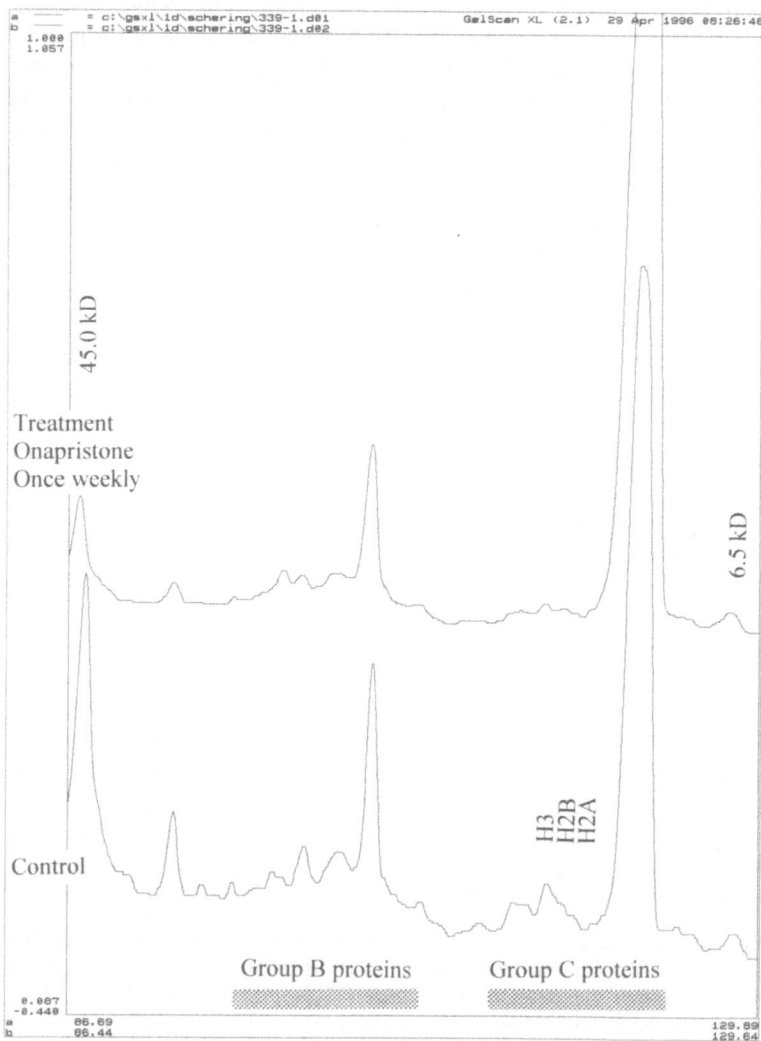

Fig. 14. Legend see p. 79

USE by laser densitometry reveals markedly changed luteal-phase patterns (obtained around day 5 after the LH peak) compared to the controls of the same patients and under the same clinical study conditions. There are considerable reductions in several protein peaks, most obviously among the low molecular weight proteins (group C of the USE pattern). In the 30 patients of each treatment group (daily and once a week) we observed two typical response categories, one exhibiting pronounced reductions in particular peaks of the pattern and the other a general quantitative diminution of distinct parts of the pattern. Nevertheless, the results of changes in the uterine protein patterns demonstrated that endometrial function under continuous progesterone antagonist administration is significantly impaired. This preliminary observation is strikingly in accord with a similar investigation just published by Gemzell-Danielsson et al. (1996) using mifepristone at low weekly doses (2.5 mg per week and 5 mg per week). In summary there are definite effects by low-dose administration of progesterone antagonists on endometrial function, in particular the delay of cellular and tissue transformation and inhibition of secretory activity, and at the same time yields no inhibition of ovulation. However, whether these effects are sufficient under the real circumstances of daily life to prevent the establishment of pregnancy awaits further clinical studies in unprotected cycles.

◀ **Fig. 14.** Laser densitometric assessment of human uterine secretion electrophoretic (USE) samples from day 4 after the luteinizing hormone (LH) peak. Treatment with the progesterone antagonist onapristone (ZK-98.299, 100 mg per week) was performed throughout the whole cycle. The control sample was assessed equally after collecting the USE sample at day 6 after the LH peak of the preceding nontreated control cycle. Significant changes appear in the histone bands H2A, H2B, and H3. There is a general quantitative dimunition, different from the changes shown in Figs. 12 and 13. Also the higher molecular weight bands are generally expressed weaker, leading to the second type of USE pattern changes after progesterone antagonist treatment (compare text). Sodium dodecyl sulfate polyacrylamide gel electrophoresis was performed in a polyacrylamide gel gradient of 8.3%–16.6%. Segment of laser densitometry is shown between 6.5 kDa and 45 kDa

3.12 Diagnostic Prediction of the Implantation Window

From animal models we have learned that a histologically normally transformed endometrium must offer an adequate lumenal secretion milieu to the preimplantational blastocyst to ensure a stage of receptivity that facilitates implantation (Beier 1973, 1978, 1982; Hegele-Hartung et al. 1992). A complete understanding of the mechanism by which receptivity acts to promote implantation is not yet available; however, several experimental approaches have presented evidence that the concept of an "implantation window" is extremely useful to understand of what happens in the uterus before and for implantation of the embryo.

When electrophoretic, chromatographic, and biological means became extremely sensitive, several research groups began independently to isolate and identify single uterine proteins that react in a way immunologically identical to the placental proteins PP12 (insulin-like growth factor binding protein 1) and PP14 (glycodelin). These two proteins were soon characterized as endometrial proteins (Bohn and Kraus 1980, 1982; Bell 1986; Huhtala et al. 1986, 1987; Koistinen et al. 1986; Than et al. 1993; Seppälä and Tiitinen 1995). Since radioimmunological determination of these endometrial proteins within peripheral blood plasma are possible, concepts have been proposed to develop blood tests for diagnostic procedures that should predict the functional stage of the endometrium. So far, however, no such reliable blood test is available, partly because other sources of synthesis and release of these proteins have been identified in the human body and partly because circumstantial evidence is against the hypothesis that peripheral blood plasma levels accurately reflect a substantial synthesis and lumenal release of endometrial proteins. All cell biological evidence on the compartmentation of epithelium, stroma, glands, and microcirculation points to the conclusion that these specific protein concentrations of the blood plasma differ from their origin in the endometrium. Interestingly, some reports in the literature suggest that there are certain conditions in which glycodelin cannot be detected in blood plasma during pregnancy (Critchley et al. 1990, 1992). These cases in patients without functional ovaries and some patients after GnRHa downregulation (Anthony et al. 1991; Todorow et al. 1993) demonstrate clearly that there is no need for glycodelin elevation in blood plasma to achieve implantation. However, investigations in GnRHa-downregulated patients demonstrate that glycodelin concentrations in uterine secretion increases normally within their luteal phase, indicating the functional significance of locally physiological amounts of the proteins in the uterine secretion, while this is not reflected in peripheral blood plasma (Todorow et al. 1995). Consequently the assessment of uterine secretion proteins for any evaluation of endometrial function requires their investigation from material obtained from the uterine cavity, not from peripheral blood, as had been demonstrated by Beier-Hellwig et al. (1988, 1989) using the one-way device Prevical.

Finally, a comparative aspect of the rabbit preimplantation model must be recalled. We are faced with the experimental fact that no single uterine protein has ever been successfully used as a marker of receptivity. It has always proved the case that several components, forming a pattern, provide the reliable information for the diagnosis of receptivity for implantation (Beier 1982, 1986; Hegele-Hartung and Beier 1986; Hegele-Hartung et al. 1992).

3.13 Conclusions for Contraceptive Medical Strategies

So far the histological evaluation of the endometrium following Noyes et al. (1950) is still the main approach for assessing endometrial quality. This bears the disadvantage of retrospective insight only, since it is usually taken at the end of a given cycle. New research approaches applying the technique of morphometric analysis according to the LH peak allow evaluation at any time within the luteal phase and promise more precision (Johannisson et al. 1982, 1987; Koninckx et al. 1977; Li et al. 1988). However, increasingly detailed information is accumulating that there is no clinical benefit in luteal-phase evaluation solely by histological dating of the endometrium. Balasch et al. (1992) have clearly shown that histological endometrial adequacy or inadequacy in the cycle of conception or in previous cycles is not related to the outcome of pregnancy in infertile patients.

The higher resolution of morphological structures by transmission or scanning electron microscopy of the epithelial surface thus far does not contribute substantially to interpretation of the adequacy of the endometrium; nor can it give a prospective judgement (Sundström et al. 1983). Consequently, reproductive biologists have searched for a

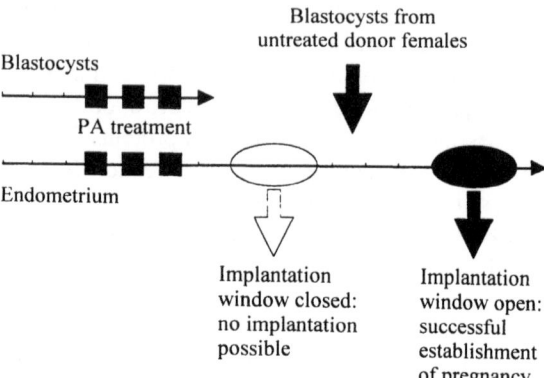

Fig. 15. Diagram of the transpositon of the implantation window (*white and black elipses*). Treatment with progestorone antagonists during the preimplantation phase of early pregnancy in the rabbit (*black squares*) results in inhibition of the progesterone-dependent endometrial transformation and inhibition of blastocyst development. The consequence of such treatment is the prevention of implantation, which corresponds to the strategy of endometrial contraception. The endometrial transformation can start again after the end of progesterone antagonist treatment, leading to a new stage of uterine receptivity after a delay of several days. Normal blastocysts of untreated donor animals may then be transferred at the appropriate stage of development and implant successfully. (Modified from Beier et al. 1994)

method to assess a receptive endometrium that goes beyond the information that is now routinely provided by ultrasound. Such a new diagnostic method should be reliable, easy, and, if necessary, repeatable to allow prospective interpretation in a therapeutic cycle.

Based on our reproductive biological research in animal models we now reply on techniques that permit protein analyses of the uterine milieu because this is the site where attachment and implantation start. Implantation succeeds only in a favorable uterine milieu as a result of an adequate endometrial transformation that yields a characteristic composition of the proteins in uterine secretion. After electrophoresis the protein patterns permit a significant prediction of implantation success. Only by means of biochemical analysis of the uterine proteins, in particular uteroglobin, have we been able to diagnose and define numerous changes of the endocrine system. For instance, the phenomenon of delayed secretion in the rabbit, initiated by postcoital injection of estrogens, revealed that the assessment of protein patterns in uterine secretion is a reliable tool (Beier 1974; Beier and Mootz 1979). This tool has made it possible to predict the time when embryo transfer of viable embryos would most likely succeed in implantation.

In addition, a further intriguing experimental approach in our rabbit model has shown the reliability of prediction by protein pattern evaluation of uterine secretion (Fig. 15). The postovulatory administration of progesterone antagonists (lilopristone, onapristone, and mifepristone) initiates a protein-biochemical alteration of uterine secretion, giving rise to a delayed secretion of 4–8 days that in turn does not permit a timely implantation. However, a reduction in the progesterone antagonists influences the secretion pattern in such a way that it gradually normalizes and, finally, is again ready for implantation after a delay of 4–5 days. The favorable point of time for embryo transfer in this experimental model could also be predicted precisely (Beier et al. 1987; Hegele-Hartung et al. 1992). We have interpreted this phenomenon clearly as a transposition of the implantation window and not as an extension of the endometrial receptive phase (Beier et al. 1994).

The strategy of endometrial contraception is based on biological interventions to prevent any receptive stage of the endometrium, which supports early preimplantational development, attachment, or implantation of the blastocyst. These biological interventions can be achieved by inhibiting progesterone at its receptor on the target cells, by preventing progesterone-dependent regulatory steps, such as cytokine-mediated paracrine effects, which control endometrial differentiation and luteal transformation. Administered in the adequate dose and at appropriate time, a pharmacologically safe progesterone antagonist will be an ideal key to keep the implantation window always closed.

Acknowledgments. The research work reported here was achieved together with my colleagues at the Department of Anatomy and Reproductive Biology, University of Aachen, Germany. In particular, I thank Dr. Karin Beier-Hellwig, Dr. Irmgard Classen-Linke, Dr. Ursula Mootz, Dr. Andreas Herrler, Ulrike Hilmes, Claudia Krusche, Joachim Alfer, Thomas Wollweber, and Michael von Wolff. Fruitful technical assistance was contributed by Barbara Bonn, Sabine Eisner, Elisabeth Theisen, Sabina Hennes, and Diana Behrend. Further, excellent scientific collaboration with Dr. Ekkehard Schillinger, Dr. Kristof Chwalisz, PD Dr. Christa Hegele-Hartung, Prof. K. Schmidt-Gollwitzer, and Dr. Sybille Beier, Schering Research Laboratories, Berlin, Germany, is gratefully acknowledged. The generous clinical cooperation of Dr. Karl Sterzik, Universitätsfrauenklinik Ulm, Germany, Prof. Christian Karl, St. Antonius-Hospital Eschweiler, Germany, Prof. Manfred Kusche, Marienhospital Aachen, Germany, Dr. Hanfried Grüne, Bethlehem-Krankenhaus Stolberg, Germany, Prof. Marc Bygdeman, Karolinska Hospital Stockholm, Sweden, and Prof. Max Elstein, University of Manchester, UK, is gratefully acknowledged. This research project was essentially supported by the Schering Aktiengesellschaft and by the Deutsche Forschungsgemeinschaft (grant Cl 88/3-1).

References

Anthony FW, Davies DW, Gadd SC, Jenkins JM, Masson GM, Chard T, Perry LA (1991) Lack of placental protein 14 production in pregnancy after frozen embryo transfer, down-regulation of anterior pituitary and administration of exogenous oestradiol and progesterone. Hum Reprod 6:737–739

Balasch FJ, Fabreugues M, Creus M, Vanrell JA (1992) The usefulness of endometrial biopsy for luteal phase evaluation in infertility. Hum Reprod 7:973–977

Bartelemez AW (1957) The phases of the menstrual cycle and their interpretation in terms of the pregnancy cycle. Am J Obstet Gynecol 74:931

Beier HM (1973) Die hormonelle Steuerung der Uterussekretion und frühen Embryonalentwicklung. Thesis, University of Kiel

Beier HM (1974) Oviductal and uterine fluids. J Reprod Fertil 37:221–237

Beier HM (1978) Physiology of uteroglobin. In: Spilman CH, Wilks JW (eds) Novel aspects of reproductive physiology, Seventh Brook Lodge Workshop. Spectrum, New York, pp 220–248

Beier HM (1982) Uteroglobin and other endometrial proteins: biochemistry and biological significance in beginning pregnancy. In: Beier HM, Karlson P (eds) Proteins and steroids in early pregnancy. Springer, Berlin Heidelberg New York, pp 38–71

Beier HM (1986) Hormone und Hormonantagonisten in der Implantationsforschung. Fortschr Fertilitätsforsch 13:2–15

Beier HM, Beier-Hellwig K (1973) Specific secretory protein of the female genital tract. Acta Endocrinol Suppl (Copenh) 180:404–425

Beier HM, Mootz U (1979) Significance of maternal uterine proteins in the establishment of pregnancy. In: Maternal recognition of pregnancy: Ciba Foundation Symposium Series 64. Excerpta Medica, Amsterdam, pp 111–140

Beier HM, Petry G, Kühnel W (1970) Endometrial secretion and early mammalian development. In: Gibian H, Plotz EJ (eds) Mammalian reproduction. Kolloquium der Gesellschaft für Biologische Chemie, Mosbach. Springer, Berlin Heidelberg New York, pp 264–285

Beier HM, Elger W, Hegele-Hartung C (1987) Effects of antiprogestins on the endometrium during the luteal phase after postovulatory treatment. In: Naftolin F, De Cherney A (eds) The control of follicle development, ovulation and luteal function: lessons from in vitro fertilization. Raven, New York, pp331–343

Beier HM, Elger W, Hegele-Hartung C, Mootz U, Beier-Hellwig K (1991) Dissociation of corpus luteum, endometrium and blastocyst in human implantation research. J Reprod Fertil 92:511–523

Beier HM, Hegele-Hartung C, Mootz U, Beier-Hellwig K (1994) Modification of endometrial cell biology using progesterone antagonists to manipulate the implantation window. Hum Reprod 9 [Suppl 1]:98–115

Beier-Hellwig K, Sterzik K, Beier HM (1988) Zur Rezeptivität des Endometriums: die Diagnostik der Proteinmuster des menschlichen Uterussekretes. Fertilität 4:128–134

Beier-Hellwig K, Sterzik K, Bonn B, Beier HM (1989) Contribution to the physiology and pathology of endometrial receptivity: the determination protein patterns in human uterine secretions. Hum Reprod 4 [Suppl 1]:115–120

Beier-Hellwig K, Sterzik K, Bonn B, Hilmes U, Bygdeman M, Gemzell-Danielsson K, Beier HM (1994) Hormone regulation and hormone antagonist effects on protein patterns of human endometrial secretion during receptivity. Ann NY Acad Sci 734:143–156

Beier-Hellwig K, Bonn B, Sterzik K, Linder D, Muller S, Bygdeman M, Beier HM (1995) Uterine receptivity and endometrial secretory protein patterns. In: Dey SK (ed) Molecular and cellular aspects of periimplantation processes, Serono Symposia USA. Springer, Berlin Heidelberg New York, pp 87–102

Bell SC (1986) Secretory endometrial and decidual proteins: studies and clinical significance of a maternally derived group of pregnancy-associated serum proteins. Hum Reprod 1:129–143

Bergh PA, Navot D (1992) The impact of embryonic development and endometrial maturity on the timing of implantation. Fertil Steril 58:537–542

Bischof P, Redard M, Gindre P, Vassilkos P, Campana A (1993) Localization of alpha 2, alpha 5, and alpha 6 integrin subunits in human endometrium, decidua and trophoblast. Eur J Obstet Gynecol Reprod Biol 51:217–226

Bohn H, Kraus W (1980) Isolierung und Charakterisierung eines neuen plazentaspezifischen Proteins (PP12). Arch Gynecol 229:279–281

Bohn H, Kraus W, Winckler W (1982) New soluble placental tissue proteins: their isolation, characterization, localization and quantification. Placenta [Suppl 4]:67–81

Breckwoldt M, Beier HM, Neumann F, Bräuer H (1994) Bildatlas zu Aspekten der Pathophysiologie des endokrinen Systems, vol 2. Medical Service, Munich

Bronson RA, Fusi FM (1996) Integrins and human reproduction. Mol Hum Reprod 2:153–168

Carson DD, Julian J, Liu S, Rohde L, Surveyor G, Wegner C (1995) Mucins and proteoglycans as modulators of embryo-uterine epithelial cell attachment. In: Dey SK (ed) Molecular and cellular aspects of periimplantation processes. Springer, Berlin Heidelberg New York, pp 103–112

Chwalisz K, Stöckemann K, Fuhrmann U, Fritzemeier KH, Einspanier A, Garfield RE (1995) Mechanism of action of the antiprogestins in the pregnant uterus. Ann NY Acad Sci 761:202–224

Classen-Linke I, Kusche M, Knauthe R, Beier HM (1995a) Expression of progesterone and estrogen receptors in human endometrial cells in culture. Exp Clin Endocrinol 103 [Suppl 1]:113

Classen-Linke I, Alfer J, Hegele-Hartung C, Chwalisz K, Kusche M, Beier HM (1995b) Hormonal regulation of β-integrin expression and its relation to immunocompetent cells in human endometrium throughout the menstrual cycle. Exp Clin Endocrinol 103 [Suppl 1]:113

Critchley HOD, Chard T, Lieberman BA, Buckley CH, Anderson DC (1990) Serum PP14 levels in a patient with Turner's syndrome pregnant after frozen embryo transfer. Hum Reprod 5:250–254

Critchley HOD, Chard T, Oladije F, Davies MC, Wang HS, Liebermann BA, Anderson DS (1992) Role of the ovary in the synthesis of placental protein 14. J Clin Endocrinol Metab 75:97–100

Crosignani PG (1988) The defective luteal phase. Hum Reprod 3:157–160

Finn CA, Martin L (1974) The control of implantation. J Reprod Fertil 39:195–206

Fischer G (1994) Über Peptidyl-prolyl-cis/trans-isomerasen und ihre Effektoren. Angewandte Chem 106:1479–1501

Forbes JA, Heinz JC (1953) Glycogen synthesis in human endometrium: a histochemical study using frozen dried material. Aust NZ J Surg 22:297

Gemzell-Danielsson K, Swahn ML, Svalander P, Bygdeman M (1993) Early luteal phase treatment with RU 486 for fertility regulation. Hum Reprod 8:870–873

Gemzell-Danielsson K, Westlund P, Johannisson E, Swahn M-L, Bygdeman M, Seppälä M (1996) Effect of low weekly doses of mifepristone on ovarian function and endometrial development. Hum Reprod 11:256–264

Glasier AF, Thong KJ, Dewar M, Mackie M, Baird DT (1992) Mifepristone (RU 486) compared with high-dose estrogen and progesterone emergency postcoital contraception. N Engl J Med 327:1041–1044

Harding MW (1991) Structural and functional features of the peptidyl prolyl cis-trans isomerase, cyclophilin. Pharmacotherapy 11:142S-148S

Hegele-Hartung C, Beier HM (1986) Distribution of uteroglobin in the rabbit endometrium after treatment with anti-progesterone (ZK 98.734): an immunocytochemical study. Hum Reprod 1:497–505

Hegele-Hartung C, Mootz U, Beier HM (1992) Luteal control of endometrial receptivity and its modification by progesterone antagonists. Endocrinology 131:2446–2460

Hey NA, Graham RA, Seif MW, Aplin JD (1994) The polymorphic epithelial mucin MUC1 in human endometrium is regulated with maximal expression in the implantation phase. J Clin Endocrinol Metab 78:337–342

Hilmes U, Beier-Hellwig K, Sterzik K, Klug J, Beier HM (1993) Identification of histones in human uterine secretion samples. J Reprod Fertil Abstr Ser 12:43

Hilmes U, Krusche C, Classen-Linke I, Karl C, Beier-Hellwig K, Beier HM (1995) Histonexpression in Korrelation zu Proliferationsaktivität und apoptotischen Vorgängen im menschlichen Endometrium. J Fertil Reprod 5:33–34

Hilmes U, Krusche C, Classen-Linke I, Karl C, Beier-Hellwig K, Beier HM (1996) Histonexpression in Korrelation zu Proliferation und Apoptose im menschlichen Endometrium. Ann Anat 178 [Suppl]:84–85

Huhtala M-L, Koistinen R, Palomäki P, Partanen P, Bohn H, Seppälä M (1986) Biologically active domain in somatomedin-binding protein. Biochem Biophys Res Commun 141:263–270

Huhtala M-L, Seppälä M, Närvänen A, Polomäki P, Julkunen M, Bohn H (1987) Amino acid sequence homology between human placental protein 14 and β-lactoglobulins from various species. Endocrinology 120:2620–2622

Ishwad PC, Katkam RR, Hinduja IN, Chwalisz K, Elger W, Puri CP (1993) Treatment with aprogesterone antagonist ZK 98.299 delays endometrial development without blocking ovulation in bonnet monkeys. Contraception 48:57–70

Johannisson E, Parker RA, Landgren B-M, Diczafalusy E (1982) Morphometric analysis of the human endometrium in relation to the peripheral hormone levels. Fertil Steril 38:564–571

Johannisson E, Landgren B-M, Diczafalusi E (1987) Endometrial morphology and peripheral hormone levels in women with regular menstrual cycles. Fertil Steril 48:401–408

Jones GS (1949) Some never aspects of the management of infertility. JAMA 141:1123

Jones GS (1976) The luteal phase defect. Fertil Steril 27:351–356

Katkam RR, Gopalkrishnan K, Chwalisz K, Schillinger E, Puri CP (1995) Onapristone (ZK 98.299): a potential antiprogestin for endometrial contraception. Am J Obstet Gynecol 173:779–787

Koistinen R, Kalkkinen N, Huhtala M-L, Seppälä M, Bohn H, Rutanen E-M (1986) Placental protein 12 is a decidual protein that binds somatomedin and has an identical N-terminal amino acid sequence with somatomedin-binding protein from human amniotic fluid. Endocrinology 118:1375–1378

Koninckx PR, Goddeeris PG, Lauweryns JM, De Hertogh RC, Brosens IA (1977) Accuracy of endometrial biopsy dating in the relation of the midcycle luteinizing hormone peak. Fertil Steril 28:443

Lebeau M-C, Baulieu EE (1994) Steroid antagonists and receptor-associated proteins. Hum Reprod 9 [Suppl 2]:11–21

Lessey BA, Damjanovich L, Coutifaris C, Castelbaum A, Albelda SM, Buck CA (1992) Integrin adhesion molecules in the human endometrium. Correlation with the normal and abnormal menstrual cycle. J Clin Invest 90:188–195

Lessey BA, Castelbaum AJ, Buck CA, Lei Y, Yowell CW, Sun J (1994) Further characterization of endometrial integrins during the menstrual cycle and in pregnancy. Fertil Steril 62:497–506

Lessey BA, Castelbaum AJ, Sawin SJ, Sun J (1995) Integrins as markers of uterine receptivity in women with primary unexplained infertility. Fertil Steril 63:535–542

Li T-C, Rogers AW, Dockery P, Lenton EA, Cooke ID (1988) A new method of histologic dating of human endometrium in the luteal phase. Fertil Steril 50:52–60

McLaren A (1973) Blastocyst activation. In: Segal SJ, Crozier R, Corfman PA, Condliffe PG (eds) The regulation of mammalian reproduction. Thomas, Springfield, pp. 321–334

Niemann LK, Choate TM, Chrousos GP, Healy DL, Morin M, Renquist D, Merriam GR, Spitz IM, Bardin CW, Baulieu EE, Loriaux DL (1987) The progesterone antagonist RU 486. A potential new contraceptive agent. N. Engl J Med 316:187–191

Nikas G, Drakakis P, Loutradis D, Mara-Skoufari C, Koumantakis E, Michalas S, Psychoyos A (1995) Uterine pinopodes as markers of the "nidation window" in cycling women receiving exogenous oestradiol and progesterone. Hum Reprod 10:1208–1213

Noyes RW, Hertig AT, Rock J (1950) Dating the endometrial biopsy. Fertil Steril 1:3–25

Parr MB, Parr EL (1974) Uterine luminal epithelium: protrusions mediate endocytosis, not apocrine secretion, in the rat. Biol Reprod 11:220–233

Psychoyos A, (1963) Precision sur l'état de "non-receptivité" de l'uterus. CR Acad Sci (Paris) 257:1153–1156

Psychoyos A (1994) The implantation window: basic and clinical aspects. In Mori T, Aono T, Tominaga T, Hiroi M (eds) Perspectives on assisted reproduction. Ares-Serono Symposium. Ser Frontiers Endocrinol 4:57

Ratajczak T, Carrello A, Mark PH et al (1993) The cyclophilin component of the unactivated estrogen receptor contains a tetratricopeptide repeat domain and shares identity with p59 (FKBP59). J Biol Chem 268:13187–13192

Rotello RJ, Lieberman RC, Purchio AF, Gerschenson LE (1991) Coordinated regulation of apoptosis and cell proliferation by transforming grwoth factor-β1 in cultured uterine epithelial cells. Proc Natl Acad Sci USA 88:3412–3415

Seppälä M, Tiitinen A (1995) Endometrial responses to corpus luteum products in cycles with induced ovulation: theoretical and practical considerations. Hum Reprod 10 [Suppl 2]:67–76

Simon C, Pellicier A, Polan ML (1995) Interleukin-1 system crosstalk between embryo and endometrium in implantation. Hum Reprod 10 [Suppl 2]:43–54

Sundström P, Nilsson O, Liedholm P (1983) Scanning electron microscopy of human preimplantation endometrium in normal and clomiphene/human chorionic gonadotropin-stimulated cycles. Fertil Steril 40:642–647

Swahn ML, Bygdeman M, Cekan S, Xing B, Mastroni B, Johannisson E (1990) The effect of RU 486 administered during the early luteal phase on bleeding pattern, hormonal parameters and endometrium. Hum Reprod 5:402–408

Swahn ML, Gemzell K, Bygdeman M (1991) Contraception with mifepristone. Lancet 338:942–943

Tabibzadeh S (1992) Patterns of expression of integrin molecules in human endometrium throughout the menstrual cycle. Hum Reprod 7:876–882

Tabibzadeh S, Sun XZ (1992) Cytokine expression in human endometrium throughout the menstrual cycle. Hum Reprod 7:1214–1221

Tabibzadeh S (1994) Cytokines and the hypothalamic-pituitary-ovarian-endometrial axis. Hum Reprod 9:947–967

Terada N, Yamamoto R, Tadada T et al (1989) Inhibitory effect of progesterone on cell death of mouse uterine epithelium. J Steroid Biochem 33:1091–1096

Than GN, Bohn H, Szabo DG (1993) Advances in pregnancy-related protein research: functional and clinical applications. CRC, Boca Raton

Todorow S, Siebzehnrübl E, Beier-Hellwig K, Meyer U, Bühner M, Tulusan A, Wildt L, Lang N (1993) PP14 and PP 12 determination in human uterine fluid: a less invasive method to monitor endometrial maturity. J Reprod Fertil Abstr Ser 12:27

Todorow S, Beier-Hellwig K, Siebzehnrübl E, Meyer U, Wildt L, Tulusan AH, Beier HM, Lang N (1995) PP14 concentration fluctuations in human uterine fluid used for monitoring endometrial function of infertility patients. Hum Reprod 10 [Abstr Book 2]:33

4 The Immune System Acting in the Human Endometrium

Y.W. Loke and A. King

4.1 Introduction

As with other organs in communication with the external environment, the uterus is subjected to and is capable of responding to a wide variety of antigenic challenge. However, what is unique to the uterus is its encounter with allogeneic placental trophoblast cells during pregnancy. It is this local immunological relationship between the early trophoblast and the uterine mucosa at the time of implantation which is the focus of the present review.

The mucosa of the human uterus, the endometrium, undergoes a series of transformations throughout the menstrual cycle, culminating in a final breakdown of the tissue at the end of the cycle at menstruation. If pregnancy occurs, the endometrium is transformed into decidua. Decidual changes occur in all the tissue compartments of the uterine mucosa including the glands, stroma and blood vessels. However, in the context of reproductive immunology, the most pertinent observation is an influx of large numbers of lymphoid cells with unusual morphology and phenotype whose lineage and function are still unclear. They have the appearance of large granular lymphocytes and possess certain characteristics of natural killer (NK) cells. We believe that these decidual lymphocytes are representative of a conserved, evolutionarily older immune system which has preceded that of the modern day adaptive immunity of T and B cells. It is this "primitive" immune system which is concerned with the control of implantation.

4.2 Evolution

When specialised organs concerned with the immune system, such as the spleen, thymus and lymph nodes began to evolve, the first specialised sites to develop were at the body surfaces. These are retained in higher vertebrates at epithelial surfaces such as skin or as mucosa-associated lymphoid tissue (MALT) such as that in the gut. The uterine mucosa has many features of MALT and is infiltrated mainly by macrophages and NK cells, both of which are cells of the innate immune system. Equivalent NK-like cells are also present in the uterus of a variety of animal species including rodents, pigs, horses and sheep, which is in line with the idea that these cells have a role to play in reproduction.

NK-like cells appeared very early in evolution and can be traced back to invertebrates. Cells with characteristics of human NK cells have been documented in the snail and the keyhold limpet. NK cells are generally considered to be the evolutionary precursors of T cells with the possible developmental sequence being NK cells $\rightarrow \gamma\delta$ T cells $\rightarrow \alpha\beta$ T cells. The immune system has probably been created in layers during evolution, with each new layer being more complex and sophisticated than the preceding one. However, the preceding layers are not replaced but either have evolved to cooperate with the newer layers or have developed some other function. Uterine NK cells could be conserved to control implantation (Loke and King 1996).

Table 1. Leucocytes in uterine mucosa. (From Loke and King 1995)

| | Nonpregnant endometrium | | Early decidua | |
	Proliferative	Secretory	Basalis (Trophoblast$^+$)	Parietalis (Trophoblast$^-$)
Granulocytes				
Neutrophils	–	–/+	–/+	–
Eosinophils	–	–	–	–
Basophils	–	–	–	–
Lymphocytes				
B cells	–(+)	–(+)	–(+)	–(+)
T cells	+	+	+	+
NK cells (LGL)	+	+++	+++++	+++
Macrophages	+	+	+++	+

4.3 Decidual Leucocytes

With the availability of monoclonal antibodies directed at leucocyte markers, the distribution of cell types within the uterine mucosa throughout the menstrual cycle and during pregnancy is now well documented (King et al. 1989; Bulmer et al. 1991). This is shown in Table 1. It can be seen that cells of the granulocyte series are absent apart from at the time of menstruation. Of the lymphoid series only a few B cells are present, while T cells are sparse. Thus, cells of the classical adaptive immune system are not a prominent feature of the uterine mucosa. In contrast, NK cells and macrophages, which are cells of the innate immune system, are the predominant populations. Furthermore, NK cells are relatively few in number during the proliferative phase of the cycle but become particularly abundant in early decidua, especially in decidua basalis where the placenta inserts. These cells therefore are temporally and spacially associated with the invading trophoblast.

4.4 T and B Cells

The few B cells present are confined to the lymphoid aggregates in the basal layer of the endometrium or decidua. Germinal centres and plasma cells are found only in uterine infections (More 1987). T cells, as defined by expression of CD3, are located at three sites: basal lymphoid aggregates, scattered throughout the stroma and intraepithelially. This pattern of distribution is similar to that seen for T cells in other mucosal sites, such as the bronchus and intestine. The proportion of T cells account for approximately 10% of all leucocytes in early decidua and remain relatively constant throughout the menstrual cycle.

4.5 Macrophages

Approximately 20% of leucocytes in endometrium and decidua are macrophages, identifiable by monoclonal antibodies to CD14. They have many features of other tissue macrophages elsewhere in the body, such as containing acid phosphatase, non-specific esterase and lysozyme, exhibit adherence to glass and are able to phagocytose opsonised red blood cells. Uterine macrophages appear not to be under hormonal control since their numbers remain relatively constant throughout the menstrual cycle. However, there are considerably larger numbers of macrophages in the decidua basalis compared to decidua parietalis.

The functions of decidual macrophages are not known. Since they express MHC class II antigen, it is possible that they are capable of antigen presentation. This would be relevant to invasion of the allogeneic placenta because antigen presentation of allogeneic proteins processed by recipient antigen-presenting cells is an indirect mechanism of graft rejection. Decidual macrophages are also capable of producing a wide range of soluble products, including the newly described cytokine vascular endothelial growth factor which has been reported to be transcribed by these cells (Charnock-Jones et al. 1993). Since the receptor for vascular endothelial growth factor (known as *flt*) is demonstrable on extravillous trophoblast (Sharkey et al. 1994), a potential mechanism by which decidual macrophages may influence trophoblast development is present. Finally, macrophages are highly phagocytic cells. Their main role at the implantation site could be to act as scavengers to remove dead and dying cells around the thin zone of necrosis (Nitabuch's layer) present at the feto-maternal interface.

4.6 Natural Killer Cells

In our view, the uterine NK cells are the leucocytes which are most likely to play a pivotal role in controlling implantation (King and Loke 1991). Morphologically, these cells contain membrane-bound granules of varying sizes and are thus known as large granular lymphocytes. These granules have been shown to contain perforin, granzymes and TIA-1, all of which are potent cytolytic enzymes (King et al. 1993). Studies with monoclonal antibodies directed at leucocyte differentiation antigens have shown that these decidual large granular lymphocytes express the leucocyte common antigen (CD45) and also the early T-lineage antigens (CD2, CD7, CD38) but not mature T cell markers (CD3, CD5, CD4, CD8). They also stain for the pan-NK cell marker (CD56) and are capable of lysing the NK cell target K562 (Starkey et al. 1988; King et al. 1989, 1991). All these properties indicate that decidual large granular lymphocytes are NK cells.

However, decidual NK cells differ from circulating classical NK cells in blood in many respects. The CD56 antigen is expressed by decidual NK cells very intensely, many more times brighter than in blood. They are thus depicted as CD56^{bright}. In blood over 90% of the CD56$^+$ NK cells also express CD16, which is the low-affinity FcγRIII for aggregated IgG. In contrast, the majority of decidual NK cells are CD16$^-$. CD57, another marker for adult NK cells, is always absent from decidual NK cells. A detailed profile of surface antigens expressed by decidual NK cells is shown in Table 2.

Although CD3 proteins are not present on the surface of CD56^{bright} decidual NK cells, there is evidence that there is expression of cytoplasmic (cy) CD3ε. Classical NK cells become cyCD3ε$^+$ only when they are activated, which suggests that decidual NK cells may be in a similar state of activation. As can be seen from Table 2, other activation markers are also present. An alternative explanation for the presence of these markers is that they may reflect the stage of development of decidual NK cells rather than their state of activation. For example, fetal CD56$^+$ NK cells isolated from fetal liver express cyCD3ε. Similarly, CD69 is also found on fetal liver CD56$^+$ cells. Indeed, there are other characteristics (Table 3) which further reveal the phenotypic and functional similarities between decidual NK cells and fetal liver NK cells.

Table 2. Phenotype of main population of CD56^{bright} decidual cells. (From Loke and King 1995)

NK cell markers	CD16$^-$
	CD57$^-$
	CD56^{bright}
Early T cell markers	CD2$^{+/-}$
	CD7$^{+/-}$
	CD38$^+$
Mature T cell markers	mCD3$^-$
	CD4$^-$
	CD6$^-$
Activation markers	CD69$^+$
	Kp43$^+$
	HLA-DR$^-$
	D45RA$^+$
Cytokine receptors	IL-1R$^-$
	IL2Rβ^+
	IL2Rα(CD25)$^{-/+}$
	c-kit^-
	IL-6R$^-$
	IL-7R$^-$
	IFN-γR$^-$
	TNF-R$^-$
	GM-CSF-R$^-$

Table 3. Characteristics of NK cells from blood, decidua and fetal liver. (From Loke and King 1995)

	Blood	Decidua	Fetal liver
NK markers	CD56^{dim}	CD56$^{bright+++}$	CD56^{bright}
	CD16^{bright}	CD16$^-$	CD16$^{-/dim}$
	CD57$^{+/-}$	CD57$^-$	CD57$^-$
Cytoplasmic CD3	cyCD3$^-$	cyCD3$^+$	cyCD3$^+$
Activation markers	CD69$^-$	CD69$^+$	CD69$^+$
NK activity	High	Low	Low
	Respond to	Respond to	Respond to
	high-dose IL-2	low-dose IL-2	low-dose IL-2
Cytokine	GM-CSF$^-$	GM-CSF$^+$	GM-CSF$^+$
production	CSF-1$^-$	CSF-1$^+$	CSF-1?

Presently very little is known about the ontogeny and developmental pathway of NK cells in contrast to the extensive studies which have been carried out on T cells. NK cells appear before T cells in early fetal life and are already present in the fetal liver before the development of the thymus, an observation which has led to the suggestion that the thymus is not necessary for the maturation of NK cells, in contrast to T cells which must undergo a period of thymic selection and differentiation. We have proposed two hypothetical NK cell differentiation pathways (Loke and King 1995). One envisages decidual NK cells and circulating adult NK cells to have a common progenitor. The former then colonise the uterine mucosa and there are subjected to tissue-specific differentiation signals resulting in a unique phenotype. In the second proposal, decidual NK cells and circulating NK cells are derived from intrinsically different progenitors and therefore use completely separate pathways of differentiation. It remains to be seen as to which of these proposals is correct.

4.7 Uterine Immune Response to Trophoblast of First Trimester Pregnancy

Unlike the villous trophoblast population in contact with maternal blood at the intervillous space which does not express any HLA class I or class II antigens, the extravillous trophoblast population which invades into the uterine decidua does express HLA class I antigens but not class II. Thus these two feto-maternal interfaces in human reproduction differ immunologically. While the maternal systemic immune response encounters a trophoblast population which is immunologically neutral, the local uterine response can potentially be stimulated by HLA class I$^+$ extravillous trophoblast. However, the trophoblast class I antigen is not the same as that expressed by other somatic cells. Extravillous trophoblast expresses the product of the non-classical HLA-G locus. Indeed, trophoblast is unique in being the only tissue to express this antigen although HLA-G mRNA has been demonstrated in some other cells but not the protein. In addition, recent studies have shown that the classical class I molecule HLA-C is also expressed by extravillous trophoblast (King et al. 1996).

It is generally agreed that HLA-G is relatively non-polymorphic (Parham 1995). Some variability has been observed at the genetic level, but few of these differences involve the peptide binding groove, and the polymorphism thus does not appear to be associated with peptide binding diversity. Extravillous trophoblast therefore is unlikely to generate any significant allogeneic signals to maternal T cells in a similar manner as a classical organ transplant. There is also less polymorphism in HLA-C than in HLA-A or HLA-B, particularly at the functional positions of the antigen recognition sites. Also, the surface expression of HLA-C is about 10% of that of HLA-A or HLA-B. This low surface expression and relative lack of diversity places HLA-C half-way between a classical and non-classical class I molecule.

The functions of HLA-G/HLA-C on trophoblast are not known. We believe that they may be important molecules by which invading trophoblast cells interact with decidual NK cells. However, the exact mechanism of recognition and its effects remain unclear. NK cells preferentially kill target cells which have low or absent HLA class I antigen expression. This observation had led to the formulation of the 'missing-self' hypothesis, which postulates that NK cells eliminate cells lacking class I molecules, in contrast to T cells which kill cells bearing foreign class I antigens. Thus the presence of class I molecules on target cells prevents NK-mediated lysis (Ljunggren and Kärre 1990). The situation has since become more complex as it is now apparent that NK cells can discriminate between different class I alleles, although they do not detect fine polymorphic differences as T cells can. Instead, NK cells appear to recognise a public, perhaps primordial, polymorphism in class I molecules. A family of human NK receptors which do recognise HLA class I antigens have recently been identified, the p58 (NKAT) family of receptors for Cw3/Cw4 and related alleles. Each NK cell can express several different receptors, some of which use class I molecules as a ligand and others of different molecular structure which use target ligands such as oligosaccharides. It seems that this is the way receptor diversity is generated in NK cells rather than by somatic recombination of a single receptor as used by T and B cells. Expression of different combinations of these receptors on each NK cell will determine its repertoire (Yokoyama 1995).

In the context of interaction with trophoblast, the expression of HLA-G/HLA-C by trophoblast could influence their susceptibility to

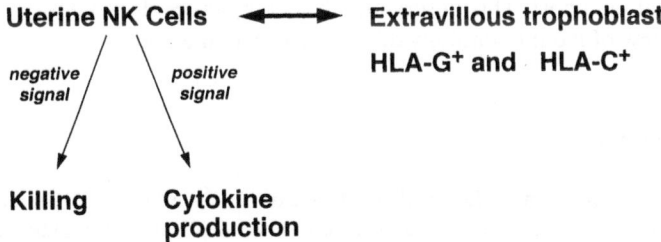

Fig. 1. A hypothetical model of the possible outcome of interaction between uterine NK cells and extravillous trophoblast at the implantation site. (From Loke and King 1995)

decidual NK cell lysis. Exposure of human trophoblast cells to exogenous IFN-γ, a cytokine which upregulates class I expression, has been observed to protect trophoblast cells against lysis by IL-2-stimulated decidual NK cells (King and Loke 1993). Similarly, HLA-G transfected into class I deficient cell lines was found to provide some protection from lysis by freshly isolated decidual NK effectors compared to the parental cell line (Chumbley et al. 1994).

The additional possibility that class I signals transmitted to decidual NK cells can affect not only cytotoxicity but also other NK cell functions such as cytokine production would need to be explored (Fig. 1). Decidual NK cells are known to produce a variety of cytokines, and trophoblast expresses appropriate receptors for many of these cytokines. Thus a potential cytokine network may be in place at the implantation site by which decidual NK cells influence trophoblast behaviour.

4.8 Conclusion

From this brief review it can be seen that the immunological relationship between the invading placenta and the uterus is not governed by the laws of classical transplantation immunology. Instead, it seems to involve a more primitive defence system whose mechanism of 'self' and 'non-self' recognition and the resultant reactions invoked are more akin to those between unrelated invertebrates than those between vertebrate allograft and host. This observation has completely altered our conceptual view of the immunology of feto-maternal interaction.

References

Bulmer J, Morrison L, Longfellow M, Ritson A, Pace D (1991) Granulated lymphocytes in human endometrium: histochemical and immunohistochemical studies. Hum Reprod 6:791–798

Charnock-Jones DS, Sharkey AM, Rajput-Williams J, Burch D, Schofield PJ, Fountain SA, Boocock CA, Smith SK (1993) Identification and localization of alternatively spliced mRNAs for vascular endothelial growth factor in human uterus and steroid regulation in endometrial carcinoma cell lines. Biol Reprod 48:1120–1128

Chumbley G, King A, Robertson K, Holmes N, Loke YW (1994) Resistance of HLA-G and HLA-A2 transfectants to lysis by decidual NK cells. Cell Immunol 155:312–322

King A, Loke YW (1991) On the nature and function of human uterine granular lymphocytes. Immunol Today 12:432–435

King A, Loke YW (1993) Effect of IFN-γ and IFN-α on killing of human trophoblast by decidual LAK cells. J Reprod Immunol 23:51–62

King A, Wellings V, Gardner L, Loke YW (1989) Immunocytochemical characterisation of the unusual large granular lymphocytes in human endometrium throughout the menstrual cycle. Hum Immunol 24:195–205

King A, Balendran N, Wooding P, Carter NP Loke YW (1991) CD3⁻ leukocytes present in the human uterus during early placentation: phenotypic and morphologic characterisation of the CD56⁺⁺ population. Dev Immunol 1:169–190

King A, Wooding P, Gardner L, Loke YW (1993) Expression of perforin, granzyme A and TIA-1 by human uterine CD56⁺ cells implies they are activated and capable of effector functions. Hum Reprod 8:2061–2067

King A, Boocock C, Sharkey AM, Gardner L, Beretta A, Siccardi AG, Loke YW (1996) Evidence for the expression of HLA-C class I mRNA and protein by human first trimester trophoblast. J Immunol 156:2068–2076

Ljunggren H-G, Kärre K (1990) In search of the 'missing self': MHC molecules and NK cell recognition. Immunol Today 11:237–244

Loke YW, King A (1995) Human implantation: cell biology and immunology. Cambridge University Press, Cambridge

Loke YW, King A (1996) Immunology of human implantation: an evolutionary perspective. Human Reprod 11:283–286

More IAR (1987) The normal human endometrium. In: Fox H (ed) Haines and
  Taylor's obstetrical and gynaecological pathology, vol 1, 3rd edn. Churchill
  Livingstone, Edinburgh, pp 302–319
Parham P (1995) Antigen presentation by class I major histocompatibility
  complex molecules: a context for thinking about HLA-G. Am J Reprod Immunol 34:10–19
Sharkey AM, Jokhi PP, King A, Loke YW, Brown KD, Smith SK (1994) Expression of *c-kit* ligand at the human materno-fetal interface. Cytokine
  6:195–205
Starkey PM, Sargent IL, Redman CWG (1988) Cell populations in human
  early pregnancy decidua: characterisation and isolation of large granular
  lymphocytes by flow cytometry. Immunology 65:129–134
Yokoyama WM (1995) Natural killer cell receptors. Curr Opin Immunol
  7:110–120

5 Cytokines and Their Receptors in the Peri-implantation Endometrium

M.J.K. Harper

5.1 Introduction

When one considers the endometrium as a target for contraception, it is necessary to survey briefly what has been achieved heretofore, and how new knowledge has expanded the potential for development of antifertility agents which could specifically disrupt the implantation process. Until recently our understanding of the events occurring in the endometrium and the signaling between the developing embryo and the endometrium was scanty. Consequently the discovery of leads that might permit identification of agents to disrupt the implantation process was limited to hormonal and antihormonal compounds. Although the various hormonal and antihormonal approaches have merit, and one can envisage combination treatments being even more effective, they all have the potential problem of lack of specificity. Now that more specific factors controlling the implantation process are being uncovered, a path to the development of more specific implantation inhibitors appears possible.

5.2 Cell Adhesion Molecules

The implantation process is composed of several events which must all occur for a successful pregnancy to occur. First, the blastocyst must attach to the uterine epithelial surface. This may be accomplished by cell adhesion molecules. Functional and structural changes occur at the apical surfaces of the endometrial epithelial cells to permit blastocyst attachment. Such changes are under hormonal control. A variety of cell adhesion molecules have been described, but those which are the most important have yet to be resolved.

One possibly important family is the integrins. Since they are to be the subject of another chapter, they are not discussed further here, except to note that changes in the expression of the various integrins may define the putative period of uterine receptivity for blastocyst attachment (Ilesanmi et al. 1993; Lessey 1994; Lessey et al. 1992, 1994; Schultz and Armant 1995).

Several carbohydrates or families of carbohydrates have been suggested as being implicated in the attachment process. Histo-blood group H type 1 antigen is expressed in the endometrial epithelium around the time of implantation in several species, including the human, and its synthesis appears to be hormonally regulated. Endometrial carbohydrates carrying the H type 1 antigen may be involved in initial blastocyst adhesion (Kimber 1994; Kimber et al. 1995). A high molecular weight glycoprotein identified by mouse ascites golgi antibodies, which involves N-acetyl-galactosamine and other determinants, is secreted from the endometrial glands in the human during the period of uterine sensitivity for implantation (Kliman et al. 1995). Mucins are O-linked glycoproteins present on the apical surface of epithelial cells (Strous and Dekker 1992), whose domains can extend for 200–500 nm from the cell surface (Jentoft 1990). MUC-1 is a mucin glycoprotein, which is expressed in the endometrial epithelial cells of the mouse uterus at a high level at proestrus and estrus. On day 4 of pregnancy (just prior to implantation) it is barely detectable. Its expression is upregulated by estrogen and downregulated by progesterone and antiestrogens (Braga and Gendler 1993; Surveyor et al. 1995). A high density of MUC-1 on apical cell surfaces could block access to the cell membrane, and therefore loss of MUC-1 may be a necessary component of the receptive state for implantation. Trophinin and tastin, recently described adhesion molecules, are associated with the cytoskeleton and have been found on monkey blastocyst trophectoderm and human endometrial luminal epithelium at the beginning of the appearance of the period of receptivity (Fukuda et al. 1995). Trophinin is an intrinsic membrane protein and tastin is a cytoplasmic protein. Tastin permits trophinin to act as a cell adhesion molecule.

Another molecule that may also be involved in blastocyst implantation is heparin-binding epidermal growth factor (HB-EGF) which binds to the EGF receptor. This binding is potentiated by heparin sulfate proteoglycans, which are present in high amount in the basal lamina of the luminal epithelium (Zhang et al. 1994a). HB-EGF shows increased expression in the uterine stromal cells and suppression in epithelial cells under progesterone dominance. Its appearance can be blocked by antiprogestins (Zhang et al. 1994b). Since the decidualizing stimulus from the blastocyst causes differentiation commencing in the stromal cells underlying the epithelial point of attachment and then is propagated to other stromal cells, HB-EGF may be important for establishing uterine receptivity for implantation and causing stromal cell proliferation (Zhang et al. 1994a).

At this time the relative importance of these various adhesion molecules for implantation, and therefore as a contraceptive target, is unknown. Some of them might prove to be suitable targets for manipulating the receptivity of the endometrial epithelium for blastocyst attachment. Premature or delayed expression of the adhesion molecules substances inhibitory to adhesion, such as the mucins, clearly might prevent blastocyst attachment.

5.3 Cytokines/Growth Factors

The most interesting new findings concerning regulation of endometrial
receptivity and blastocyst implantation involve cytokines and growth
factors. A variety of experimental approaches have been used to show
the importance of such molecules in implantation. The exact role that
each plays, and whether the role is permissive or obligate has not yet
been determined. In addition, many of the experiments with cytokines
have been performed only in the mouse, since production of transgenic
animals with genes "knocked out" or mutated are easiest in this species.
This raises several important questions regarding the general applicability of findings from such paradigms to other species. Regulation of
blastocyst implantation appears to be different in ruminants compared to
rodents and primates. Interferons are important signaling molecules for
maternal recognition of pregnancy in the former, whereas other factors
may be critical in the latter. Thus, much work on comparative aspects of
the implantation process still needs to be carried out.

However, from such experiments three cytokines have been implicated as important for implantation in the mouse and are discussed here.

5.3.1 Colony-Stimulating Factor-1

A mutant inbred mouse strain has been constructed with undetectable
levels of colony-stimulating factor (CSF) 1 expression (Pollard et al.
1991). It was determined that when homozygous males and females
were bred, implantation failed. This was, however, not an effect specific
to the maternal environment, since when homozygous females were
bred with heterozygous males, a modest improvement in the pregnancy
rate was observed. This suggests that the embryo can play a role in
compensating for the lack of maternal CSF-1 (Pollard et al. 1991).
CSF-1 has been shown to induce synthesis of another cytokine, tumor
necrosis factor-α (TNFα). However, TNFα expression in the reproductive tract of the homozygous mutants was not different from that in
normal mice (Hunt et al. 1993). Interestingly, an excess of CSF-1 is also
deleterious to pregnancy. Administration of exogenous CSF-1 causes
defective embryonic development, which can be reversed by administration of TNFα or granulocyte-macrophage CSF, but not by transforming

growth factor-β_1 (Tartakovsky and Ben-Yair 1991). In cultured human endometrial stromal cells secretion of macrophage CSF is progesterone dependent (Kariya et al. 1994; Hatayama et al. 1994), and TNFα inhibits decidualization of such cells (Inoue et al. 1994) and decidual cell prolactin production (Jikihara and Handwerger 1994). TNFα is a potent stimulator of prostaglandin (PG; both PGF and PGE) release from human luteal-phase endometrial cell cultures, epithelial cells responding better than stromal cells. This stimulation was blocked both by a protein synthesis inhibitor (cycloheximide) and a transcription inhibitor (actinomycin D), implying that TNFα acts through gene transcription and translation (Chen et al. 1995b). Taken together these findings suggest that the balance between CSF-1 and TNFα may be critical for normal progression of the implantation process and decidualization.

5.3.2 Interleukin-1

A second cytokine implicated in implantation for which the evidence seems more compelling is interleukin (IL)-1α. IL-1α and IL-1β are two structurally related proteins with a molecular mass of about 17 kDa, but with different isoelectric points (Dower et al. 1986; Oppenheim et al. 1986). The two forms bind to the same receptor (IL-1R) which also exists in two forms, the IL-1 type I and type II (Dower et al. 1986). In the mouse IL-1α and IL-1β mRNA and IL-1 bioactivity increase from day 3 of pregnancy to peak at the time of implantation on day 4 and are then decreased on days 7 and 8 (De et al. 1993). IL-1α is secreted from polarized, but not apparently from nonpolarized monolayer, mouse endometrial epithelial cell cultures (Robertson et al. 1992; Jacobs and Carson 1993). In the rabbit uterus IL-1α protein is at a high level between days 3 and 6 of pregnancy but, unlike the mouse, declines significantly in the 24 h prior to implantation (Yang et al. 1995a). IL-1β mRNA has been found in human endometrium and IL-1β bioactivity localized to endometrial macrophages (Kauma et al. 1990; Simón et al. 1993b). Presumably the changes seen in the endometrium are hormonally regulated, and in human and rabbit are presumably due to progesterone.

High-affinity receptors for IL-1α are present on human endometrial epithelial cells and IL-1R type I mRNA is expressed in the same cells throughout the menstrual cycle reaching a peak in the luteal phase (Tabibzadeh et al. 1990; Simón et al. 1993a,b). Furthermore, IL-1β which is increased during endometrial decidualization also acts as a modulator of the degree of decidualization (Frank et al. 1995). In this regard IL-1 acts in an opposite manner to TNFα and yet as TNFα, IL-1α, at similar doses, stimulates PGF and PGE secretion from human luteal-phase endometrial cell cultures, and similarly this stimulation is blocked by both actinomycin D and cycloheximide (Chen et al. 1995b). Similar results using rat endometrial stromal cell cultures have been demonstrated for stimulation of PGE by IL-1α (Bany and Kennedy 1995). Part of the IL-1 regulatory system is a naturally occurring IL-1R antagonist. Blockade of the endometrial, but not embryonic, IL-1R type I with the IL-1R antagonist during the preimplantation period prevents implantation in mice (Simón et al. 1994). In addition, IL-1α promotes embryonic development and implantation in two different models of pregnancy failure in mice (Tartakovsky and Ben-Yair 1991) and human embryos secrete both IL-1α and IL-1β (Sheth et al. 1991; Zolti et al. 1991). Whether only maternal or embryonic and maternal sources of IL-1 are important for implantation remains to be definitively established. Also, how IL-1 fits into the regulatory scheme proposed above for CSF-1 and TNFα is not clear, but all three cytokines appear to regulate endometrial function in different ways prior to and during implantation.

5.3.3 Leukemia Inhibitory Factor

Leukemia inhibitory factor (LIF) is a 38- to 67-kDa glycoprotein, which exerts pleiotropic actions on a variety of different cell types, including embryonic stem cells, primordial germ cells, myeloid cell lines, adipocytes, hepatocytes and peripheral neurons. LIF is usually secreted, but in mice two different LIF mRNAs have been found to be transcribed with two different promoters, producing two forms of LIF protein, one of which is secreted, and one which remains extracellular matrix associated (Rathjen et al. 1990). LIF is expressed in the tissues of neonatal and adult mice, with the most abundant mRNA expression seen in the uterine endometrial glands on day 4 of pregnancy (the day of implantation). A similar level was seen in the day 4 pseudopregnant uterus. Much reduced levels were present on days 1–3 and 5–19 of pregnancy. No expression was seen in the nonpregnant uterus, the uterus experiencing delayed implantation or the 8- to 17-day-old fetus (Bhatt et al. 1991). As a consequence of these experiments it was suggested that "LIF may be acting in some manner to stimulate the blastocyst, whether directly or indirectly, to implant" (Bhatt et al. 1991). To test this hypothesis further Stewart and colleagues mutated the LIF gene in the third exon which resulted in a truncated LIF protein without biological activity (Stewart et al. 1992). This construct was used to produce by targeted mutagenesis of embryonic stem cells and homologous recombination blastocysts and embryos heterozygous for the mutation. The heterozygous mice were mated to produce homozygous animals which appeared phenotypically normal except that they were some 25%–35% lighter than wild-type animals (Stewart et al. 1992). Homozygous males were fertile and produced offspring from both wild-type and heterozygous females. In contrast, homozygous females mated to wild-type, heterozygous, or homozygous males did not become pregnant. These females were not sterile because normal blastocysts were found in the uterus both on day 4 (the day of implantation) and on day 7, which implies induction of delayed implantation. These blastocysts when transplanted to wild-type females on day 3 of pseudopregnancy implanted normally. Wild-type blastocysts also failed to implant in the homozygous transgenic females, even after incubation in recombinant LIF prior to transfer or when transferred in medium containing LIF. However, a modest degree of implantation was produced in homozygous mice given LIF by minipump (Stewart et al. 1992). These experiments definitively established that LIF production by, and action on, the uterus rather than the embryo is a critical factor for initiation of implantation in the mouse, although it does not address exactly how LIF works at the cellular level.

In the mouse estrogen is required for blastocyst implantation (Psychoyos 1974), and in the mouse uterus both LIF message and protein show two distinct peaks of expression coincident with elevated estrogen levels: one at proestrus/estrus during which time ovulation occurs; and the second on day of pregnancy, just preceding blastocyst implantation (Bhatt et al. 1991; Shen and Leder 1992; Yang et al. 1995b). In untreated ovariectomized mice the level of LIF protein observed by immunohistochemistry was low in uterine epithelium and glands but was upregulated by estradiol alone or estradiol and progesterone combined. Progesterone alone had no effect (Yang et al. 1996a). LIF mRNA is also upregulated by estrogen (Bhatt et al. 1991). These results clearly demonstrate that in the mouse LIF is regulated by estrogen.

The importance of LIF in the implantation process in other species, especially in ones not requiring estrogen, has not been established, and this is of crucial importance for relevance to the human. However, the importance of LIF is underscored by the high degree of conservation in the coding regions and high degree of similarity of the protein across species (Willson et al. 1992). In the rabbit, LIF protein is localized in the endometrial epithelium, endometrial glands and myometrium. The level of LIF is low in the uterus of nonestrous and estrous rabbits, and reaches its highest level on days 5 and 6 of pregnancy, declining on day 7, significantly at the nonimplantation areas and modestly at the implantation sites. As in the mouse a similar level of LIF protein is seen on day 5 of pregnancy and pseudopregnancy (Yang et al. 1994). These results suggest that also in this species uterine LIF is hormonally regulated. However, since the rabbit, unlike the mouse, does not require estrogen for induction of implantation (Kwun and Emmens 1974), it seems likely that LIF in this species is hormonally regulated differently from the mouse. Indeed this has proved to be the case. In unmated rabbits LIF protein is at a low level in the uterine epithelium and glands and is upregulated by progesterone alone or progesterone combined with estradiol. Addition of an antiprogestin blocks the increase in LIF induced by progesterone plus estrogen, while addition of an antiestrogen has no such effect (Yang et al. 1996a). These results clearly demonstrate that in the rabbit uterus LIF is regulated by progesterone, which is why there is, unlike in the mouse, no obvious peak of expression at estrus. In pigs, in which blastocyst attachment occurs about day 14 of pregnancy, LIF mRNA is highest on day 11, and LIF protein secreted into the luminal fluid is highest on day 12 of pregnancy and day 13 of the estrous cycle (Anegon et al. 1994).

The situation in women is not so clear-cut as in the mouse and rabbit. In endometrial specimens from women during nonconception cycles, both LIF message and protein are low or absent during the proliferative phase and high during the secretory phase and remain high to the end of the cycle (Kojima et al. 1994; Charnock-Jones et al. 1994; Yang et al. 1996b). In contrast, secretion of LIF protein from human endometrial cell cultures, shows a peak at the midluteal phase (around the time of implantation in a conception cycle), followed by a marked decline towards menstruation (Chen et al. 1995a). Thus, LIF protein secretion in culture throughout the cycle has a different temporal pattern to that of its localization in the tissue by immunohistochemistry. A possible explanation for this discrepancy is that if both cell-associated and secretory forms of LIF occur in the human as in the mouse, the secreted form is present only at the midluteal phase, with the cell associated form predominating thereafter. The continued elevation of LIF mRNA and protein to the end of the luteal phase in the human is quite different to that in the mouse and rabbit in which levels fall rapidly after implantation. However, no conception cycles have been studied in the human, and in the mouse and rabbit studies samples taken from pseudopregnant animals at times after the appropriate time for implantation in pregnant animals have not been studied. It may be that the occurrence of implantation itself downregulates LIF mRNA and protein. Recombinant LIF has no effect on basal or estrogen stimulated prostaglandin release from human luteal-phase endometrial cell cultures (Chen et al. 1995a). In contrast, both TNFα and IL-1α stimulate both PGE and PGF release from similar cultures in a dose-dependent fashion (Chen et al. 1995b). Thus these results indicate that the lack of effect of LIF to stimulate PG release is a real phenomenon, and all the more curious since both IL-1α and TNFα upregulate LIF expression (Hamilton et al. 1993). Clearly there are interesting interactions in the endometrium between these various cytokines which have yet to be resolved.

LIF is a member of a family of helix bundle peptides, which comprise a diverse class of cytokines that have broad, overlapping physiological and molecular actions (Horseman and Yu-Lee 1994). The overlapping functions of these cytokines suggest that one cytokine could substitute for another if the latter is expressed at subnormal levels. It has been shown that there are significant similarities in primary amino acid sequences and predicted secondary structures of LIF, oncostatin M (OSM), IL-6 and granulocyte-CSF (G-CSF). It has thus been proposed that these structurally related members of a cytokine family modulate differentiation in a variety of cells (Rose and Bruce 1991). LIF is more closely related to OSM than to IL-6 or G-CSF. The percentage scores for amino acid similarities, including conservative amino acid changes, between human LIF, mouse LIF, human OSM, human IL-6 and human G-CSF are 86, 30, 19, and 23, respectively (Rose and Bruce 1991).

Thus, there is clearly the possibility that in some cells OSM could substitute for LIF. For example, OSM inhibits proliferation of mouse M1 myeloid leukemic cells, and the dose-response curve for LIF is essentially identical, while the half-maximal dose of IL-6 is tenfold higher, and G-CSF is ineffective (Rose and Bruce 1991). However, this question has recently been examined in greater detail and it was concluded that "OSM and LIF act on human cells through different receptors... [and] that none of the factors [OSM, LIF, IL-6 or ciliary neurotrophic factor (CNTF)] examined... are precisely interchangeable in terms of their biological actions" (Piquet-Pellorce et al. 1994). Thus, it is unlikely that such substitution actually occurs in the implantation process, since only the LIF gene was "knocked out."

The actions of these various cytokines on cells are mediated through membrane-bound receptors, which show the same overlapping of function as the helix bundle peptides (Horseman and Yu-Lee 1994). Specificity of response may be ensured by intracellular structure of the cytokine receptor dictating which signaling molecules are activated and expression levels of signaling molecules in the different cell types (Taniguchi 1995). Binding of these cytokines to their receptor complexes activates a signal transduction pathway, resulting in rapid tyrosine phosphorylations, followed by activation of a protein kinase cascade and early gene responses (Nakajima and Wall 1991; Lord et al. 1991; Murakami et al. 1991). Similarities between the signal receptor transducing components of IL-6, LIF, G-CSF, and CNTF have been recently reported. Equilibrium analysis of the binding of radioiodinated LIF in the mouse has led to the classification of two receptor types, low and high affinity (Yamamoto-Yamaguchi et al. 1986). On hemopoietic cells the low-abundance high-affinity form had a dissociation constant K_d of 10–200 pM and a binding capacity of 150–400 receptors/cell while the abundant low-affinity form had a K_d of 1–3 nM and 2000–6000 receptors/cell (Yamamoto-Yamaguchi et al. 1986; Williams et al. 1988; Rodan et al. 1990; Tomida et al. 1990; Hilton et al. 1991). Recently it has been suggested that the receptors for all these cytokines involve the IL-6 transduction component gp130: For IL-6 the receptor complex comprises two gp130 units, and for LIF and CNTF one gp130 and one LIF receptor β-unit. All are complexed with a third element a cytokine-specific α-subunit, which may be membrane-bound or act as a soluble factor, and regulate the binding of factors to the β-subunits (Ip et al. 1992). The cloned LIF receptor (LIFR) only binds LIF with low affinity, but binding of gp130 to the LIFR, transforms LIFR into a high-affinity form (Gearing et al. 1991, 1992). OSM does not bind to the LIF low-affinity receptor but does to the high-affinity form (Gearing et al. 1992). Receptor activation of this cytokine family results from homo- or heterodimerization of gp130, which converts the low-affinity α:β- complexes to a high-affinity form. The receptor components gp130 and LIF-Rβ constitutively associate with Jak-Tyk kinases, which are activated by dimerization of the receptor-β components (Murakami et al. 1993; Lütticken et al. 1994; Stahl et al. 1994; Hirano et al. 1994). A family of proteins known as signal transduction and activation of transcription proteins (Stat) are involved in the actions of many polypeptide ligands on cells. Stat3 is activated through phosphorylation on tyrosine as a DNA binding protein by the LIF–IL-6–CNTF family of ligands (Zhong et al. 1994). Selection of the particular substrate Stat3 is specified not by the particular Jak activated, but by the tyrosine-based motifs in the receptor components gp130 and LIFR (Stahl et al. 1995). Use of the relatively specific tyrosine kinase inhibitor staurosporine effectively prevents phosphorylation of the receptor subunits by either CNTF or LIF and also prevents gene induction (Stahl et al. 1994), thus confirming the need for activation of tyrosine kinase for signal transduction and gene expression. LIF can trigger differentiation-induction, differentiation-suppression, proliferation, or activation, depending on the cell type.

Some information is available on the temporal and spatial immuno-histochemical localization of the LIFR by binding of biotinylated mouse LIF and gp130 in the uterus of mouse and rabbit. In the mouse LIFR, as the LIF protein, was highest at ovulation and on day 4 of pregnancy, and localized to the luminal and glandular epithelium. gp130 was highest on days 3 and 4 of pregancy, also in the epithelium. There was little staining for LIFR or gp130 in the stroma until day 5 when epithelial staining for LIF, LIFR, and gp130 were reduced (Yang et al. 1995b). The presence of LIFR and gp130 in the luminal epithelium on day 4 and the stroma on day 5 may indicate the presence of the high-affinity form of the LIFR. Significant staining of the myometrium for LIF, LIFR, and gp130 was also observed but showed little change with stage of pregnancy. The coexistence of high levels of LIF protein, LIFR, and gp130 in the day 4 endometrium is consistent with the previously observed high expression of mRNA in the uterus on the same day and the importance of LIF for the implantation process. In the rabbit binding of LIF (LIFR) was also mainly localized to the myometrium, endometrial glands, and epithelium. LIFR was low in unmated animals and on days 1 and 2 of pregnancy. Binding of LIF to luminal epithelium increased from day 3 and to glandular epithelium from day 5 of pregnancy. Highest levels of LIFR in the epithelium were seen on days 5 and 6, with a slight decline observed on day 7, with little difference between the mesometrial and antimesometrial regions of the implantation site. There was no difference in LIFR level between day 6 of pregnancy or pseudopregnancy. gp130 showed a slightly different pattern of distribution, being absent from the stroma and almost absent from the myometrium and glandular epithelium at all stages. It was present in luminal epithelium, reaching maximal levels on day 6 of pregnancy and pseudopregnancy, but diminishing on day 7 of pregnancy, particularly at the antimesometrial area of the implantation site (Yang et al. 1995c). Whether LIFR and gp130 appear in the stroma after implantation, as in the mouse, is not known. As in the mouse, the coexistence of high levels of LIF protein and LIFR on day 6 of pregnancy, just prior to implantation in the rabbit, again suggests the importance of LIF in the implantation process in this latter species. The different patterns of distribution of LIFR and gp130 suggest that LIF function may be regulated by the relative amount of LIFR with high and low affinities or the presence of other cytokines. Coexpression of LIFR and gp130 suggests the presence of the high-affinity receptor form, while high gp130 levels, not so coexpressed, might indicate the presence of IL-6 receptors (which contain two gp130 units). Theoretically blockade of the LIFR receptor should, as in the gene "knock-out" mouse, prevent implantation. However, since LIFRβ subunit is a component of the receptor for other cytokines, it will be necessary to target the blockade to the LIFRα subunit which is specific to the LIFR.

5.4 Other Growth Factors

In nonhuman primates a variety of other growth factors whose secretion by the endometrium is hormonally regulated have been described. There are cell-specific changes in expression of the receptors for insulin-like growth factor (IGF) I and EGF, and for secreted proteins IGF binding protein 1 and retinol binding protein (Fazleabas et al. 1994). In human endometrial cell cultures IGF-I, its receptor, and the IGF binding proteins 1–4 are all localized to the epithelial cells and are highest at the early/mid secretory phase of the cycle (Tang et al. 1994). These changes are thought to be modulated by the embryo, and thus may be important for implantation. However, at present the data are purely correlative.

Fibroblast growth factors (FGFs) are involved in angiogenesis, cell growth, and differentiation. In the mouse disruption of the gene for one of these, FGF-4, causes severe inhibition of the growth of the inner cell mass (the cells that form the embryo) of the blastocyst and failure of pregnancy just after implantation (Feldman et al. 1995). FGFs have a dual receptor system; one component is the FGF receptor with an extracellular ligand binding domain and an intracellular tyrosine kinase domain, and the other is a series of heparin or heparan sulfate proteoglycans required for FGF binding. There are several binding sites for these proteoglycans on FGF (Ornitz et al. 1995).

5.5 Conclusions

This brief review of present knowledge about cytokines/growth factors shows that several molecules may be involved in the implantation process, and that there are significant interactions between many of them. It seems probable that as work proceeds, more cytokines/growth factors that also play a role will be identified. Thus there are likely to be several targets for specific interference with the implantation process. Nevertheless, several important questions need to be resolved, not the least of which is the applicability of findings in the mouse to the human situation. If we are considering the endometrium as a target for contraception, and this implies blocking the implantation process, we should pursue only those leads applicable to the human. Already with the present imperfect state of knowledge, there appear to be promising approaches which could form the basis for a once-a-month contraceptive pill. Critical experiments will be needed to bring these possibilities to the proof of concept stage. Even then questions will remain concerning the specific time that the agent must be given and how often. There may also be a problem of shortening of the menstrual cycle, thus causing difficulties in determining the time for optimal dosing in the next cycle. These new leads do, however, show promise of more specificity than the existing hormonally based approaches and thus worthy of further study.

References

Anegon I, Cuturi MC, Godard A, Moreau M, Terqui M, Martinat-Botté F, Soulillou JP (1994) Presence of leukaemia inhibitory factor and interleukin 6 in porcine uterine secretions prior to conceptus attachment. Cytokine 6:493–499

Bany BM, Kennedy TG (1995) Interleukin-1α regulates prostaglandin production and cyclooxygenase activity in sensitized rat endometrial stromal cells in vitro. Biol Reprod 53:126–132

Bhatt H, Brunet LJ, Stewart CL (1991) Uterine expression of leukemia inhibitory factor coincides with the onset of blastocyst implantation. Proc Natl Acad Sci USA 88:11408–11412

Braga VMM, Gendler SJ (1993) Modulation of Muc-1 mucin expression in the mouse uterus during the estrus cycle, early pregnancy and placentation. J Cell Sci 105:397–405

Charnock-Jones DS, Sharkey AM, Fenwick P, Smith SK (1994) Leukemia inhibitory factor mRNA concentration peaks in human endometrium at the time of implantation and the blastocyst contains mRNA for the receptor at this time. J Reprod Fertil 101:421–426

Chen D-B, Hilsenrath R, Yang Z-M, Le S-P, Kim S-R, Chuong CJ, Poindexter AN III, Harper MJK (1995a) Leukaemia inhibitory factor in human endometrium during the menstrual cycle: cellular origin and action on production of glandular epithelial cell prostaglandin in vitro. Hum Reprod 10:911–918

Chen D-B, Yang Z-M, Hilsenrath R, Le S-P, Harper MJK (1995b) Stimulation of prostaglandin (PG) F$_{2\alpha}$ and PGE$_2$ release by tumour necrosis factor-α and interleukin-1α in cultured human luteal phase endometrial cells. Hum Reprod 10:2773–2780

De M, Sandford TR, Wood GW (1993) Expression of interleukin 1, interleukin 6 and tumor necrosis factor α in mouse uterus during the peri-implantation period of pregnancy. J Reprod Fertil 97:83–89

Dower SK, Kronheim SR, Hopp TP, Cantrell M, Deeley M, Gillis S, Henney CS, Urdal DL (1986) The cell surface receptors for interleukin-1α and interleukin-1β are identical. Nature 324:266–268

Fazleabas AT, Hild-Petito S, Verhage HG (1994) Secretory proteins and growth factors of the baboon (Papio anubis) uterus: potential roles in pregnancy. Cell Biol Intl 18:1145–1153

Feldman B, Poueymirou W, Papaioannou VE, DeChiara TM, Goldfarb M (1995) Requirement of FGF-4 for postimplantation mouse development. Science 267:246–249

Frank GR, Brar AK, Jikihara H, Cedars MI, Handwerger S (1995) Interleukin-1β and the endometrium: an inhibitor of stromal cell differentiation and possible autoregulator of decidualization in humans. Biol Reprod 52:184–191

Fukuda MN, Sato T, Nakayama J, Klier G, Mikami M, Aoki D, Nozawa S (1995) Trophinin and tastin, a novel cell adhesion molecule complex with potential involvement in embryo implantation. Genes Dev 9:1199–1210

Gearing DP, Thut CJ, VandenBos T, Gimpel SD, Delaney PB, King J, Price V, Cosman D, Beckmann MP (1991) Leukemia inhibitory factor is structurally related to the IL-6 signal transducer, gp130. EMBO J 10:239–248

Gearing DP, Comeau MR, Friend DJ, Gimpel SD, Thut CJ, McGourty J, Brasher KK, King JA, Gillis S, Mosley B, Ziegler SF, Cosman D (1992) The IL-6 signal transducer, gp130: an oncostatin M receptor and affinity converter for the LIF receptor. Science 255:1434–1437

Hamilton JA, Waring PM, Filonzi EL (1993) Induction of leukemia inhibitory factor in human synovial fibroblasts by IL-1 and tumor necrosis factor-α. J Immunol 150:1496–1502

Hatayama H, Kanzaki H, Iwai M, Kariya M, Fujimoto M, Higuchi T, Kojima K, Nakayama H, Mori T, Fujita J (1994) Progesterone enhances macrophage colony-stimulating factor production in human endometrial stromal cells in vitro. Endocrinology 135:1921–1927

Hilton DJ, Nicola NA, Metcalf D (1991) Distribution and comparison of receptors for leukemia inhibitory factor on murine hemopoietic and hepatic cells. J Cell Physiol 146:207–215

Hirano T, Matsuda T, Nakajima K (1994) Signal transduction through gp130 that is shared among the receptors for the interleukin 6 related cytokine subfamily. Stem Cells 12:262–277

Horseman ND, Yu-Lee L-Y (1994) Transcriptional regulation by the helix bundle peptide hormones: growth hormone, prolactin and hematopoietic cytokines. Endocr Rev 15:627–649

Hunt JS, Chen H-L, Hu X-L, Pollard JW (1993) Normal distribution of tumor necrosis factor-α messenger ribonucleic acid and protein in the uteri, placentas, and embryos of osteopetrotic (op/op) mice lacking colony-stimulating factor-1. Biol Reprod 49:441–452

Ilesanmi AO, Hawkins DA, Lessey BA (1993) Immunohistochemical markers of uterine receptivity in the human endometrium. Microsc Res Technique 25:208–222

Inoue T, Kanzaki H, Iwai M, Imai K, Narukawa S, Higuchi T, Katsuragawa H, Mori T (1994) Tumor necrosis factor α inhibits in-vitro decidualization of human endometrial stromal cells. Hum Reprod 9:2411–2417

Ip NY, Nye SH, Boulton TG, Davis S, Taga T, Li Y, Birren SJ, Yasukawa K, Kishimoto T, Anderson DJ, Stahl N, Yancopoulos GD (1992) CNTF and LIF act on neuronal cells via shared signaling pathways that involve the IL-6 signal transducing receptor component gp130. Cell 69:1121–1132

Jacobs AL, Carson DD (1993) Uterine epithelial cell secretion of interleukin-1α induces prostaglandin E_2 (PGE_2) and $PGF_{2\alpha}$ secretion by uterine stromal cells in vitro. Endocrinology 132:300–308

Jentoft N (1990) Why are proteins O-glycosylated? Trends Biochem Sci 15:291–294

Jikihara H, Handwerger S (1994) Tumor necrosis factor-α inhibits the synthesis and release of human decidual cell prolactin. Endocrinology 134:353–357

Kariya M, Kanzaki H, Hanamura T, Imai K, Narukawa S, Inoue T, Hatayama H, Mori T (1994) Progesterone-dependent secretion of macrophage colony-stimulating factor by human endometrial stromal cells of nonpregnant uterus in culture. J Clin Endocrinol Metab 79:86–90

Kauma S, Matt D, Strom S, Eierman D, Turner T (1990) Interleukin-1β (IL-1β), human leukocyte antigen HLA-DR α, and transforming growth factor-β (TGF-β) expression in endometrium, placenta and placental membranes. Am J Obstet Gynecol 163:1430–1436

Kimber SJ (1994) Carbohydrates as low affinity binding agents involved in initial attachment of the mammalian embryo at implantation. In: Ward RHT, Smith SK, Donnai D (eds) Early fetal growth and development. Royal College of Obstetricians and Gynecologists Press, London, pp 75–102

Kimber SJ, Illingworth IM, Glasser SR (1995) Expression of carbohydrate antigens in the rat uterus during early pregnancy and after ovariectomy and steroid replacement. J Reprod Fertil 103:75–87

Kliman HJ, Feinberg RF, Schwartz LB, Feinman MA, Lavi E, Meaddough EL (1995) A mucin-like glycoprotein identified by MAG (mouse ascites golgi) antibodies. Menstrual cycle-dependent localization in human endometrium. Am J Pathol 146:166–181

Kojima K, Kanzaki H, Iwai M, Hatayama H, Fujimoto M, Inoue T, Horie K, Nakayama H, Fujita J, Mori T (1994) Expression of leukemia inhibitory factor in human endometrium and placenta. Biol Reprod 50:882–887

Kwun JK, Emmens CW (1974) Hormone requirements for implantation and pregnancy in the ovariectomized rabbit. Aust J Biol Sci 27:275–283

Lessey BA (1994) The use of integrins for the assessment of uterine receptivity. Fertil Steril 61:812–814

Lessey BA, Damjanovich L, Coutifaris C, Castelbaum A, Albelda SM, Buck CA (1992) Integrin adhesion molecules in the human endometrium. Correlation with the normal and abnormal menstrual cycle. J Clin Invest 90:188–195

Lessey BA, Castelbaum AJ, Buck CA, Lei Y, Yowell CW, Sun J (1994) Further characterization of endometrial integrins during the menstrual cycle and in pregnancy. Fertil Steril 62:497–506

Lord KA, Abdollahi A, Thomas SM, DeMarco M, Brugge JS, Hoffman-Liebermann B, Liebermann DA (1991) Leukemia inhibitory factor and interleukin–6 trigger the same immediate early response, including tyrosine phosphorylation, upon induction of myeloid leukemia differentiation. Mol Cell Biol 11:4371–4379

Lütticken C, Wegenka UM, Yuan J, Buschmann J, Schindler C, Ziemiecki A, Harpur AG, Wilks AF, Yasukawa K, Taga T, Kishimoto T, Barbieri G, Pellegrini S, Sendtner M, Heinrich PC, Horn F (1994) Association of transcription factor APRF and protein kinase Jak1 with the interleukin-6 signal transducer gp130. Science 263:89–92

Murakami M, Narazaki M, Hibi M, Yawata H, Yasukawa K, Hamaguchi M, Taga T, Kishimoto T (1991) Critical cytoplasmic region of the interleukin-6 signal transducer gp130 is conserved in the cytokine receptor family. Proc Natl Acad Sci USA 88:11349–11353

Murakami M, Hibi M, Nakagawa N, Nakagawa T, Yasukawa K, Yamanishi Y, Taga T, Kishimoto T (1993) Il-6-induced homodimerization of gp130 and associated activation of a tyrosine kinase. Science 260:1808–1810

Nakajima K, Wall R (1991) Interleukin-6 signals activating junB and tis11 gene transcription in a B-cell hybridoma. Mol Cell Biol 11:1409–1418

Oppenheim JJ, Kovacs EJ, Matsushima K, Durum SK (1986) There is more than one interleukin-1. Immunol Today 7:45–56

Ornitz DM, Herr AB, Nilsson M, Westman J, Svahn C-M, Waksman G (1995) FGF binding and FGF receptor activation by synthetic heparan-derived di- and trisaccharides. Science 268:432–436

Piquet-Pellorce C, Grey L, Mereau A, Heath JK (1994) Are LIF and related cytokines functionally equivalent? Exp Cell Res 213:340–347

Pollard JW, Hunt JS, Wiktor-Jedrzejczak W, Stanley ER (1991) A pregnancy defect in the osteopetrotic (op/op) mouse demonstrates the requirement for CSF-1 in female fertility. Dev Biol 148:273–283

Psychoyos A (1974) Hormone control of ovo-implantation. Vitam Horm 32:201–256

Rathjen PD, Toth S, Willis A, Heath JK, Smith AG (1990) Differentiation inhibition activity is produced in matrix associated and soluble forms that are generated by alternate promoter usage. Cell 62:1105–1114

Robertson SA, Mayrhofer G, Seamark RF (1992) Uterine epithelial cells synthesize granulocyte-macrophage colony stimulating factor and interleukin-6 in pregnant and non-pregnant mice. Biol Reprod 46:1069–1079

Rodan SB, Wesolowski G, Hilton DJ, Nicola NA, Rodan GA (1990) Leukemia inhibitory factor binds with high affinity to preosteoblastic RCT-1 cells and

120   M.J.K. Harper

potentiates the retinoic acid induction of alkaline phosphatase. Endocrinology 127:1602–1608

Rose TM, Bruce AG (1991) Oncostatin M is a member of a cytokine family that includes leukemia-inhibitory factor, granulocyte colony-stimulating factor, and interleukin-6. Proc Natl Acad Sci USA 88:8641–8645

Schultz JF, Armant DR (1995)β_1- and β_3-class integrins mediate fibronectin binding activity at the surface of developing mouse peri-implantation blastocysts. J Biol Chem 270:11522–11531

Shen MM, Leder P (1992) Leukemia inhibitory factor is expressed by the preimplantation uterus and selectively blocks primitive ectoderm formation in vitro. Proc Natl Acad Sci USA 89:8240–8244

Sheth KV, Roca GL, Al-Sedairy ST, Parhar RS, Hamilton CJCM, Al-Abdul Jabbar F (1991) Prediction of successful embryo implantation by measuring interleukin-1α and immunosuppressive factor(s) in preimplantation embryo culture fluid. Fertil Steril 55:952–957

Simón C, Piquette GN, Frances A, Westphal LM, Heinrichs WL, Polan ML (1993a) Interleukin-1 type I receptor messenger ribonucleic acid (mRNA) expression in human endometrium throughout the menstrual cycle. Fertil Steril 59:791–796

Simón C, Piquette GN, Frances A, Polan ML (1993b) Localization of interleukin-1 type I receptor and interleukin-1β in human endometrium throughout the menstrual cycle. J Clin Endocrinol Metab 77:549–555

Simón C, Frances A, Piquette GN, El-Danasouri I, Zurawski G, Dang W, Polan ML (1994) Embryonic implantation in mice is blocked by interleukin-1 receptor antagonist. Endocrinology 134:521–528

Stahl N, Boulton TG, Faruggella T, Ip NY, Davis S, Witthun BA, Quelle FW, Silvennoinen O, Barbieri G, Pellegrini S, Ihle JN, Yancopoulos GD (1994) Association and activation of Jak-Tyk kinases by CNTF-LIF-OSM-IL-6β receptor components. Science 263:92–95

Stahl N, Faruggella T, Boulton TG, Zhong Z, Darnell JE Jr, Yancopoulos GD(1995) Choice of STATs and other substrates specified by modular tyrosine-based motifs in cytokine receptors. Science 267:1349–1353

Stewart CL, Kaspar P, Brunet LJ, Bhatt H, Gadi I, Köntgen F, Abbondanzo SJ (1992) Blastocyst implantation depends on maternal expression of leukemia inhibitory factor. Nature 359:76–79

Strous GJ, Dekker J (1992) Mucin-type glycoproteins. Crit Rev Biochem Mol Biol 27:57–92

Surveyor GA, Gendler SJ, Pemberton L, Das SK, Chakraborty I, Julian J, Pimental RA, Wegner CC, Dey SK, Carson DD (1995) Expression and steroid hormonal control of Muc-1 in the mouse uterus. Endocrinology 136:3639–3647

Tabibzadeh S, Kaffka KL, Satyaswaroop PG, Kilian PL (1990) Interleukin-1 (IL-1) regulation of human endometrial function: presence of IL-1 receptor correlates with IL-1-stimulated prostaglandin E_2 production. J Clin Endocrinol Metab 70:1000–1006

Tang X-M, Rossi MJ, Masterson BJ, Chegini N (1994) Insulin-like growth factor I (IGF-I), IGF-I receptors, and IGF binding proteins 1-4 in human uterine tissue: tissue localization and IGF-I action in endometrial stromal and myometrial smooth muscle cells in vitro. Biol Reprod 50:1113–1125

Taniguchi T (1995) Cytokine signaling through nonreceptor protein tyrosine kinases. Science 268:251–255

Tartakovsky B, Ben-Yair E (1991) Cytokines modulate preimplantation development and pregnancy. Dev Biol 146:345–352

Tomida M, Yamamoto-Yamaguchi Y, Hozumi M, Holmes W, Lowe DG, Goeddel DV (1990) Inhibition of development of (Na^+)-dependent hexose transport in renal epithelial LLC-PK1 cells by differentiation-stimulating factor for myeloid leukemia cells/leukemia inhibitory factor. FEBS Lett 268:261–264

Williams RL, Hilton DJ, Pease S, Willson TA, Stewart CL, Gearing DP, Wagner EF, Metcalf D, Nicola NA, Gough NM (1988) Myeloid leukemia inhibitory factor maintains the developmental potential of embryonic stem cells. Nature 336:684–687

Willson TA, Metcalf D, Gough NM (1992) Cross-species comparison of the sequence of the leukaemia inhibitory factor gene and its protein. Eur J Biochem 204:21–30

Yamamoto-Yamaguchi Y, Tomida M, Hozumi M (1986) Specific binding of a factor inducing differentiation to mouse myeloid leukemic M1 cells. Exp Cell Res 164:97–102

Yang Z-M, Le S-P, Chen D-B, Harper MJK (1994) Temporal and spatial expression of leukemia inhibitory factor in rabbit uterus during early pregnancy. Mol Reprod Dev 38:148–152

Yang Z-M, Chen D-B, Le S-P, Harper MJK (1995a) Interleukin-1α in the rabbit uterus during early pregnancy. Early Pregn Biol Med 1:201–205

Yang Z-M, Le S-P, Chen D-B, Cota J, Siero V, Yasukawa K, Harper MJK (1995b) Leukemia inhibitory factor (LIF), LIF receptor and gp130 in the mouse uterus during early pregnancy. Mol Reprod Dev 42:407–414

Yang Z-M, Le S-P, Chen D-B, Yasukawa K, Harper,M.J.K. (1995c) Expression patterns of leukemia inhibitory factor receptor (LIFR) and the gp130 receptor component in rabbit uterus during early pregnancy. J Reprod Fertil 103:249–255

Yang Z-M, Chen D-B, Le S-P, Harper MJK (1996a) Differential hormonal regulation of leukemia inhibitory factor (LIF) in rabbit and mouse uterus. Mol Reprod Dev 43:470–476

Yang Z-M, Chen D-B, Le S-P, Brown RW, Chuong CJ, Harper MJK (1996b) Localization of leukemia inhibitory factor in human endometrium during the menstrual cycle. Early Pregn Biol Med 2:18–22

Zhang Z, Funk C, Roy D, Glasser SR, Mulholland J (1994a) Heparin-binding epidermal growth factor-like growth factor is differentially regulated by progesterone and estradiol in rat uterine epithelial and stromal cells. Endocrinology 134:1089–1094

Zhang Z, Funk C, Glasser SR, Mulholland J (1994b) Progesterone regulation of heparin-binding epidermal growth factor-like factor gene expression during sensitization and decidualization in the rat uterus: effects of the antiprogestin ZK 98.299. Endocrinology 135:1256–1263

Zhong Z, Wen Z, Darnell JE Jr (1994) Stat3: a STAT family member activated by tyrosine phosphorylation in response to epidermal growth factor and interleukin-6. Science 264:95–98

Zolti M, Ben-Rafael Z, Meirom R, Shemesh M, Bider D, Mashiach S, Apte R (1991) Cytokine involvement in oocytes and early embryos. Fertil Steril 56:265–272

6 Metalloproteinases and Regulation of Endometrial Function

P. Bischof

6.1 Matrix Metalloproteinases and Their Inhibitors

Matrix metalloproteinases (MMP) form a family of homologous enzymes (Table 1) which have a Zn^{2+} atom in their active site (see Matrisian 1990 for review). They are secreted as inactive pro enzymes (zymogens) which become activated upon partial hydrolysis whereby they loose their propeptide. They are classified in three subfamilies according to their substrate specificity: *Gelatinases* are represented by two enzymes, gelatinase A and B (72 and 92 kDa gelatinases, or MMP-2 and MMP-9, respectively). These proteases digest collagen type IV (the major constituent of basement membranes) and denatured collagen (gelatin). *Collagenases* include three proteases: the interstitial collagenase (MMP-1 or collagenase), the neutrophil collagenase (MMP-8), and collagenase 3 (MMP-13). These enzymes digest collagen types I, II, III, VII, and X. They are thus directed at digesting the collagen of the extracellular matrix of the interstitium. *Stromelysins* form a subfamily

Table 1. Biochemical Properties of MMP and their inhibitors

	MMP-1	MMP-2	MMP-3	MMP-7	MMP-8
Other names	Interstitial collagenase Fibroblast collagenase	Gelatinase A 72-kDa gelatinase	Stromelysin 1 Transin-1	PUMP-I Matrilysin	Neutophil collagenase PMNL collagenase
Enzyme No.	3.4.24.7	3.4.24.24	3.4.24.17	3.4.24.23	3.4.24.34
M.W.	54007	73882	53977	29677	53412
Number of a.a.	469	660	477	267	46
Signal peptide	1–19	1–29	1–17	1–17	1–20
Propepetide	20–99	30–109	18–99	18–94	81–100
Catalytic domain	100–274	110–465	100–286	95–267	101–275
Hemopexinlike	275–469	466–660	287–477		276–467
Position of zinc	218	403	218	214	217
Position of carbohydrates	120	573, 642	120		54,73,112, 204,246
Position of disulfide bonds	278–466	469–660	290–477		279–464
Substrates	Col I,II,III, VII,X MMP-5, entactin α1-plasmin inhibitor α1-anti-chymotrypsin	Col IV,V, VII,X gelatin I fibronectin elastin	Col III,IV, IX,X gelatin I,II, IV,V laminin proteogly-cans fibronectin elastin, casein α1-plasmin inhibitor α1-anti-chymotrypsin	Casein, Fibronectin gelatin I,II, IV,V proteoglycans MMP-2	Col I,III
Proform MW (kDa)	54	72	57	28	53
Active form MW (kDa)	42 (24)	66(21)	48,28	19	65
Activators	APMA, trypsin	APMA, MMP-7	APMA, trypsin		APMA, plasmin
Activators	MMP-3, plasmin	MT-MMP	plasmin, heat		MMP-3
Location of gene	Chr 11	Chr16	Chr 11		
Number of exons	10	13			

Table 1 (continued)

MMP-9	MMP-10	MMP-11	MMP-13	TIMP-1	TIMP-2	TIMP-3
Gelatinase B 92-kDa gelatinase	Stromelysin 2 Transin-2	Stromelysin 3	Collagenase 3	Erytroid potentiating activity EPA		
3.4.24.35	3.4.24.22	3.4.24.-	3.4.24.-			
78427	54151	54595	53819	23171	24399	24145
707	476	488	471	207	220	211
1–19	1–17	1–31	1–23	1–23	1–26	1–23
20–106	18–98	32–97	24–103			
107–510	99–285	98–286	104–280	24–207	27–220	24–211
511–707	286–476	287–488	281–471			
401	217	215	222			
38,120,127			117,152	53,101		
516–704	289–476	294–180	284–471	6 altogether	6 altogether	6 altogether
Col IV,V gelatin I,V	Col II,IV,V Gelatin I,III, IV,V fibronectin	Col IV	Col I α1-anti-trysin			
92,125,220 88 trypsin, APMA	53 47 (28) trypsin, APMA	53		28	20	
Chr 16 13	Chr 11					

of four enzymes (MMP-3, 7, 10, and 11; also called stromelysin-1, matrilysin or putative metalloproteinase, stromelysin-2, and strome-lysin-3, respectively). These proteases have a relatively broad substrate specificity and digest collagen type IV, V, VII as well as laminin, fibronectin, proteoglycans, and gelatin. Activation of the pro-MMP into active MMP can be reproduced in vitro by the addition of different agents such as mercurial salts, plasmin, or trypsin. Although the physi-ological activators of the different MMP are unknown, it has been shown that plasmin (Murphy et al. 1992) and MMP-3 (Ogata et al. 1992) are potent activators of several MMP. This means that MMPs most probably act in cascade such as the enzymes involved in blood coagulation. Activated enzymes digest the extracellular matrices with-out damaging the cells. For all except one MMP (MMP-2) it is consid-ered that the active enzymes are secreted into the extracellular space where they digest the matrix components, and where they are under the control of local inhibitors. For MMP-2, however, Emonard and cowork-ers (1992) reported on the existence of an MMP-2 binding site on human breast cancer cells. This and other observations led Cockett et al. 1994 to propose a model for MMP-2 dependent tumor cell invasion. According to their model, pro-MMP-2 is bound via its C terminus to the cell surface through a binding site located at the invading front of a tumour. This exposes the fibronectinlike collagen binding domain which interacts with the surrounding collagen. Upon activation, possi-bly through a cell-membrane associated mechanism, MMP-2 degrades collagen and facilitates invasion.

So far 3 tissue inhibitors of metalloproteinases (TIMP-1, -2, and -3) have been described. These are homologous, cystein-rich proteins se-creted locally in the extracellular space where they control the activity of MMP. TIMPs inhibit tumor cell invasion in vitro and in vivo (Gold-berg and Eisen 1990) by binding to the MMP. TIMP-2 specifically inhibits MMP-2 by binding to the C terminus of the pro-MMP-2 and inhibits activation possibly by competing with the binding site of pro-MMP-2 on the cell surface.

6.2 Endometrial MMP

6.2.1 Cellular Origin of Endometrial MMP

The human endometrium is a tissue where intense remodeling takes place. Every month during the reproductive years of a women the endometrium proliferates, differentiates, and is shed. It is thus not surprising to find in this tissue enzymes capable of digesting the different components of the extracellular matrix.

Ovine endometrial cells (stromal and epithelial) produce stromelysin-1 (MMP-3; Salamonsen et al. 1991), gelatinase B (MMP-2) and interstitial collagenase (MMP-1: Salamonsen et al. 1993) when cultured in vitro. Similarly, stromelysin-2 (MMP-10), TIMP-1, and TIMP-2 mRNA have been shown to be expressed by decidualized mouse endometrium (Waterhouse et al. 1993). Decidual TIMP-1 mRNA levels are specifically increased between 6 and 10 days of pregnancy whereas TIMP-2 and stromelysin-2 mRNA levels steadily increase throughout gestation.

Human endometrial explants cultured in vitro for 48 h release gelatinase A and B (MMP-2, MMP-9) and interstitial collagenase (MMP-1; Marbaix et al. 1992). Both human endometrial stromal and epithelial cells when cultured separately release several metalloproteinases (Martelli et al. 1993). The activity of the released enzymes does not depend on the histology (proliferative or secretory) of the endometrium where the cells originate but on the type of substrate on which the cells attach when cultured in vitro. Interestingly, we have observed that the collagenolytic activity released by both types of endometrial cells is much higher when cells are purified from endometria bearing a Gravigard IUD than from normal endometria (Martelli et al. 1993). Studies using immunohistochemistry (Rodgers et al. 1993; Polette et al. 1994), or in situ hybridization (Rodgers et al. 1993; Polette et al. 1994; Hampton and Salamonsen 1994) have clearly shown that endometrial cell produce gelatinases A and B, interstitial collagenase, matrilysin (MMP-7), stromelysin-1, TIMP-1, and TIMP-2. Matrilysin mRNA is expressed only in epithelial cells whereas interstitial collagenase and TIMP-1 mRNA are found only in stromal cells (Rodgers et al. 1994). The expression of matrilysin, interstitial collagenase, and stromelysin-1 mRNA is clearly related to menses since these are not detectable on days

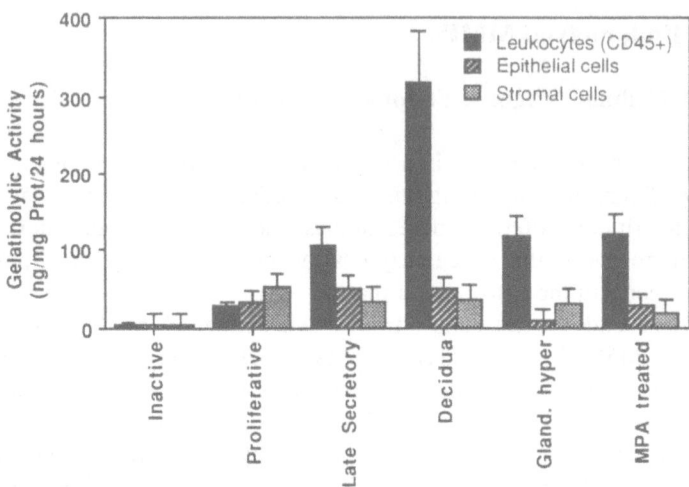

Fig. 1. Gelatinolytic activity released in vitro by endometrial leukocytes, epithelial and stromal cells isolated from endometria in different physiological conditions

5–25 of the cycle but are increased from day 26 to day 4 of the following cycle. In contrast, TIMP-1 and TIMP-2 mRNA is expressed throughout the cycle (Rodgers et al. 1994; Hampton and Salamonsen 1994).

Besides the glandular epithelial and stromal cells, the endometrium contains several other cell types. Various authors have shown that bone marrow derived cells such as macrophages, T cells, B cells, and granulocytes colonize the endometrium at each cycle (Bulmer and Sunderland 1984; King and Loke 1991). These leukocytes represent an increasing proportion of endometrial cells as the menstrual cycle progresses, increasing from 8% in the proliferative phase to 23% in the secretory phase and up to 30% in early pregnancy decidua (Bulmer et al. 1988). Large granular lymphocytes (LGL) are a particular leukocyte subset quite unique to the endometrium (King and Loke 1990). LGL are natural killer cells expressing the antigen CD56. They represent the largest proportion (up to 75%, Bulmer et al. 1991) of all endometrial leukocytes, and their function is unknown.

Using an immunoadsorbtion technique on enzymatically dispersed endometrial cells, we separated and cultured different endometrial cell

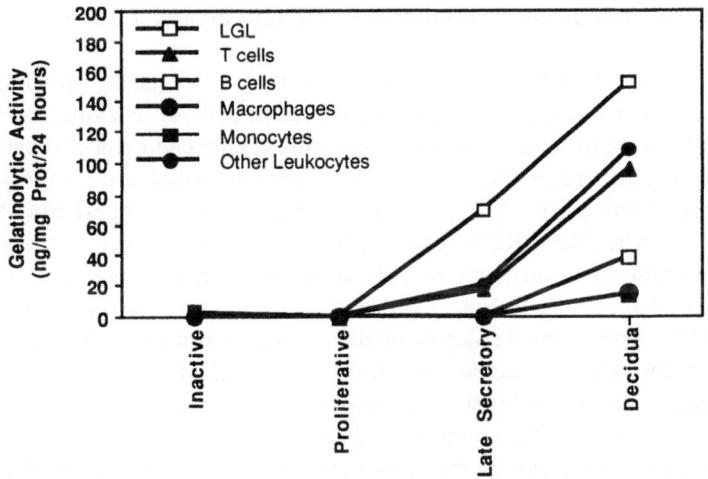

Fig. 2. Gelatinolytic activity released in vitro by endometrial leukocyte subsets isolated from endometria in different physiological conditions

subsets obtained at different phases of the cycle and early pregnancy (Shi et al. 1995). The supernatants from the cell cultures were analyzed for gelatinolytic activity by an assay that has been published previously (Bischof et al. 1995a). Figure 1 shows that after ovulation, but not before, the CD 45 positive endometrial leukocytes secrete considerably more gelatinolytic enzymes than epithelial or stromal cells. Among the various endometrial leukocyte subsets LGL release the highest gelatinolytic activity, followed by the macrophages, T cells, B cells, and monocytes (Fig. 2). For all types of cells the secretion of gelatinolytic enzymes is higher in decidua than in other endometria. These results show quite clearly that the endometrial leukocytes and particularly the LGL contribute massively to the overall proteolytic activity of the endometrium. One might thus wonder whether their role in endometrial remodeling and in implantation is not more important than epithelial or stromal cells.

6.2.2 Regulation of Endometrial MMP and Potential Role

The activity of MMP is tightly controlled at three levels: the production and secretion of the proenzyme, the activation of the proenzyme, and the inhibition of the active enzyme. The regulators are endocrine and paracrine or autocrine. Estradiol stimulates interstitial collagenase activity in cervical fibroblasts of pregnant guinea pigs whereas progesterone has the opposite effect (Rajabi et al. 1990). The stimulatory effect of estradiol seems to be mediated by prostaglandins since indomethacin abolishes the estradiol-induced MMP-1 activity. Progesterone inhibits MMP-1 activity by a receptor-mediated mechanism (since RU-486 inhibits the progesterone effect). The inhibitory effect of progesterone on cervical fibroblasts MMP-1 activity is probably due to an increase in TIMP-1 and TIMP-2 activity (Imada et al. 1994). These animal data on the effects of steroids on the proteolytic potential of cervical fibroblasts fit very well the known effects of antigestagens on cervical ripening in humans (Radestad et al. 1993).

Ovarian steroids modulate also endometrial MMP. Marbaix and colleagues (1992) convincingly showed that progesterone in physiological concentrations totally abolishes the release of MMP-1 and MMP-9 by endometrial explants. RU-486 antagonizes these effects of progesterone. Similar data were generated by cell culture studies in which progesterone inhibits MMP-3 production (protein and mRNA; Schatz et al. 1994) and the gelatinases (Bischof et al., unpublished observation) in endometrial stromal and decidual cells. Since MMP-3 is a known activator of other MMP, one can speculate that at the end of the cycle when progesterone withdrawal occurs, the inhibitory effect of progesterone gradually declines, allowing the endometrial cells including the bone marrow derived ones, to secrete MMP and to digest the endometrial extracellular matrix, thus starting the process of menstruation. This speculation would explain why the expression of endometrial mRNA for MMP-1 and MMP-3 can be visualized by northern blot only in menstrual and perimenstrual endometria (Hampton and Salamonsen 1994).

In addition to the endocrine regulators, the human endometrium is also subjected to autocrine/paracrine regulations. Leukocytes and the other endometrial cells produce and secrete an array of cytokines (see Tabibzadeh 1991 for review), and this chapter considers only interleukin-1 (IL-1), transforming growth factor-β (TGF-β), and leukemia inhibitory factor (LIF).

IL-1 consists of two distinct but related molecules (IL-1α, IL-1β) which mediate similar effects. IL-1 is a known product of monocytes and macrophages but is also produced by endometrial cells. Human endometrial epithelial, stromal cells, and trophoblast express IL-1 receptors (Tabibzadeh 1991). IL-1 has been shown to increase the activity of MMP-1, MMP-3, and TIMP in human fibroblasts (Unemori et al. 1994) and of gelatinase activity and invasive behavior in human cytotrophoblast cells (Librach et al. 1994). It is very interesting to note that while IL-1 inhibits decidualization of stromal cells in vitro (Kariya et al. 1991) it stimulates the production of MMP-1, MMP-3, and MMP-9 but not MMP-2 in the same cells (Rawdanowicz et al. 1994). One might therefore speculate that trophoblast derived IL-1 stimulates the release of stromal cells MMP, thereby promoting trophoblast invasion of the endometrium.

TGFβ is represented by five homodimeric polypeptides which share 70%–80% structural homologies. TGFβ1, TGFβ2, and TGFβ3 are produced by many mammalian cells including macrophages, fibroblasts, activated T cells, decidual cells, endometrial stromal and epithelial cells, and cytotrophoblast cells (Graham et al. 1992). In human fibroblasts and in keratinocytes it has been shown that TGFβ increases MMP-2 and MMP-9 activity while it decreases that of TIMP-2 (Salo et al. 1991; Overall et al. 1991). In contrast, the inhibitory effect that decidual cell conditioned medium exerts on the invasive behavior of cytotrophoblast cells seems to be due to TGFβ since antibodies to this cytokine inhibit its effect (Graham and Lala 1991). TGFβ exerts this anti-invasive effect by stimulating the secretion of TIMP by cytotrophoblastic cells. Thus here again, TGFβ could be an endometrial signal which controls trophoblast invasion during implantation and placentation.

LIF is a pleiotropic cytokine which was initially identified as a factor promoting differentiation and inhibiting proliferation of the murine myeloid leukemia cell line M1 (Tomida et al. 1984). In mice LIF expression appears in the endometrium on the 4th day of pregnancy, just before implantation of the blastocyst (Bhatt et al. 1991). This transient expression of LIF is essential for pregnancy since in transgenic female mice lacking the LIF gene implantation does not occur. Furthermore, when the blastocysts of these transgenic mice are transferred to wild-

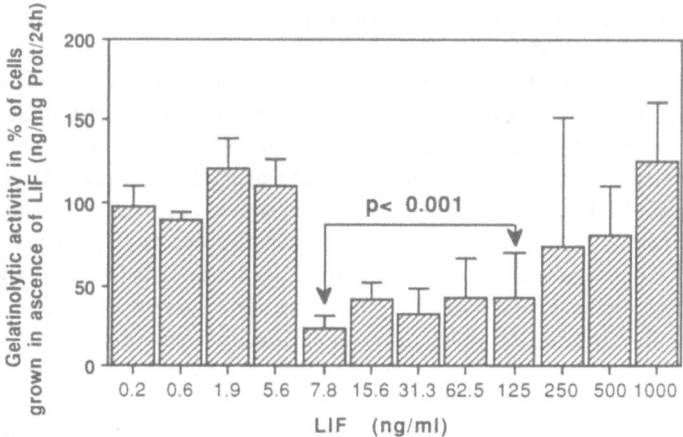

Fig. 3. Effect of recombinant human LIF on the gelatinolytic activity of purified (leukocyte free) human cytotrophoblastic cells cultured in vitro

type pseudopregnant recipients, the blastocysts implant and lead to a
normal pregnancy (Stewart et al. 1992). The human endometrium also
produces LIF (Kojima et al. 1994), and LIF mRNA is more abundant in
a secretory endometrium than a proliferative one (Kojima et al. 1994).
Since LIF can also be a regulator of trophoblast invasion in the human
(Kojima et al. 1995), we examined the effects of LIF on the gelatinolytic
activity of cytotrophoblastic cells (Bischof et al. 1995b). As shown in
Fig. 3, recombinant human LIF inhibits the gelatinolytic activity secreted by cytotrophoblastic cells. LIF exerts profound effects on cytotrophoblast differentiation since at the same time that this cytokine
inhibits MMP it also inhibits hCG secretion (Bischof et al. 1995b). We
therefore conclude that endometrial LIF inhibits differentiation of cytotrophoblastic cells in syncytium (decrease in human chorionic gonadotropin), inhibiting at the same time the acquisition of an invasive phenotype (inhibition of gelatinases) by cytotrophoblast cells. If this is true in
vivo, the net result of LIF activity would be to maintain the cytotrophoblastic cells in an undifferentiated state.

6.3 Conclusions

The secretion of endometrial MMP is due not only to epithelial and stromal cells but also to the bone marrow derived cells which colonize the endometrium at each cycle. The contribution of these latter cells to the total proteolytic potential of the endometrium is quantitatively superior to the epithelial and stromal cells. This implies that bone marrow derived cells play a much more important role in endometrial remodeling than suspected. Although the evidence is still circumstantial, it is highly probable that endometrial MMP are involved in the mechanism of uterine bleeding. That fact that their expression is inhibited by progesterone and stimulated by antigestagens constitutes another explanation for the menses inducing effect of these new drugs.

MMP are probably also involved in the regulation of trophoblast invasion during implantation and placentation. The in vitro experimental evidences point to two possible mechanisms: (a) trophoblast-derived factors (e.g., IL-1) can stimulate the release of endometrial MMP which digest the endometrial extracellular matrix and favor trophoblast invasion. (b) On the other hand, endometrial factors such as TIMP, TGFβ, or LIF can control trophoblast invasion by inhibiting directly the proteolytic potential of trophoblastic cells.

Since angiogenesis also involves extracellular matrix degradation, and since MMP are involved in this digestion process, it is conceivable that endometrial MMP secretion also influence (regulate?) endometrial angiogenesis. This remains to be explored.

Acknowledgments. The author wishes to thank the Swiss National Science Foundation for their generous support over the last 6 years.

References

Bhatt H, Brunet LJ, Stewart CL (1991) Uterine expression of leukemia inhibitory factor coincides with the onset of blastocyst implantation. Proc Natl Acad Sci 88:11402–11412

Bischof P, Martelli M, Campana A, Itoh Y, Ogata Y, Nagase H (1995a) Importance of metalloproteinases (MMP) in human trophoblast invasion early pregn. Biol Med 1:263–269

Bischof P, Haenggeli L, Campana A (1995b) Effect of leukemia inhibitory factor on human cytotrophoblast differentition along the invasive pathway. Am J Reprod Immunol 34:225–230

Bulmer JN, Sunderland CA (1984) Immunohistological characterisation of lymphoid cell populations in early human placental bed. Immunology 52:349–357

Bulmer JN, Lunny DP, Hagin SV (1988) Immunohistochemical characterisation of stromal leukocytes in non pregnant endometrium. Am J Reprod Immunol Microbiol 17:83–90

Cockett MI, Birch ML, Murphy G, Hart IR, Docherty AJP (1994) Metalloproteinase domain structure, cellular invasions and metastasis. Biochem Soc Transact 22:55–57

Emonard HP, Remacle AG, Noel AC, Grimaud JA, Stetler-Stevenson WG, Foidart JM (1992) Tumor cell surface-associated binding site for the M(r) 72,000 type IV collagenase. Cancer Res 52:5845–5848

Goldberg GI, Eisen AZ (1990) Regulatory mechanisms in breast cancer. In: Lipman MK, Dickso RB (eds) Regulatory mechanisms in breast cancer. Kluwer, Dordrecht, pp 421–440

Graham CH, Lala PK (1991) Mechanism of control of trophoblast invasion in situ. J Cell Physiol 148:228–234

Graham CH, Lysiak JJ, Mc Crae KR, Lala PK (1992) Localisation of transforming growth factor at the human fetal-maternal interface: role in trophoblast growth and differentiation. Biol Reprod 46:561–572

Hampton AL, Salamonsen LA (1994) Expression of messenger ribonucleic acid endoding matrix metalloproteinases and their tissue inhibitors is related to menstruation. J Endocrinol 141:R1–R3

Imada K, Ito A, Itoh Y, Nagase H, Mori Y (1994) Progesterone increases the production of tissue inhibitor of metalloproteinases-2 in rabbit uterine cervical fibroblasts. Febs Lett 341:109–112

Kariya M, Kanzaki H, Takakura K, Imai K, Okamoto N, Emi N, Kariya Y, Mori T (1991) Interleukin 1 inhibits in vitro decidualization of human endometrial stromal cells. J Clin Endocrinol Metab 73:1170–1174

King A, Loke YW (1991) On the nature and function of human uterine granular lymphocyte. Immunol Today 12:432–435

Kojima K, Kanzaki H, Iwai M, Hatayama H, Fujimoto M, Inoue T, Horie K, Nakayama H, Fujita J, Mori T (1994) Expression of leukemia inhibitory factor in human endometrium and placenta. Biol Reprod 50:882–887

Kojima K, Kanzaki H, Iwai M, Hatayama H, Fujimoto M, Narukawa S, Higuchi T, Kaneko Y, Mori T, Fujita J (1995) Expresion of leukaemia inhibitory factor (LIF) receptor in human placenta: a possible role for LIF in the growth and differentiation of trophoblasts. Mol Hum Reprod 10:1907–1911

Librach CL, Feigenbaum SL, Bass KE, Cui TY, Verastas N, Sadovsky Y, Quigley JP, French DL, Fisher SJ (1994) Interleukin-1 beta regulates human cytotrophoblast metalloproteinase activity and invasion in vitro. J Biol Chem 269:17125–17131

Marbaix E, Donnez J, Courtoy PJ, Eeckhout Y (1992) Progesterone regulates the activity of collagenase and related gelatinases A and B in human endometrial explants. Proc Natl Acad Sci USA 8:17789–11793

Martelli M, Campana A, Bischof P (1993) Secretion of matrix metalloproteinase by human endometrial cells in vitro. J Reprod Fertil 98:67–76

Matrisian L (1990) Metalloproteinases and their inhibitors in matrix remodelling. Trends Genet 6:121–125

Murphy G, Atkinson S, Ward R, Gavrilovic J, Reynolds JJ (1992) The role of plasminogen activators in the regulation of connective tissue metalloproteinases. Ann NY Acad Sci 667:1–12

Ogata Y, Enghild JJ, Nagase H (1992) Matrix metalloproteinase 3 (stromelysin) activates the precursor for human matrix metalloproteinase 9. J Biol Chem 267:3581–3584

Overall CM, Wrana JL, Sodek J (1991) Transcriptional and post transcriptional regulation of 72 kDa gelatinase type IV collagenase by transforming growth factor β1 in human fibroblasts. J Biol Chem 266:14064–14071

Polette M, Nawrocki B, Pintiaux A, Massenat C, Maquoi E, Volders L, Schaaps JP, Birembaut P, Foidart JM (1994) Expression of gelatinases A and B and their tissue inhibitors by cells of early and term human placenta and gestational endometrium. Lab Invest 71:838–846

Radestad A, Thyberg J, Christensen N (1993) Cervical ripening with mifepristone (RU 486) in first trimester abortion. An electron microscope study. Hum Reprod 8:1136–1142

Rajabi M, Solomon S, Poole AR (1990) Hormonal regulation of interstitial collagenase in the uterine cervix of pregnant guinea pig. Endocrinology 128:863–871

Rawdanowicz TJ, Hampton AL, Nagase H, Wooley DE, Salamonsen LA (1994) Matrix metalloproteinase production by cultured human endometrial stromal cells: identification of interstitial collagenase, gelatinase-A, gelatinase-B, and stromelysin-1 and their differential regulation by interleukin-1 alpha and tumor necrosis factor-alpha. J Clin Endocrinol Metab 79:530–536

Rodgers WH, Osteen KG, Matrisian LM, Navre M, Giudice L, Gorstein F (1993) Expression and localisation of matrylysin, a matrix metalloproteinase, in human endometrium during the reproductive cycle. Am J Obstet Gynecol 168:253–260

Rodgers WH, Matrisian LM, Giudice LC, Dsupin B, Cannon P, Svitek C, Gorstein F, Osteen KG (1994) The pattern of matrix metalloproteinase expres-

sion in cycling endometrium imply differential functions and regulation by
steroid hormones. J Clin Invest 94:946–953

Salamonsen LA, Nagase H, Woolley DE (1991) Production of matrix metalloproteinase 3 (stromelysin) by cultured ovine endometrial cells. J Cell Sci
100:381–385

Salamonsen LA, Nagase H, Suzuki R, Woolley DE (1993) Production of matrix metalloproteinase-1 (interstitial collagenase) and matrix metallopro-
tease-2 (gelatinase A: 72 kDa gelatinase) by ovine endometrial cells in vitro: different regulation and preferential expression by stromal fibroblasts. J
Reprod Fertil 98:583–589

Salo T, Lyons JG, Rahemtulla F, Birkedal-Hasen H, Larjava H (1991) Transforming growth factor-1 Up-regulates type IV collagenase expression in
cultured human keratinocytes. J Biol Chem 266:11436–11441

Schatz F, Papp C, Toth-Pal E, Lockwood CJ (1994) Ovarian steroid-modulated
stromelysin-1 expression in human endometrial stromal and decidual cells.
J Clin Endocrinol Metab 78:1467–1472

Shi WL, Mognetti B, Campana A, Bischof P (1995) Metalloproteinase secretion by endometrial leukocyte subsets. Am J Reprod Immunol 34:299–310

Stewart CL, Kaspar P, Brunet LJ, Bhatt H, Gadi I, Ksntgen F, Abbondanzo S
(1992) Blastocyst implantation depends on maternal expression of leukemia
inhibitory factor. Nature 359:76–79

Tabibzadeh S (1991) Human endometrium: an active site of cytokine production and action. Endocr Rev 12:272–290

Tomida M, Yamamoto-Yamaguchi Y, Hozumi, M (1984) Purification of a factor inducing differentiation of mouse myeloid leukemic M1 cells from conditioned mouse fibroblast L929 cells. J Biol Chem 259:10978–10982

Unemori EU, Ehsani N, Wang M, Lee S, McGuire J Amento EP (1994) Interleukin 1 and transforming growth factor alpha synergistic stimulation of
metalloproteinases, PGE2 and proliferation in human fibroblasts. Exp Cell
Res 210:166–171

Waterhouse P, Denhardt DT, Khokha R (1993) Temporal expression of tissue
inhibitor of metalloproteinases in mouse reproductive tissues during gestation. Mol Reprod Dev 35:219–226

7 Novel Cell Adhesion Molecules: Roles in Implantation?

C.D. MacCalman, A. Omigbodun, X.C. Tian, J.E. Fortune,
E.E. Furth, C. Coutifaris, and J.F. Strauss III

7.1 Introduction

Implantation of the embryo is a critical event in pregnancy. Peri-implantation pregnancy loss may contribute to more than 20% of unexplained infertility (American Society for Reproductive Medicine 1995). Only one in five women undergoing in vitro fertilization and embryo transfer establish a viable pregnancy. A limiting factor in the success of the assisted reproductive technologies is thought to be the ability of the blastocyst to attach to and/or invade into the endometrium. Despite the recognition that implantation is a key step in pregnancy, the basic cell biology of this process remains poorly understood.

The first step in human implantation involves the attachment of the trophoblast of the blastocyst to the surface epithelium of the endometrium (Aplin 1991; Tabibzadeh and Babknia 1995). After this initial interaction the trophoblast cells proliferate, invade the underlying stroma, and subsequently differentiate into chorionic villi which are composed of two layers: the inner cell layer which is comprised of mitotically active cytotrophoblasts and the outer syncytial trophoblast which is a terminally differentiated multinucleated cell formed by the fusion of postmitotic cytotrophoblasts. Subsequently the cytotrophoblasts at the tips of the villi acquire a highly invasive phenotype. These cells form columns which extend through the syncytial trophoblast layer and invade the decidua (Boyd and Hamilton 1967). The extravillous trophoblasts are believed to be involved in anchoring the placenta to the decidua. Furthermore, some of the extravillous trophoblasts penetrate the basal lamina of the uterine arterioles and line these vessels to form the endovascular trophoblasts, ensuring a continuous blood supply to the placenta (Loke 1990). In doing so the trophoblast cells must interact not only with one another but with the diverse populations of cells that constitute the endometrium. Thus implantation can be described as a precise series of membrane-mediated events.

The process of implantation is dependent on the trophoblast cells interacting with the endometrium during a defined period (the window of implantation; Psychoyos 1976, 1986). Outside of this receptive period the endometrium discourages implantation. Progesterone (P_4) and estradiol (E_2) play a central role in preparing the endometrium for implantation (Psychoyos 1976, 1986). In the postovulatory phase, under the influence of P_4, glandular secretion and stromal decidualization become the dominant features of the endometrium.

The decidualization of the endometrium involves the differentiation of the stromal cells, which acquire distinct morphological and functional features (Noyes et al. 1950). Morphological decidualization is associated with an increase in cell size and shape, development of the organelles involved in protein synthesis (rough endoplasmic reticulum) and secretion (Golgi apparatus), and the formation of gap junctions and desmosomes (Wynn 1974). Decidual cells are believed to anchor trophoblast cells and consequently arrest their invasive migration (Pijenborg et al. 1980; Flamigni et al. 1991). The depth of trophoblast invasion is precisely controlled and errors have extreme consequences on the health of the mother and fetus (Buster and Carson 1995). For example, shallow invasion is associated with significant maternal and fetal morbidity and mortality. In contrast, the absence of decidua allows trophoblasts to invade deep into the underlying tissue as is the case in ectopic pregnancy.

Cytotrophoblast invasion encompasses dynamic changes in cell-cell and cell-matrix interactions (reviewed by Tabibzadeh and Babaknia 1995). Cytotrophoblasts detach from the tips of the anchoring villi and interact with the cells of the maternal decidua and vasculature. During invasion the matrix is remodeled by trophoblasts and the repertoire of cell surface receptors for matrix components expressed on the surface of the trophoblasts changes in concert with the invasion process. Most of the recent trophoblast invasion studies have focused on the role of proteinases in matrix degradation and the ability of the family of cell-substrate adhesion molecules, known as the integrins, to mediate trophoblast-matrix interactions. The adhesive mechanisms involved in mediating cell-cell interactions in trophoblast invasion and trophoblast-endometrial cell interactions have been relatively neglected. As a first step in identifying the adhesion molecules involved in mediating the complex cellular interactions, we have focused our studies on the family of calcium-dependent cell adhesion molecules, known as the cadherins.

7.2 The Cadherins

The cadherins are members of a gene superfamily of integral membrane glycoproteins that mediate calcium-dependent cell adhesion (Takeichi 1991). Recent studies using the polymerase chain reaction (PCR) have identified a number of new members of this supergene family (Suzuki et al. 1990; Tanihara et al. 1994; Hoffmann and Balling 1995). Cloning studies have revealed that some of these cadherin subtypes have unique structural features indicating that the cadherins are composed of two evolutionary distinct subfamilies: type 1 cadherins (also known as classical cadherins) and type 2 cadherins (Suzuki et al. 1990; Tanihara et al. 1994; Takeichi 1995).

The subfamily of classical cadherins, which includes the three originally described cadherins, E-cadherin (E-cad), N-cadherin (N-cad), and P-cadherin (P-cad; Suzuki et al. 1990; Tanihara et al. 1994; Takeichi 1995) mediate cell adhesion through homotypic interactions (Takeichi 1991, 1995). The classical cadherins are composed of five extracellular domains, a single transmembrane domain, and two cytoplasmic domains (Ozawa et al. 1990; Magee and Buxton 1991). Each of the first four extracellular domains contain the putative calcium binding regions. In addition, the first extracellular domain of each classical cadherin harbors the cell adhesion recognition (CAR) sequence HAV (Blaschuk et al. 1990; Overduin et al. 1995). The nonconserved amino acid residues immediately adjacent to the HAV site modulate the ability of cadherins to interact with one another in a homotypic manner (Nose et al. 1990; Overduin et al. 1995).

The cytoplasmic domains are the most highly conserved regions of the classical cadherins (Kemler 1993). These domains are associated with three intracellular proteins known as α-, β-, and γ-catenin (K.R. Johnson et al. 1993; Piepenhagen and Nelson 1993). The catenins are thought to mediate the interaction between the classical cadherins and the microfilaments of the cytoskeleton. The classical cadherins cannot promote cell adhesion unless they are complexed with catenins (Kintner 1992; Kemler 1993).

The cadherins are key morphoregulators (Takeichi 1991). The spatiotemporal expression of the classical cadherins is tightly regulated during development. Embryonic cells displaying different classical cadherins segregate from one another. Thus it is believed that these cell adhesion molecules provide the molecular basis for the segregation of populations of cells and the subsequent formation of tissues during development.

In the adult the classical cadherins have been localized to the membrane domains of adherens junctions and are believed to maintain the differentiated state of the cell (Geiger and Ayalon 1992; Grunwald 1993). For example, the loss of E-cad expression has been found to be correlated with the neoplastic transformation of epithelial cells in vivo and in vitro (Birchmeier et al. 1991; Behrens 1993).

Type 2 cadherins, like the classical cadherins are comprised of five extracellular domains, a transmembrane domain, and two cytoplasmic domains (Suzuki et al. 1990; Tanihara et al. 1994; Hoffmann and Balling 1995). Similar to classical cadherins, the first four extracellular domains of the type 2 cadherins contain the conserved putative calcium-binding sites. These cadherin subtypes also contain the highly conserved cytoplasmic domains specific for most cadherins. However, type 2 cadherins show low overall amino acid homology with the classical cadherins and share common sequence features, such as characteristic amino acid deletions or additions and distinctive amino acid substitutions at various sites which are not found in classical cadherins. In particular, type 2 cadherins do not contain the cadherin specific CAR sequence. Although the CAR sequence of type 2 cadherins has not been determined, recent studies indicate that type 2 cadherins are capable of mediating cell adhesion in a homotypic manner (Okazaki et al. 1994; Kimura et al. 1995). It has not been determined whether type 2 cadherin function is dependent on an interaction between the conserved cytoplasmic domains and the catenins.

The function of the type 2 cadherins has not yet been determined. However, there is increasing evidence to suggest that this subfamily of cadherins plays a key role in development. Recent studies indicate that the type 2 cadherin, known as cadherin-11 (cad-11) is spatiotemporally expressed during rat and mouse embryogenesis (Hoffmann and Balling 1995; Kimura et al. 1995; Simmoneau et al. 1995). Cad-11 has been localized to mesenchymal tissues and specific regions of the neural tube. Similar to the classical cadherins, the expression of cad-11 appears to be associated with various morphogenetic events, such as somitogenesis. Further evidence to support the hypothesis that cad-11 is a key morphoregulator is that cad-11 expression is complementary to the expression pattern of both E- and N-cad (Kimura et al. 1995).

7.3 Cadherins Present in the Female Reproductive Tract

In view of the central role that cadherins play in embryonic development and in maintaining the integrity of tissues in the adult, it is likely that members of this supergene family are involved in mediating the cyclic remodeling processes that occur in the endometrium in preparation for embryo implantation. E-cad and P-cad have been localized to the surface and glandular epithelium of the human endometrium at all stages of the menstrual cycle (Van der Linden et al. 1994; Tabibzadeh et al. 1995). E-cad and P-cad have also been detected in endometrial tissue found in menstrual effluent and in endometriosis (Van der Linden et al. 1995). However, the cadherin subtype(s) present in the stroma or the decidua of the human endometrium have not been identified.

The constitutive expression of both E-cad and P-cad in the epithelial cell layers of the human endometrium during the menstrual cycle suggests that these cell adhesion molecules do not define the putative window of implantation and are therefore not likely to play a central role in implantation in the human. Further evidence that E-cad and P-cad do not mediate human trophoblast-endometrial cell interactions has been provided by studies examining the cadherin subtypes present in trophoblast cells. E-cad has been localized to the villous cytotrophoblasts but not the highly invasive extravillous cytotrophoblast cells or the differentiated syncytial trophoblast of the human placenta (Coutifaris et al. 1991; Campbell et al. 1995). As the extravillous cytotrophoblasts and syncytial trophoblasts form intimate interactions with both the epithelial and stromal cells of the endometrium, it seems unlikely that E-cad is involved in trophoblast-endometrial cell interactions. Furthermore, P-cad which is involved in trophoblast-endometrium interactions in the mouse (Kadokawa et al. 1989), has not been detected in human trophoblast cells (Shimoyama et al. 1989). One conclusion emerging from the evaluation of these observations is that other, yet unidentified, cadherin subtypes are present in the human endometrium and placenta, and that these cell adhesion molecules are likely to be involved in mediating trophoblast-endometrium interactions in the human. In view of these observations, we have undertaken a comprehensive survey of the cadherin subtypes expressed in the endometrium, trophoblast , and ovary.

7.4 Materials and Methods

7.4.1 Cell Preparation and Culture

Trophoblast Cells. The b30 clone of BeWo cells (a gift from Dr. A.I. Schwartz, Washington University, St. Louis, Mo.) were maintained in Dulbecco's modified Eagle's medium containing 25 mM glucose, 25 mM HEPES and 50 μg/ml gentamicin and supplemented with 10% heat-inactivated fetal calf serum. Cells were harvested after 0 or 72 h of culture in the presence or absence of 8-bromo-cAMP (1.5 mM).

Stroma Cells. Human stroma cells were isolated from the endometrium of hysterectomy specimens from premenopausal women, using methods modified from Satyaswaroop et al. (1979). Briefly, the endometrium was minced and subjected to collagenase digestion (0.25%). The stromal cells were isolated from the epithelial cells by passing the supernatant through a sieve (38 μm). Isolated glands were retained on the sieve and the stroma cells, which passed through the sieve, were collected in a 15-ml tube. The stroma cells were further purified by layering the supernatant on a Ficoll-Paque gradient and centrifuging the columns at 400 g for 10 min.

Granulosa Cells. Human granulosa cells obtained from patients undergoing in vitro fertilization and embryo transfer were isolated and cultured as described by Golos and Strauss (1987). The cells were isolated from follicles prepared by stimulation with purified urinary follicle-stimulating hormone 34 h after injection of 5000 IU chorionic gonadotropin.

Corpora Lutea. Luteolysis was induced in 20 regularly cycling Holstein heifers from the research heard at Cornell University by a single injection of prostaglandin (PG) F$_{2\alpha}$ (25 mg Lytalyse, i.m.; Upjohn, Kalamazoo, Mich.) on the evening of day 6 or the morning of day 7 (day 0=onset of estrus). The animals were assigned at random to be ovariectomized at 0 (n=6), 2 (n=4), 12 (n=4), or 24 (n=6) h after PGF$_{2\alpha}$ treatment. Ovariectomy was performed per vaginum under local anesthesia (2% procaine, epidural). The ovarian pedicle was clamped and cut with an écraseur; the écraseur was left in place for an additional 10 min to prevent bleeding from the pedicle. Within 15 min of surgery ovaries were transported to the laboratory in ice-cold Eagle's minimum essential medium containing 25 mM HEPES buffer (GIBCO, Grand Island, N.Y.). Luteal tissue was dissected from the ovaries, trimmed of all visible connective tissue surrounding the corpus luteum, and cut into 5- to 7-mm cubes.

7.4.2 RNA Preparation

Total RNA was prepared by the phenol-chloroform method of Chomczynski and Sacchi (1987).

7.4.3 Reverse Transcriptase PCR and DNA Sequence Analysis

Reverse transcriptase (RT) PCR was performed using the method described by Suzuki et al. (1990). Degenerate oligonucleotides encoding amino acid sequences that are conserved among all of the known cadherins (forward primer 5'-GATTCACNGCNCCNCCNTAYGA-3', reverse primer 5'-GATTCTCNGCNARYTTYTTAAR-3'; where R is either A or G, Y is either C or T, and N is either A, C, G, or T) were used as primers in the RT-PCR (Suzuki et al. 1990; Tanihara et al. 1994). Template cDNAs were synthesized from total RNA extracted from either BeWo cells, a choriocarcinoma cell line which undergoes terminal differentiation in the presence of cAMP, or isolated populations of endometrial stroma cells, ovarian theca cells, or granulosa cells.

The resultant RT-PCR products, 160 bp in size, were subcloned into the PCR II vector by a blunt-end ligation for subsequent DNA sequence analysis using an automated DNA sequencer (Applied Biosystems) employing the Taq DyeDeoxy sequencing reagents.

A pair of oligonucleotides encoding amino acid sequences that are specific to cad-11 (forward primer 5'-CTCCTCCGTAT-TACTCCATTCAA -3', reverse primer 5'-ATTTGCTCCAGGTGTC-AAGACAT-3') were used as RT-PCR primers. The cycling program used for this set of primers consisted of denaturation at 95°C for 1 min, annealing at 65°C for 1.5 min, and polymerization at 72°C for 3 min. The cycling programs were repeated 35 times.

7.4.4 Northern Blot Analysis

The RNA species were resolved by electrophoresis in 1% agarose gels containing 3.7% formaldehyde. Approximately 20 mg total RNA was loaded per lane. The fractionated RNA species were then transferred onto charged nylon membranes.

The northern blots were probed with either human cad-11, cadherin-6 (cad-6), or N-cad cDNA probes according to the methods of MacCalman and Blaschuk (1994). The blots were then washed twice with 2X SSPE at room temperature, twice with 2X SSPE containing 1% SDS at 55°C and twice with 0.2X SSPE at room temperature. To standardize the amounts of total RNA in each lane the blots were then reprobed with a radiolabeled synthetic oligonucleotide specific for 18S rRNA according to the protocols described by MacCalman et al. (1992). The blots were again subjected to radioautography to detect the hybridization of the radiolabeled probe to the 18S rRNA.

7.4.5 Immunohistochemistry

Immunohistochemistry was performed using a mouse monoclonal antibody directed against human cad-11, previously described by MacCalman et al. (1996). Sequential incubations were performed according to the method of Cartun and Pedersen (1989), and included 10% normal horse serum for 30 min, primary antiserum at 37°C for 1 h, secondary biotinylated antibody at 37°C for 45 min, streptavidin-biotinylated horseradish peroxidase complex reagent at 37°C for 30 min, and three 5-min washes in PBS. The slides were then exposed to chromagen reaction solution (0.035% diaminobenzidine and 0.03% H_2O_2) for 10 min, washed in tap water for 5 min, counterstained in hematoxylin, dehydrated, cleared, and mounted.

Table 1. Analysis of the cadherin subtypes present in BeWo cells cultured in the presence or absence of 8-bromo cAMP

Time in culture (h)	cAMP	No. of clones analyzed	Cadherin subtype	% of clones analyzed
0	–	10	E-cadherin	100
	+	10	E-cadherin	100
72	–	10	E-cadherin	100
	+	10	E-cadherin	10
			Cadherin-11	90

7.5 Results and Discussion

7.5.1 Identification of the Cadherin Subtypes Present in Human Trophoblast Cells

RT-PCR was performed using RNA prepared from BeWo cells which had been cultured in the presence or absence of cAMP for 0 or 72 h. DNA sequence analysis of the RT-PCR products identified two major cadherin subtypes: E-cad and cad-11 (Table 1). E-cad was found to be the major cadherin subtype present in the undifferentiated trophoblast cells. In contrast, cad-11 expression was detected only in BeWo cells which had undergone cAMP-induced differentiation. Taken together, these observations suggest that cad-11 and E-cad are coordinately regulated during trophoblast differentiation in vitro. E-cad, which mediates cytotrophoblast-cytotrophoblast interactions, is downregulated as the mononuclear trophoblast cells differentiate and fuse to form syncytium. In contrast, cad-11 mRNA levels increase as the trophoblast cells undergo terminal cellular differentiation (MacCalman et al. 1996).

Cad-11 was further localized to the placenta extravillous cytotrophoblasts and syncytial trophoblast using immunohistochemistry

---

Fig. 1A–C. Immunolocalization of Cad-11 in the human placenta and endometrium. Immunostaining was observed in the syncytial and extravillous cytotrophoblasts of the human placenta (**A**), the glandular epithelium of the endometrium during the proliferative phase (**B**) and the decidual stroma of early pregnancy (**C**)

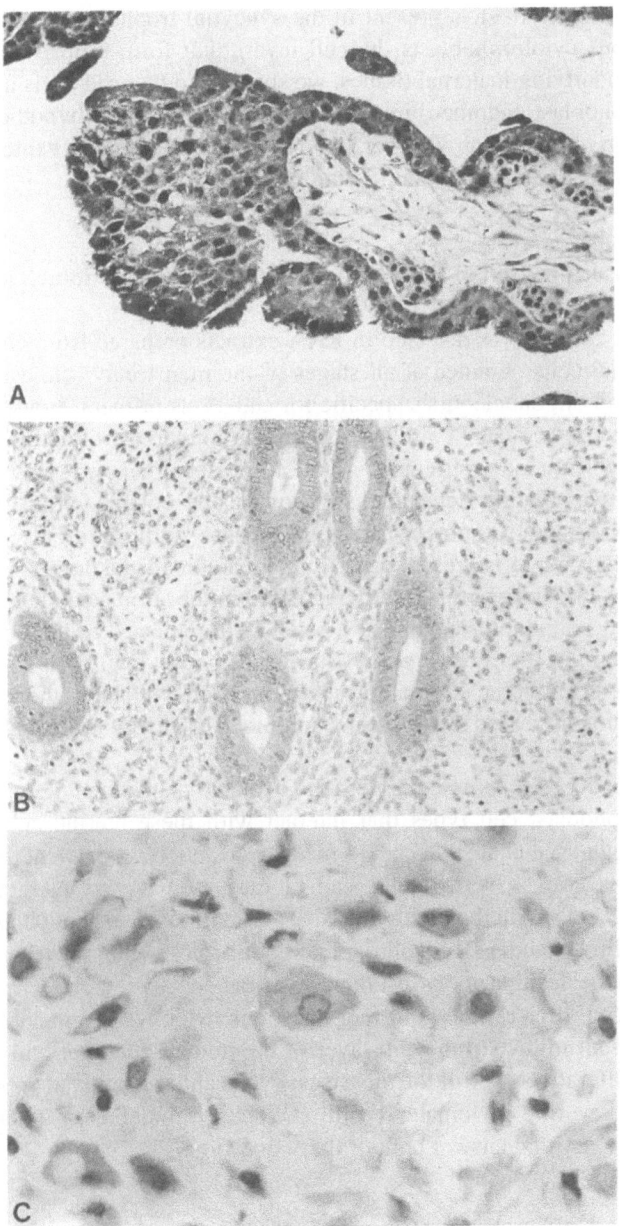

Fig. 1. Legend see p. 146

(Fig. 1). As cad-11 is present in the syncytial trophoblast and the extravillous cytotrophoblasts the cell layers that form intimate contacts with underlying maternal tissues, we speculated that cad-11 is involved in trophoblast-endometrium interactions. To test this hypothesis we went on to determine whether cad-11 is spatiotemporally expressed in the human endometrium during the menstrual cycle.

7.5.2 Localization of Cadherin-11 in the Human Endometrium

Cad-11 mRNA was detected in RNA extracts prepared from glandular epithelial cells obtained at all stages of the menstrual cycle using RT-PCR and oligonucleotides specific for cad-11 as primers. However, we failed to detect cad-11 mRNA in extracts prepared from stroma cells obtained from the proliferative stage of the menstrual cycle. In contrast, cad-11 was readily detectable in stroma cells obtained from the late secretory stage of the menstrual cycle. These studies not only demonstrate that cad-11 is present in the human endometrium but also suggest that cad-11 expression is tightly regulated in the stroma cell layer.

Using immunohistochemistry, cad-11 was detected in the glandular epithelium of the endometrium (Fig. 1). Although low levels of cad-11 were detected in the stroma during the proliferative phase, the levels of expression increased as the stroma continued to undergo decidualization (Fig. 1).

As cad-11 is expressed in both the decidual cells of the uterus and in the trophoblast cell types that interact with these uterine cells, it is tempting to speculate that cad-11 mediates trophoblast cell–endometrial cell interactions. In particular, cad-11 may mediate the interaction of decidual cells with the highly invasive extravillous cytotrophoblasts in a homophilic manner. This cellular interaction may anchor the trophoblast cells to the decidua and arrest their invasion.

These results raise two further questions: which cadherin subtype(s) are present in the stroma cell layer of the human endometrium during the proliferative stage of the menstrual cycle, and, secondly, does cad-11 play a key role in female fertility? We have undertaken a series of studies to try and answer both of these questions.

Table 2. Analysis of the cadherin subtypes present in endometrial stroma cells during the proliferative stage of the menstrual cycle

Stage	No. of clones analyzed	Cadherin subtype	% of clones analyzed
Proliferative	12	Cadherin-6	80
		Cadherin-4	10
		E-cadherin	10

7.5.3 Identification of the Cadherin Subtypes Present in Stromal Cells of the Endometrium

RT-PCR was performed using RNA extracted from stroma cells obtained from the proliferative stage of the menstrual cycle and the degenerate oligonucleotides corresponding to the conserved cytoplasmic domain of the cadherins as primers.

DNA sequence analysis of the resultant PCR products suggest that three cadherin subtypes are present in the stroma cell layer during the proliferative stage of the menstrual cycle (Table 2).

Cad-6 appears to be the predominant cadherin subtype present in stroma cells. Previous studies had failed to detect E-cad in the endometrial stroma (Van der Linden et al. 1994; Tabibzadeh et al. 1995) using immunohistochemistry. Although we detected E-cad in isolated stroma cells using RT-PCR, we cannot determine whether the E-cad mRNA is present in the stroma cells or in the small number of glandular epithelial cells present in these cell preparations. In addition, the cadherin subtypes present in the stroma appear to be tightly regulated. Cad-11 was not detected in stroma cells isolated during the proliferative phase but was readily detectable in cells isolated from the secretory phase.

Table 3. Analysis of the cadherin subtypes present in isolated human granulosa cells

Time in culture	No. of clones analyzed	Cadherin subtype	% of clones analyzed
0	10	N-cadherin	80
		Cadherin-6	20
		Cadherin-11	0
72	10	Cadherin-11	80
		N-cadherin	20
		Cadherin-6	0

7.5.4 Cadherin Subtypes Present in the Ovary

To determine whether cad-11 is expressed in other reproductive tract tissues that undergo cyclic differentiation we examined the ovary.

RT-PCR was performed using RNA extracted from freshly isolated human granulosa cells or granulosa cells that were allowed to undergo spontaneous luteinization in culture and the degenerate oligonucleotides corresponding to the conserved cytoplasmic domain of cadherins as primers. DNA sequence analysis of the resultant PCR products demonstrated that N-cad and cad-6 are the two major cadherin subtypes present in freshly isolated granulosa cells (Table 3). We failed to detect cad-11 in extracts prepared from freshly isolated granulosa cells. In contrast, cad-11 and N-cad but not cad-6 were detected in luteinized granulosa cells.

In order to determine the expression pattern of these three cadherin subtypes in human granulosa cells we performed northern blot analysis using RNA extracted from freshly isolated and luteinized granulosa cells and the PCR products as probes. Northern blot analysis demonstrated that cad-11 was not present in freshly isolated granulosa cells but was readily detectable in cells which had undergone luteinization (Fig. 2). In contrast, the mRNA levels of N-cad and cad-6 mRNA transcripts were high in freshly isolated granulosa cells and declined as the cells underwent luteinization.

These studies demonstrate that the cadherin subtypes expressed by human granulosa cells are tightly regulated and also suggest that cad-11 may be involved in the formation and organization of the corpus luteum.

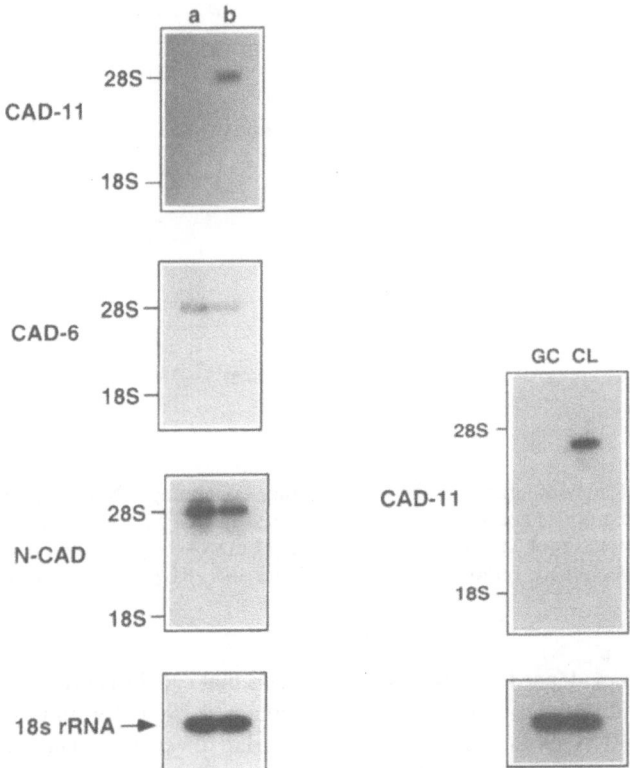

Fig. 2 *(left).* Radioautograms of a northern blot containing RNA extracted from isolated human granulosa cells cultured for 0 h *(lane A)* or 72 h *(lane B).* The blot was probed with radiolabeled cad-11, cad-6, or N-cad, and a radiolabeled synthetic oligonucleotide specific for 18S rRNA

Fig. 3 *(right).* Radioautograms of a northern blot containing RNA extracted from isolated bovine granulosa cells *(GC)* or corpus luteum *(CL).* The blot was probed with radiolabeled cad-11 cDNA, and a radiolabeled synthetic oligonucleotide specific for 18S rRNA

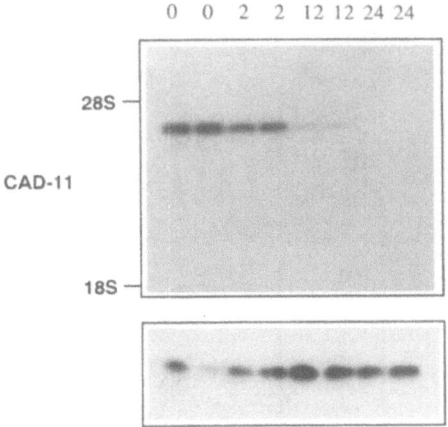

Fig. 4. Radioautograms of the northern blot containing RNA extracted from bovine corpora lutea which had been exposed to PGF$_{2\alpha}$ for 0, 2, 12, or 24 h. The blot was probed with radiolabeled cad-11 cDNA *(upper panel)* and a radiolabeled synthetic oligonucleotide specific for 18S rRNA *(lower panel)*

Further evidence to support the hypothesis that cad-11 is involved in the formation of the corpus luteum was obtained by performing RT-PCR using RNA extracted from human ovarian theca cells and oligonucleotides specific for cad-11 as primers. Cad-11 mRNA transcripts were readily detectable in theca cells. As both theca cells and luteinized granulosa cells are present in the corpus luteum (Bloom and Fawcett 1978; Kamat et al. 1995), it is tempting to speculate that cad-11 mediates the interactions between these two cell types and thus plays a central role in the formation of the corpus luteum.

Cad-11 mRNA was readily detectable in total RNA extracts prepared from bovine corpora lutea but not granulosa cells isolated from preovulatory follicles, using northern blot analysis (Fig. 3). The levels of cad-11 mRNA declined as the corpora lutea underwent luetislysis induced by prostaglandin F$_{2\alpha}$ (Fig. 4). The levels of cad-11 mRNA transcripts in bovine corpora lutea were reduced after being exposed to PGF$_{2\alpha}$ for 2 h and after, 48 h, were not detected. These findings suggest a correlation between cad-11 expression and the functional status of the corpus luteum. The formation and organization of the corpus luteum also has a direct effect on endometrial function and early implantation.

The corpus luteum acts as the major source of P_4 in early pregnancy (Csapo and Pulkkinen 1978; M.R. Johnson et al. 1993). This steroid hormone has been shown to act directly on the stroma cells of the endometrium and is believed to be a key regulator of decidualization (Bourgain et al. 1994). Failure to establish a functional corpus luteum leads to endometrial dysfunction and implantation loss (Bourgain et al. 1994).

7.6 Summary and Future Directions

It is tempting to propose that cad-11 regulates endometrial function and implantation at two distinct levels. Firstly, if cad-11 plays a central role in the formation of the corpus luteum, failure to upregulate cad-11 expression in granulosa cells during luteinization would result in the formation of a dysfunctional corpus luteum. This in turn would have a direct effect on endometrial function and implantation. Secondly, cad-11 may mediate trophoblast–decidual cell interactions. Cad-11 expression may be necessary to anchor the invading trophoblast cells to the decidua and consequently regulate trophoblast invasion in the endometrium.

Our studies suggest that the type 2 cadherin, known as cad-11, may play a central role in maintaining fertility. We have examined cad-11 mRNA levels in the human placenta, endometrium, and ovary. In all three tissues the expression of this cell adhesion molecule appears to be tightly regulated. Furthermore, the expression of cad-11 is correlated with cellular differentiation; in the placenta cad-11 expression increases as trophoblast cells undergo terminal differentiation and fusion, in the uterus cad-11 levels increase as the stroma cells undergo decidualization in preparation for the implanting embryo, and in the ovary cad-11 expression in granulosa cells is upregulated as the granulosa cells undergo luteinization in the postovulatory phase. The spatiotemporal expression pattern of cad-11 suggests that this cell adhesion molecule may mediate trophoblast–endometrial cell interactions and may play a central role in the formation of the corpus luteum.

154   C.D. MacCalman et al.

References

American Society for Reproductive Medicine (1995) Assisted reproductive techniques in the United States and Canada: 1993 results generated from the American Society for Reproductive Medicine/Society for Assisted Reproductive Technology Registry. Fertil Steril 64:13–21

Aplin JD (1991) Implantation, trophoblast differentiation and haemochorial placentation: mechanistic evidence in vivo and in vitro. J Cell Sci 99:681–692

Behrens J (1993) The role of cell adhesion molecules in cancer invasion and metastasis. Breast Cancer Res Treat 24:175–184

Birchmeier W, Behrens J, Weidner KM, Frixen UH, Schipper, J (1991) Dominant and recessive genes involved in tumor cell invasion. Curr Opin Cell Biol 3:832–840

Blaschuk OW, Pouliot Y, Holland PC (1990) Identification of a conserved region common to cadherins and influenza strain A hemagglutinins. J Mol Biol 211:679–681

Bloom W, Fawcett D (1975) A textbook of histology. Saunders, Philadelphia, p 855

Bourgain C, Smitz J, Camus M, Erard P, Devroey P, Van Steirteghem AC, Kloppel G (1994) Human endometrial maturation is markedly improved after luteal supplementation of gonadotropin releasing hormone analogue/human menopausal gonadotropin stimulated cycles. Hum Reprod 9:32–40

Boyd JD, Hamilton WJ (1967) Development and structure of the human placenta from the end of the 3rd month of gestation. J Obstet Gynaecol Br Commonw 74:161–226

Buster JE, Carson SA (1995) Ectopic pregnancy-new advances in diagnosis and treatment. Curr Opin Obstet Gynecol 3:168–175

Campbell S, Swann HR, Seif MW, Kimber SJ, Aplin J. (1995) Cell adhesion molecules on the oocyte and perimplantation human embryo. Mol Hum Reprod 1:1571–1578

Cartun RW, Pedersen CA. (1989) An immunocytochemical technique offering increased sensitivity and lowered cost with streptavidin-horseradish peroxidase conjugate. J Histotechnol 12:273–280

Chomczynski P, Sacchi N (1987) Single-step method of RNA isolation by acid guanidine thiocyanate-phenol chloroform extraction. Anal Biochem 162:156–159

Coutifaris C, Kao LC, Sehdev HM, Chin U, Babalola GO, Blaschuk OW, Strauss JF III (1991) E-cadherin expression during the differentiation of human trophoblasts. Development 113:767–777

Csapo AI, Pulkkinen M (1978) Indispensibility of the human corpus luteum in the maintenance of early pregnancy. Obstet Gynecol Surv 33:69–81

Flamigni C, Bulleti C, Polli V, Ciotti PM, Prefetto RA, Galassi A, Di Cosmo E (1991) Factors regulating interaction between trophoblast and human endometrium. Ann NY Acad Sci 662:176–190

Geiger B, Ayalon O (1992) Cadherins. Annu Rev Cell Biol 8:307–322

Golos TG, Strauss JF III (1987) Regulation of low density lipoprotein receptor gene expression in cultured human granulosa cells: roles of human chorionic gonadotropin, 8-bromo-3',5'-cyclic adenosine monophosphate, and protein synthesis. Mol Endocrinol 1:321–326

Grunwald GB (1993) The structural and functional analysis of cadherin calcium-dependent cell adhesion molecules. Curr Opin Cell Biol 5:797–805

Hoffmann I, Balling R (1995) Cloning and expression of a novel mesodermally expressed cadherin. Dev Biol 169:337–346

Johnson KR, Lewis JE, Li D, Wahl J, Soler AP, Knudsen KA, Wheelock MJ (1993) P- and E- cadherin are in separate complexes in cells expressing both cadherins. Exp Cell Res 207:252–260

Johnson MR, Riddle AF, Grudzinskas JG, Sharma V, Campbell S, Collins WP, Lightman SL, Mason B, Nicolaides KH (1993) Endocrinology of IVF pregnancies during the first trimester. Hum Reprod 8:316–325

Kadokawa Y, Fuketa I, Nose A, Takeichi M, Nakatsuji N (1989) Expression pattern of E- and P-cadherin in mouse embryos during the periimplantation period. Dev Growth Differ 31:23–30

Kamat BR, Bronn LF, Manseau EJ, Senger DR, Dvorak HF (1995) Expression of vascular permeability factor/vascular endothelial growth factor by human granulosa and theca lutein cells. Role in corpus luteum development. Am J Pathol 146:157–165

Kemler R (1993) From cadherins to catenins: cytoplasmic protein interactions and regulation of cell adhesion. Trends Genet 9:317–321

Kimura Y, Matsunami H, Inoue T, Shimamura K, Uchida N, Ueno T, Miyazaki T, Takeichi M (1995). Cadherin-11 expressed in association with mesenchymal morphogenesis in the head, somite, and limb bud of early mouse embryos. Dev Biol 169:347–358

Kintner C (1992) Regulation of embryonic cell adhesion by the cadherin cytoplasmic domain. Cell 69:225–236

Loke YW (1990) Experimenting with human extravillous trophoblast: a personal view. Am J Reprod Immunol 24:22–28

MacCalman CD, Blaschuk OW (1994) Gonadal steroids regulate N-cadherin mRNA levels in the mouse testis. Endocrine 2:157–163

MacCalman CD, Bardeesy N, Holland PC, Blaschuk OW (1992) Noncoordinate developmental regulation of N-cadherin, N-CAM, integrin and fibronectin mRNA levels during myoblast terminal differentiation. Dev Dynam 195:127–132

MacCalman CD, Bronner M, Omigbodun A, Coutifaris C, Strauss JF III (1995) Identification of the cadherin subtypes present in the human placenta. Soc Gynecol Invest (abstract)

MacCalman CD, Omigbodun A, Furth EE, Bronner M, Coutifaris C, Strauss JF III (1996) Regulated expression of cadherin-11 in human epithelial cells: a role for cadherin-11 in trophoblast endometrium interactions. Dev Dynam 206:201–211

Magee AI, Buxton RS (1991) Transmembrane molecular assemblies regulated by the greater cadherin family. Curr Opin Cell Biol 3:854–861

Nose A, Tsuji K, Takeichi M (1990) Localization of specificity determining sites in cadherin cell adhesion molecules. Cell 61:147–155

Noyes RW, Hertig AT, Rock J (1950) Dating the endometrial biopsy. Fertil Steril 1:3–25

Okazaki M, Takeshita S, Kawai S, Kikuno R, Tsujimara A, Kudo A, Amman E (1994) Molecular cloning and characterization of OB-cadherin, a new memeber of the cadherin family expressed in osteoblasts. J Biol Chem 269:12092–12098

Overduin M, Harvey TS, Bagby S, Tong KI, Yau P, Takeichi M, Ikura M (1995) Solution structure of the epithelial cadherin domain responsible for selective cell adhesion. Science 267:386–389

Ozawa M, Ringwald M, Kemeler R (1990) Uvomorulin-catenin complex formation is regulated by a specific domain in the cytoplasmic region of the cell adhesion molecule. Proc Natl Acad Sci USA 87:4226–4250

Piepenhagen PA, Nelson WJ (1993) Defining E-cadherin-associated protein complexes in epithelial cells: plakoglobin, β- and γ- catenin are distinct componenets. J Cell Sci 104:751–762

Pijenborg F, Dixon G, Robertson WB, Brosens I (1980) Trophoblastic invasion of the human decidua from 8–18 weeks of pregnancy. Placenta 1:3–19

Psychoyos A (1976) Hormonal control of uterine receptivity for nidation. J Reprod Fertil 25 [Suppl]:17–28

Psychoyos A (1986) Uterine receptivity of nidation. Ann NY Acad Sci 476:36–42

Satyaswaroop PG, Bressler RS, De La Pena, MM, Gurpide E (1979) Isolation and culture of human endometrial glands. J Clin Endocrinol Metab 48:639–641

Shimoyama Y, Yoshida T, Terada M, Shimatsato Y, Aba O, Hirohashi S (1989) Molecular cloning of the human Ca2+-dependent cell-cell adhesion molecule homologous to mouse placental cadherin: its low expression in human placental tissues. J Cell Biol 109:1787–1794

Simmoneau L, Kitagawa M, Suzuki S, Thiery JP (1995). Cadherin-11 expression marks the mesenchymal phenotype-towards new functions for cadherins. Cell Adhes Commun 3:115–130

Suzuki S, Sano K, Tanihara H (1990) Diversity of the cadherin family: evidence for eight new cadherins in nervous tissue. Cell Regul 2:261–270

Tabibzadeh S, Babaknia A (1995) Signals and molecular pathways involved in implantation, a symbiotic interaction between blastocyst and endometrium involving adhesion and tissue invasion. Mol Human Reprod 1:1579–1602

Tabibzadeh S, Babknia A, Kong QF, Kapur S, Zupi E, Marconi D, Romanini C, Satyaswaroop PG (1995) Menstruation is associated with disordered expression of desmoplakin I/II and cadherin catenins and conversion of F-actin to G-actin in endometrial epithelium. Hum Reprod 10:776–784

Takeichi M (1991) Cadherin cell adhesion receptors as morphogenetic regulators. Science 251:1451–1455

Takeichi M (1995) Morphogenetic roles of classical cadherins. Curr Opin Cell Biol 7:619–627

Tanihara H, Sano K, Heimark R, St John TS, Suzuki S (1994) Cloning of five human cadherins clarifies characteristic features of cadherin extracellular domain and provides further evidence for two structurally different types of cadherins. Cell Adhes Commun 2:15–26

Van der Linden PJQ, de Goeij AFPM, Dunselman GAJ, Arends JW, Evers JLH (1994) P-cadherin expression in human endometrium and endometriosis. Gynecol Obstet Invest 38:183–185

Van der Linden PJQ, de Goeij AFPM, Dunselman GAJ (1995) Expression of cadherins and integrins in human endometrium throughout the menstrual cycle. Fertil Steril 62:1210–1216

Wynn RM (1974) Ultrastructural development of the human decidua. Am J Obstet Gynecol 118:652–670

8 The Glycoprotein MUC1 and Extracellular Matrix Molecules as Markers of Endometrial Differentiation

J.D. Aplin

8.1 Endometrial Epithelium

8.1.1 Glycoprotein Biosynthesis and Secretion

Remarkable alterations occur in the ultrastructure of epithelial cells in the human endometrium during the period from ovulation to implantation (Warren et al. 1994). This applies to both glandular and luminal cell compartments, but the changes are more pronounced in the former. At the time of ovulation the cytoplasm contains free and bound ribosomes, mitochondria and golgi apparatus. The distribution of organelles is not obviously polarised. Proliferation is evident in the epithelial population. By 3 days after the luteinising hormone peak (day LH+3) the fraction of proliferating cells has dropped sharply, and very significant differentiative changes are already apparent, though their extent is at this stage somewhat variable within the cell population. Morphological changes include the appearance of glycogen deposits in the basal cytoplasm, of giant mitochondria enveloped in rough or semi-rough endoplasmic reticulum and of increasingly abundant golgi apparatus in the apical cytoplasm. Stacks of golgi cisternae are visible lying parallel to the apical cell surface; these then expand and reorient parallel to the lateral cell border. By day LH+6 they have become dilated. The apical cytoplasm is now rich in secretory vesicles. Both cilated and microvillous cells are present, and both show secretory capacity (Campbell et al. 1988). The gland lumens increase in diameter and secretory material appears in amounts that increase to day LH+6 and remain high for several days thereafter (Noyes et al. 1950; Li et al. 1988a). Embryo transfer data suggest implantation occurs approximately in the period between days LH+7 and 11 (Bergh and Navot 1992).

Glycoproteins are abundant in this secretory pathway. Staining of endometrium with lectins indicates that a variety of different glycan structures are abundant in the epithelial cells and their apical secretions. Many of the glycans that have been studied are present in both the proliferative and secretory phase epithelium, but with a trend to increasing abundance and release from the cells in the secretory phase (Aplin 1991; Jones, Stoddart and Aplin, unpublished). However, there are several glycan structures recognised by lectins or monoclonal antibodies that have more specificity for the secretory phase epithelium. These include blood group A-related structures (terminal α-linked N-acetyl galactosamine) recognised by the lectin from dolichus biflorus (DBA; Aplin 1991) or monoclonal antibodies (Kliman et al. 1995), the sialyl Tn structure recognised by monoclonal antibody B72.3 (Thor et al. 1987; Soisson et al. 1989), sialyl Lewis x (Hey and Aplin 1996), the sialokeratan sulphate chain terminus recognised by monoclonal antibody D9B1 (Smith et al. 1989; Hoadley et al. 1990; Aplin 1991) and keratan sulphate itself (Hoadley et al. 1990; Aplin 1991; Graham et al. 1994). All these structures are the products of transferase enzymes–sialyl transferases, α-N-acetyl galactosamine transferase and sulphotransferase – whose activity is associated with the trans-golgi and post-golgi secretory compartments (Taatjes et al. 1988). The D9B1-, B72.3- and DBA-binding moieties are absent in normal proliferative phase tissue and strongly expressed in the secretory phase, while keratan sulphate and sialyl Lewis x are strongly upregulated in the secretory phase.

8.1.2 MUC1: Structure and Endometrial Expression

One highly glycosylated cell surface and secretory component of endometrial epithelium is MUC1. Immunoblotting and immunoprecipitation experiments have suggested that several glycan structures that have been shown to be cycle-regulated – sialokeratan sulphate, sialyl Tn, sialyl Lewis x and blood group A — are associated with MUC1 (Hoadley et al. 1990; Kliman et al. 1995; Hey and Aplin 1996; Graham, Hey and Aplin, unpublished).

MUC1 is a large type 1 cell surface glycoprotein with a short cytoplasmic domain (56 residues), transmembrane domain and a large extracellular domain containing a variable number tandem repeat (VNTR) sequence (Fig. 1; Gendler et al. 1990; Lan et al. 1990; Ligtenberg et al. 1990; Wreschner et al. 1990). The TR is a sequence of 20 amino acid residues with five potential O-glycosylation sites (S,T). The number of

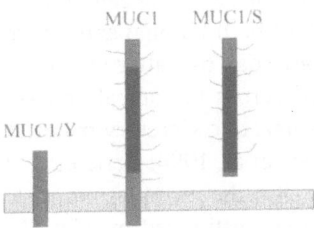

Fig. 1. Isoforms of MUC1 identified in endometrium. *Horizontal bar*, apical epithelial cell surface; *black bar*, VNTR region of the ectodomain of MUC1, absent from the short form MUC1/Y. MUC1/Y has only been identified as a transcript. The ectodomain contains a high proportion of serine, threonine and proline residues and is highly O-glycosylated. In addition, the membrane-proximal region contains several N-glycosylation sites. The ectodomain is predicted to assume a highly extended conformation

repeats present varies from 20 to more than 80, with each individual expressing two codominant alleles. In addition to O-glycosylation, there are also N-glycosylation sites in the membrane-proximal region. The cytoplasmic domain may be phosphorylated (Zrihan-Licht et al. 1994a). The molecular mass of the mature product varies in the range 200–500 kDa.

Immunochemical investigations of human endometrium have been carried out using monoclonal antibodies that recognise peptide sequences containing the immunodominant motif PDTRP from the MUC1 TR (Hey et al. 1994). The corresponding mRNA has been examined by probing with a cDNA that corresponds to sequence in the TR region of the ectodomain. MUC1 is expressed throughout the cycle in glandular and luminal epithelial cells. Inactive (postmenopausal) endometrium contains low but detectable levels of polypeptide in the glandular epithelium. In the proliferative phase levels of polypeptide and mRNA expression are again low but detectable. Interglandular heterogeneity is evident at the polypeptide level. Most of the product is cell-associated, either within the cytoplasm or at the apical cell surface; little secretory material is evident.

Beginning at about the time of ovulation there is a significant (six-fold) increase in the abundance of the mRNA. Polypeptide first accumulates in the epithelial cytoplasm where it is very abundant by 3–4 days after ovulation. At this stage immunoreactivity can be detected throughout the cytoplasm, but there is also a concentration of immunoreactivity at the apical cell surface of both luminal and glandular epithelial cells. In the mid secretory phase (day 6–7 after ovulation) these intracellular reserves are translocated across the apical cell surface as a result of which a mass of immunoreactive secretory material accumulates in the gland lumens (Fig. 2; Hey et al. 1994; Serle et al. 1994). This product lacks immunoreactivity for the cytoplasmic C-terminal domain of MUC1. The molecular mass estimated by SDS-PAGE is in excess of 250 kDa, with multiple banding and band broadening arising as the result of glycan microheterogeneity and allelic variation of polypeptide length. Later in the secretory phase extracellular MUC1 can still be detected; however, cellular heterogeneity is more evident, with some cytoplasmic immunoreactivity remaining, other cells having apparently stopped producing. Correspondingly, mRNA levels start to decline in the late secretory phase.

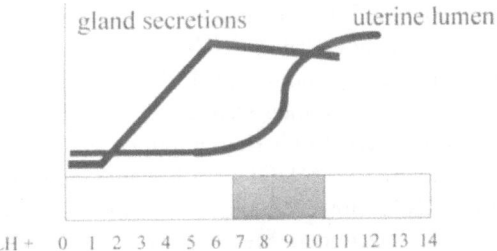

Fig. 2. MUC1 in endometrial secretions (gland secretions measured as extracellular immunoreactivity in tissue sections; uterine luminal levels measured by immunoassay of flushings) as a function of the evolving secretory phase (days following the LH peak). The probable implantation phase is indicated (*hatched sector*) based on the data of Bergh and Navot (1992). (MUC1 data based on Hey et al. 1994, 1995)

Secretory products are predicted to diffuse from the mouths of the glands into the uterine lumen. However, immunohistochemical analysis is less informative about this compartment because the contents are lost during tissue processing. As an alternative approach, secretory MUC1 in the uterine cavity was followed in uterine flushings (Fig. 2; Hey et al. 1995). Low levels of the product are detectable in the early secretory phase; about a week after ovulation the concentration starts to rise, and this increase continues into the late secretory phase, consistent with a progressive release from the glandular compartment into the uterine cavity. These data indicate that the expression of MUC1 is hormonally regulated.

The observations raise questions as to the mechanism of MUC1 secretion in endometrium. The rather rapid mobilisation of large amounts of product from intracellular reserves to the gland lumens may be accomplished by translocation of full-length membrane-intercalated MUC1 to the cell surface followed by release of a proteolytically cleaved ectodomain into the gland lumen (Ligtenberg et al. 1992a). Alternatively, differential mRNA splicing could give rise to a form of the molecule lacking the transmembrane and cytoplasmic regions (Williams et al. 1990).

MUC1 mRNA sequences were investigated using an RT-PCR protocol focusing on the region between the 3' end of the TR domain and the transmembrane domain. The data indicate the existence of a splice form of MUC1 mRNA in endometrium (MUC1/S) that lacks the transmembrane and cytoplasmic sequences (Fig. 1). The MUC1/S mRNA can be detected in all phases of the menstrual cycle as well as in endometrial cell lines (Aplin and Hey 1995; Hey, unpublished data). Thus the secreted form of endometrial MUC1 may be generated from an alternatively spliced mRNA. However, the quantitative significance of this event remains to be determined. Messenger RNA encoding a short form of the molecule (MUC1/Y) that lacks the VNTR domain (Zrihan-Licht et al. 1994b) is also present in endometrium (Fig. 1; Aplin and Hey 1995), but it is currently unclear whether this is translated.

8.1.3 MUC1: Involvement in Implantation and Inter-species Comparisons

As it approaches the epithelial surface, the attaching embryo would be expected to make an initial encounter with the epithelial glycocalyx, which in human seems to become more abundant in the implantation phase (Jansen et al. 1985; Smith et al. 1989; Hoadley et al. 1990; Aplin et al. 1994). In certain other species, such as the mouse, the glycocalyx thins at this time (Enders and Schlafke 1974). The cell surface form of MUC1 is particularly abundant on the microvilli and cilia that extend from the apical surface of endometrial epithelial cells (Aplin et al. 1994; Campbell et al. 1988). Experiments in transfected cell lines indicate that high levels of cell surface MUC1 can inhibit cell-cell interactions by simple steric hindrance of ligand access to the cell surface (Ligtenberg et al. 1992b); the large ectodomain and highly extended conformation of the mucin mean that it projects much farther from the surface than conventional receptors such as integrins.

Thus it appears surprising that MUC1 is expressed at relatively high levels in implantation phase human endometrial epithelium (Hey et al. 1994, 1995); this is the case both in glandular and luminal epithelial cells though most studies have focused on the gland cells and more detailed studies of the luminal epithelial cell surface are required. In the baboon, a species in which the anatomy of implantation is similar to that in humans, the level of MUC1 is high at the apical luminal epithelial cell surface at the time of implantation (Hild-Petito et al. 1996). In contrast, the mouse downregulates its homologue Muc1 in preparation for implantation (Braga and Gendler 1993; Surveyor et al. 1995). It is interesting in this light that implantation is usually successful in the mouse while in human a high proportion of replaced embryos fail. Could the uterus be imposing a barrier to the implanting embryo? One reason this might be the case is the relatively high proportion of abnormal embryos observed in human. It is not in the female's interest to invest resources or time in pregnancies that are destined to fail. Implantation could be a selection process in which only healthy embyos succeed. *How* they succeed remains an open question. One possibility is that factors released by a healthy embryo may effect local modifications to the endometrium. If so, our ingenuity in devising experimental models to test the function of MUC1 in human implantation will be tested to the full.

In baboons interesting differences have been observed in reproductive performance between females at different levels of the social hierarchy. High-ranking females appear to conceive more easily, but this is correlated with increased pregnancy loss (Packer et al. 1995; Wasser 1995). In humans defective endometrial differentiation is observed in endometrium from recurrent spontaneous miscarriage. This includes a reduction in the abundance of MUC1 (Serle et al. 1994; Hey et al. 1995). Such data might imply that the selection process is deficient, allowing implantation of embryos that are not competent to develop to term. One important consequence of this line of argument is that an abnormal maternal environment leads to the survival of embryos in which *intrinsic* abnormalities are present.

8.1.4 MUC1 and Its Associated Glycans as Markers of Steroid and Anti-steroid Action

The observation that MUC1 is transcriptionally upregulated in the early secretory phase suggests that progesterone may stimulate its expression in endometrium. Genomic 5' noncoding sequences have been obtained in human, and possible progesterone (and estrogen and glucocorticoid) regulatory elements have been identified, as well as an E-box and SP1, AP1 and AP2 sites (Lancaster et al. 1990; Abe and Kufe 1993). However, there is no current evidence to support direct action of the progesterone–progesterone receptor complex on MUC1 transcription. Alternative models are possible in which the action of progesterone on the endometrial stroma leads to paracrine effects on epithelial phenotype. In either case, MUC1 might well be useful as a molecular marker of anti-progestin effects on epithelial differentiation. However, it will be important to match very carefully the assay measurement with the timing of biopsy or fluid retrieval. Peri-ovulatory differentiation events might be monitored by measuring mRNA or intracellular core protein levels. The increase several days later of secretory MUC1 in uterine flushings is a good marker of epithelial function in the peri-implantation phase.

Alternatively, MUC1-associated glycans are attractive as markers of progesterone-driven epithelial differentiation, and also therefore of anti-progestin effects on the target tissue. There is evidence that glycan structures are altered in a range of endometrial pathologies (Aplin 1991; Serle et al. 1994). Furthermore it has been shown that the secretory phase expression of the D9B1 and B72.3 epitopes and DBA-binding glycan structures are inhibited by post-ovulatory administration of RU486 (Graham et al. 1991; Gemzell-Danielsson et al. 1994; Aplin and Wiehle, unpublished). RU486 administered on day LH+2 also suppresses the formation of secretory vesicles and a reduction is observed in the amount of luminal secretory material (Li et al. 1988b).

Using glycan structures diagnostically has both advantages and disadvantages. The main advantage is that because these are added late in biosynthesis they report pharmacological effects at any one of a number of steps: transcription, core protein translation, intracellular translocation, glycosyl transferase expression, etc. Set against this is the fact that within the normal epithelial cell population there is a considerable heterogeneity of glycan expression, leading to mosaicism (Campbell et al. 1988). MUC1 is itself a spectrum of glycoforms (Hey and Aplin 1996). Specific structures may be relatively abundant in some cells or glands but absent from others. If small biopsies (e.g. Sharman or pipelle) are to be used, this can lead to sampling errors.

8.2 Stromal Extracellular Matrix

8.2.1 ECM Remodelling During Decidualisation

Early secretory phase endometrial stroma is densely populated by elongated and undifferentiated fibroblasts. In the narrow intercellular spaces is found a collagenous extracellular matrix mainly comprising bundles of uniform diameter banded collagen fibrils with associated microfibrils (Aplin 1989, 1994; Aplin and Jones 1989). In the midsecretory phase oedematous patches appear in which the cell density is diminished. Around the glands and vessels the cell density remains high (Buckley and Fox 1989; Mylona et al. 1995). The ultrastructure of the cells at this time is largely unchanged. Thus, at the time implantation occurs, the stromal cells remain undifferentiated. However, decidualisation occurs within a few days, beginning around the vessels and beneath the luminal epithelium and extending throughout the tissue. Resident stromal cells differentiate from fibroblasts to become enlarged, sometimes binucleate decidual cells (Enders 1991). A greatly increased proportion of bone marrow derived cells is apparent, consisting mainly of macrophages, large granulated lymphocytes and a few T cells (Bulmer 1994). This reaction is to progesterone and occurs entirely independent of embryonic influence (Buckley and Fox 1989). Decidual changes are also apparent in the perivascular stroma in the late secretory phase of the cycle (Noyes et al. 1950; Buckley and Fox 1989).

During decidualisation there is a dramatic alteration in the architecture of the extracellular matrix (ECM). Collagen fibril density is reduced with a concomitant reduction in the mass ratio of collagen and abundance of three major collagen types, I, III and V (Hurst et al. 1994). In decidua of first trimester there is a much more abundant amorphous ground substance and the fibrillar components are anisotropic, of variable diameter and not bundled (Aplin and Jones 1989; Aplin 1989, 1994). Decidual cells also produce an unusual capsular basal lamina (Wynn 1974; Aplin and Jones 1989; Aplin 1989; Enders 1991).

RAT/coll VI

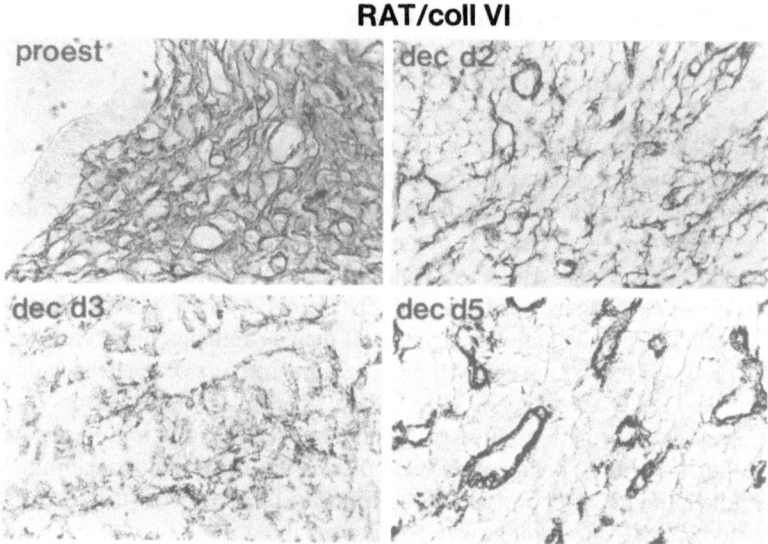

Fig. 3. Loss of collagen type VI from steroidally primed rat stroma during decidualisation in response to a mechanical stimulus. Immunoperoxidase histochemistry. In proestrous (*proest*) the stromal ECM is abundantly immunoreactive. By 5 days after the stimulus (*dec d5*) the stromal cells are unreactive, but strong reactivity is evident in the blood vessels. Days 2 (*dec d2*) and 3 (*dec d3*) show intermediate levels of immunoreactivity. (Reprinted with permission from Mulholland et al. 1992)

8.2.2 Collagen Type VI

The major collagens I, III and V are present in ECM of both endometrium and decidua. However, reorganisation can be deduced from the observation that cryptic epitopes on collagen type V are unmasked (Aplin et al. 1988). Collagen type VI forms microfibrils that associate with bundles of fibrillar collagen and appear to cross-link these with macrostructures such as cells, glands and vessels in the tissue. It is abundant in proliferative and early secretory phase stroma, but during decidualisation it disappears from all locations except the walls of vessels (Aplin et al. 1988; Mylona et al. 1995). Similar observations have been made in rats (Fig. 3; Mulholland et al. 1992; Dziadek et al.

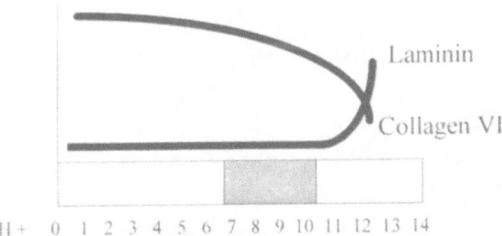

Fig. 4. Human stromal ECM differentiates in middle to late secretory phase with the loss of collagen VI and de novo expression of laminin. The implantation phase is indicated by a hatched sector. (Based on data from Aplin et al. 1988; Mylona et al. 1995; Church et al. 1996a)

1995). In humans a two-stage mechanism appears to operate: initially, extracellular breakdown is observed coinciding with the appearance of stromal oedema in the mid secretory phase (Fig. 4). At this stage mRNA for the three subunits of collagen VI is still abundant in stromal cells. Later mRNA levels drop so that in decidua of first trimester message is abundant only in perivascular cells. A different splice variant of the $\alpha3(VI)$ mRNA also appears (Ball, Kielty and Aplin, unpublished). The mechanism of extracellular breakdown of collagen VI is unknown; it is resistant to matrix metalloproteinases but cleaved by the mast cell derived enzymes tryptase and chymase and the neutrophil enzymes cathepsin G and elastase (Kielty et al. 1993). Interestingly, mast cells in the endometrium are observed to degranulate in the middle and late secretory phases (Jeziorska et al. 1995). It has previously been suggested that mast cells may play a role in decidualisation (Shelesnyak 1986).

8.2.3 Laminins

The decidual cell basement membrane contains laminin (Fig. 5), collagen type IV, heparan sulphate proteoglycan (perlecan) and osteonectin (Wewer et al. 1985; Faber et al. 1986; Kisalus et al. 1987; Kisalus and Herr 1988; Aplin et al. 1988; Wewer et al. 1988). Laminin exists in several isoforms and it is interesting that different laminins are ex-

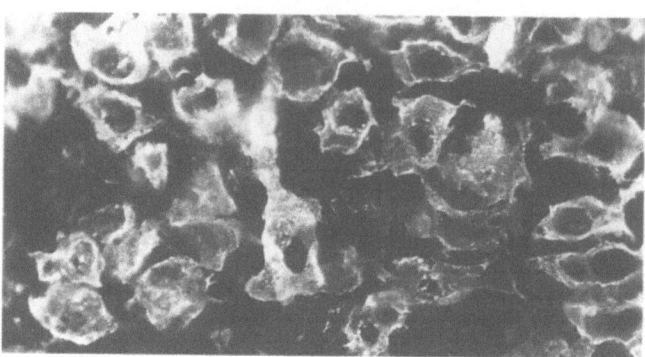

Fig. 5. Laminin γ_1 chain in human first trimester decidual cells detected by immunofluorescence with a specific monoclonal antibody. Note the delicate pericellular reactivity associated with each decidual cell

pressed in the different cell compartments of endometrium: in the vessels and glands laminins 1 ($\alpha_1\beta_1\gamma_1$) and 3 ($\alpha_1\beta_2\gamma_1$) are found and this varies neither during the menstrual cycle nor in pregnancy. In decidual cells, laminins 2 ($\alpha_2\beta_1\gamma_1$) and 4 ($\alpha_2\beta_2\gamma_1$) are expressed (Fig. 5) and the constituent subunits are absent from the stroma until decidualisation occurs (Church et al. 1996a; Fig. 4). Thus the α_2-subunit is characteristic of decidual cells. The α_4-chain is also present in these cells (Church et al. 1996b). Thus laminin presents a complex picture of steroidal regulation. Some members of its family of subunits (β_1, β_2 and γ_1) are coexpressed in the epithelial, vascular and stromal compartments. These chains are regulated in the stroma, but not in epithelial or vascular cells. In contrast, the α_2-subunit is found only in stromal cells where its expression is regulated; the polypeptide appears to be absent from proliferative phase stroma but present in decidual cells. The α_1-subunit is strongly and constitutively expressed by both epithelial and vascular cells. It is also weakly present in decidualised stromal cells.

Laminin is not known to exhibit regulated expression in any other normal adult tissue and it presents an interesting model of coordinated gene regulation in the context of a multi-subunit protein. Further studies are required to understand how this is achieved. It is possible that maternal stromal differentiation plays an important role in trophoblast access to, and transformation of, maternal blood vessels in early pregnancy. Therefore novel contraceptive or contragestational strategies, rather than focussing on the closure of an epithelially defined implantation window, might instead target the stroma to inhibit the establishment of hemochorial contact.

Acknowledgements. I am grateful to Ros Graham, Neil Hey, Carolyn Jones, Yiota Mylona, TC Li, Anna Charlton, Mourad Seif and Heather Church for their contributions to the studies reviewed herein. Financial support for the studies reported was received from MRC, Wellcome and WellBeing.

References

Abe M, Kufe D (1993) Characterisation of cis-acting elements regulating transcription of the human DF3 breast carcinoma-associated antigen. Proc Natl Acad Sci USA 90:282–286

Aplin JD (1989) Cellular biochemistry of the endometrium. In: Wynn RM, Jollie WP (eds) Biology of the uterus. Plenum, New York, pp 89–129

Aplin JD (1991) Glycans as biochemical markers of human endometrial secretory differentation. J Reprod Fertil 91:525–541

Aplin JD (1994) Products of endometrial differentiation. In: Chard T, Grudzinskas JG (eds) The uterus. Cambridge reviews in human reproduction. Cambridge University Press, Cambridge, pp 125–147

Aplin JD, Hey NA (1995) MUC1 and endometrium and embryo implantation. Biochem Soc Transact 28:826–831

Aplin JD, Jones CJP (1989) Extracellular matrix in endometrium and decidua. In: Genbacev O, Klopper A, Beaconsfield R (eds) Placenta as a model and source. Plenum, New York, pp 115–128

Aplin JD, Charlton AK, Ayad S (1988) An immunohistochemical study of human endometrial extracellular matrix during the menstrual cycle and first trimester of pregnancy. Cell Tissue Res 253:235–240

Aplin JD, Seif MW, Graham RA, Hey NA, Behzad F, Campbell S (1994) The endometrial cell surface and implantation: expression of the polymorphic mucin MUC-1 and adhesion molecules during the endometrial cycle. Ann NY Acad Sci 734:103–121

Bergh PA, Navot D (1992) The impact of embryonic development and endometrial maturity on the timing of implantation. Fertil Steril 58:537–542

Braga VMM, Gendler SJ (1993) Modulation of Muc-1 mucin expression in the mouse uterus during the estrus cycle early pregnancy and placentation. J Cell Sci 105:397–405

Buckley CH, Fox H (1989) Biopsy pathology of the endometrium. Chapman and Hall Medical, London

Bulmer JN (1994) Human endometrial lymphocytes in normal pregnancy and pregnancy loss. Ann NY Acad Sci 734:185–192

Campbell S, Seif MW, Aplin JD, Richmond SJ, Haynes P, Allen TD (1988) Expression of a secretory product by microvillous and ciliated cells of the human endometrial epithelium in vivo and in vitro. Hum Reprod 3:927–934

Church HJ, Vicovac LJ, Williams JDL, Hey NA, Aplin JD (1996a) Human decidual cells express laminins 2 and 4. Lab Invest 74:21–32

Church HJ, Richards AJ, Aplin JD (1996b) Laminins in decidua placenta and choriocarcinoma cells. Trophoblast Res (in press)

Dziadek M, Darling P, Zhang R-Z, Pan TC, Tillet E, Timpl R, Chu M-L (1995) Expression of collagen 1(VI) 2(VI) and 3(VI) chains in the pregnant mouse uterus. Biol Reprod 52:885–894

Enders AC (1991) Current topic: structural responses of the primate endometrium to implantation. Placenta 12:309–325

Enders AC, Schlafke S (1974) Surface coats of the mouse blastocyst and uterus during the preimplantation period. Anat Rec 180:31–46

Faber M, Wewer UM, Berthelsen JG, Liotta LA, Albrechtsen R (1986) Laminin production by human endometrial stromal cells relates to the cyclic and pathological state of the endometrium. Am J Pathol 124:384–391

Gemzell-Danielsson K, Svalander P, Swahn M-L, Johannisson E, Brygdeman M (1994) Effects of a single post-ovulatory dose of RU486 on endometrial maturation in the implantation phase. Hum Reprod 9:2398–2404

Gendler SJ, Lancaster CA, Taylor-Papadimitriou J, Duhig T, Peat N, Burchell J, Pemberton L, Lalani E, Wilson D (1990) Molecular cloning and expression of human tumour-associated polymorphic epithelial mucin. J Biol Chem 265:15286–15293

Graham RA, Li T-C, Seif MW, Aplin JD, Cooke ID (1991) The effects of the antiprogesterone RU486 (Mifepristone) on an endometrial secretory glycan: an immunocytochemical study. Fertil Steril 55:1132–1136

Graham RA, Li T-C, Cooke ID, Aplin JD (1994) Keratan sulphate as a secretory product of human endometrium: cyclic expression in normal women. Hum Reprod 9:926–930

Hey NA, Aplin JD (1996) Sialyl Lewis x and Sialyl Lewis a are expressed by human endometrial MUC1. Glycoconjugate J (in press)

Hey NA, Graham RA, Seif MW, Aplin JD (1994) The polymorphic epithelial mucin MUC1 in human endometrium is regulated with maximal expression in the implantation phase. J Clin Endocrinol Metab 78:337–342

Hey NA, Li T-C, Devine PL, Graham RA, Aplin JD (1995) MUC1 in secretory phase endometrium: expression in precisely dated biopsies and flushings from normal and recurrent miscarriage patients. Hum Reprod 10:2655–2662

Hild-Petito S, Carson DD, Fazleabas A (1996) Muc1 expression is differentially regulated in uterine lumenal and glandular epithelia of the baboon. Biol Reprod (in press)

Hoadley ME, Seif MW, Aplin JD (1990) Menstrual cycle-dependent expression of keratan sulphate in human endometrium. Biochem J 266:757–763

Hurst PR, Gibbs RD, Clark DE, Myers DB (1994) Temporal changes to uterine collagen types I III and V in relation to early pregmancy in the rat. Reprod Fertil Dev 6:669–677

Jansen RP, Turner M, Johannisson E, Landgren B-M, Diczfalusy E (1985) Cyclic changes in human endometrial surface glycoproteins: a quantitative histochemical study. Fertil Steril 44:85–91

Jeziorska M, Salamonsen LA, Wooley DE (1995) Mast cell and eosinophil distribution and activation in human endometrium throughout the menstrual cycle. Biol Reprod 53:312–320

Kielty CM, Lees M, Shuttleworth CA, Woolley D (1993) Catabolism of intact type VI collagen microfibrils: susceptibility to degradation by serine proteinases. Biochem Biophys Res Commun 191:1230–1236

Kisalus LL, Herr JC (1988) Immunocytochemical localisation of heparan sulphate proteoglycan in human decidual cell secretory bodies and placental fibrinoid. Biol Reprod 39:419–430

Kisalus LL, Herr JC, Little CD (1987) Immunolocalisation of extracellular matrix proteins and collagen synthesis in first-trimester human decidua. Anat Rec 218:402–415

Kliman HJ, Feinberg RF, Schwarz LB, Feinman MA, Lavi E, Meaddough EL (1995) A mucin-like glycoprotein identified by MAG antibodies Menstrual cycle-dependent localisation in human endometrium. Am J Pathol 146:166–181

Lan MS, Batra SK, Qi W-N, Metzgar RS, Hollingsworth MA (1990) Cloning and sequencing of a human pancreatic tumor mucin cDNA. J Biol Chem 265:15294–15299

Lancaster CA, Peat N, Duhig T, Wilson D, Taylor-Papadimitriou J, Gendler SJ (1990) Structure and expression of the human polymorphic epithelial gene: an expressed VNTR unit. Biochem Biophys Res Commun 173:1019–1029

Li T-C, Rogers AW, Dockery P, Lenton EA, Cooke ID (1988) A new method of histologic dating of human endometrium in the luteal phase. Fertil Steril 50:52–60

Li T-C, Dockery P, Thomas P, Rogers AW, Lenton EA, Cooke ID (1988b) The effects of progesterone receptor blockade in the luteal phase of normal fertile women. Fertil Steril 50:732–742

Ligtenberg MJL, Vos HL, Gennissen AMC, Hilkens J (1990) Episialin a carcinoma-associated mucin is generated by a polymorphic gene encoding splice variants with alternative amino termini. J Biol Chem 265:5573-5578

Ligtenberg MJL, Kruijshaar L, Buijs F, van Meijer M, Litvinov SV, Hilkens J (1992a) Cell-associated episialin is a complex containing two proteins derived from a common precursor. J Biol Chem 267:6171–6177

Ligtenberg MJL, Buijs F, Vos HL, Hilkens J (1992b) Suppression of cellular aggregation by high levels of episialin. Cancer Res 52:2318–2324

Mulholland J, Aplin JD, Ayad S, Hong L, Glasser SR (1992) Loss of type VI collagen from rat endometrium during decidualisation. Biol Reprod 46:1136–1143

Mylona P, Kielty CM, Hoyland J, Aplin JD (1995) Expression of type VI collagen in human endometrium and decidua. J Reprod Fertil 103:159–167

Noyes RW, Hertig AT, Rock J (1950) Dating the endometrial biopsy. Fertil Steril 1:3–25

Packer C, Collins DA, Sindimwo A, Goodall J (1995) Reproductive constraints on aggressive competition by female baboons. Nature 373:60–63

Serle E, Li T-C, Graham RA, Cooke ID, Seif MW, Warren MA, Aplin JD (1994) A morphological and immunohistochemical study of endometrial development in the peri-implantation phase of women with recurrent miscarriage. Fertil Steril 62:989–996

Shelesnyak MC (1986) A history of research on nidation. Ann NY Acad Sci 476:5–24

Smith RA, Seif MW, Rogers AW, Li T-C, Dockery P, Cooke ID, Aplin JD (1989) The endometrial cycle: the expression of a secretory component correlated with the luteinising hormone peak. Hum Reprod 4:236–242

Soisson AP, Berchuck A, Lessey BA, Soper JT, Clarke-Pearson DL, McCarty KS, Bast RC (1989) Immunohistochemical expression of TAG-72 in normal and malignant endometrium: correlation of antigen expression with estrogen receptor and progesterone receptor levels. Am J Obstet Gynecol 161:1258–1263

Surveyor GA, Gendler SJ, Pemberton L, Das SK, Chakraborty I, Julian J, Pimental RA, Wegner CC, Dey SK, Carson DD (1995) Expression and steroid hormonal control of Muc1 in the mouse uterus. Endocrinology 136:3639–3647

Taatjes DJ, Roth J, Weinstein J, Paulson JC (1988) Post-Golgi localisation and regional expression of rat intestinal sialyltransferase detected by immunoelectron microscopy with polypeptide epitope-purified antibody. J Biol Chem 263:6302–6309

Thor A, Viglione MJ, Muraro R, Ohuchi N, Schlom J, Gorstein F (1987) Monoclonal antibody B723 reactivity with human endometrium: a study of normal and malignant tissues. Int J Gynecol Pathol 6:235–247

Warren MA, Li T-C, Klentzeris LD (1994) Cell biology of the endometrium: histology cell types and menstrual changes. In: Chard T, Grudzinskas JG (eds) The uterus. Cambridge University Press, Cambridge, pp 94–124

Wasser SK (1995) Costs of conception in baboons. Nature 376:219–220

Wewer UM, Faber M, Liotta LA, Albrechtsen R (1985) Immunochemical and ultrastructural assessment of the nature of the pericellular basement membrane of human decidual cells. Lab Invest 53:624–633

Wewer UM, Albrechtsen R, Fisher LW, Young MF, Termine JD (1988) Osteonectin/SPARC/BM-40 in human decidua and carcinoma tissues characterised by de novo formation of basement membrane. Am J Pathol 132:345–355

Williams CJ, Wreschner DH, Tanaka A, Tsarfaty I, Keydar I, Dion AS (1990) Multiple protein forms of the human breast tumor-associated epithelial membrane antigen (EMA) are generated by alternative splicing and induced by hormonal stimulation. Biochem Biophys Res Commun 170:1331–1338

Wreschner DH, Hareuveni M, Tsarfaty I, Smorodinsky N, Horev J, Zaretsky J, Kotkes P, Weiss M, Lathe R, Dion A, Keydar I (1990) Human epithelial tumor antigen cDNA sequences Differential splicing may generate multiple protein forms. Eur J Biochem 189:463–473

Wynn RM (1974) Ultrastructural development of the human decidua. Am J Obstet Gynecol 118:652–670

Zrihan-Licht S, Baruch A, Elroy-Stein O, Keydar I, Wreschner DH (1994a) Tyrosine phosphorylation of the MUC1 breast cancer membrane proteins Cytokine receptor-like molecules. FEBS Lett 356:130–136

Zrihan-Licht S, Vos HL, Baruch A, Elroy-Stein O, Sagiv D, Keydar I, Hilkens J, Wreschner DH (1994b) Characterization and molecular cloning of a novel MUC1 protein devoid of tandem repeats expressed in human breast cancer tissue. Eur J Biochem 224:787–795

9 Intrinsic and Extrinsic Hormonal Influences Contributing to Endometrial Receptivity in Normal Reproduction and After Ovum Donation

D. de Ziegler

9.1 The Egg Donation Lesson

In vitro fertilization (IVF) was originally designed to help women conceive whose tubes are damaged or absent. However, IVF soon opened the possibility of women who lack ovarian function becoming pregnant with the help of donated oocytes (IVF-OD) and giving birth (Rosenwaks 1987). To succeed, however, IVF-OD requires that the endometrium of recipient women be receptive to embryos with the sole help of exogenous hormones. Originally this task appeared complex. The first regimens designed for recipients of IVF-OD attempted closely to mimic the pattern of hormonal levels normally encountered in the menstrual cycle (Lutjen et al. 1984; Navot et al. 1984). Soon, however,

D. de Ziegler

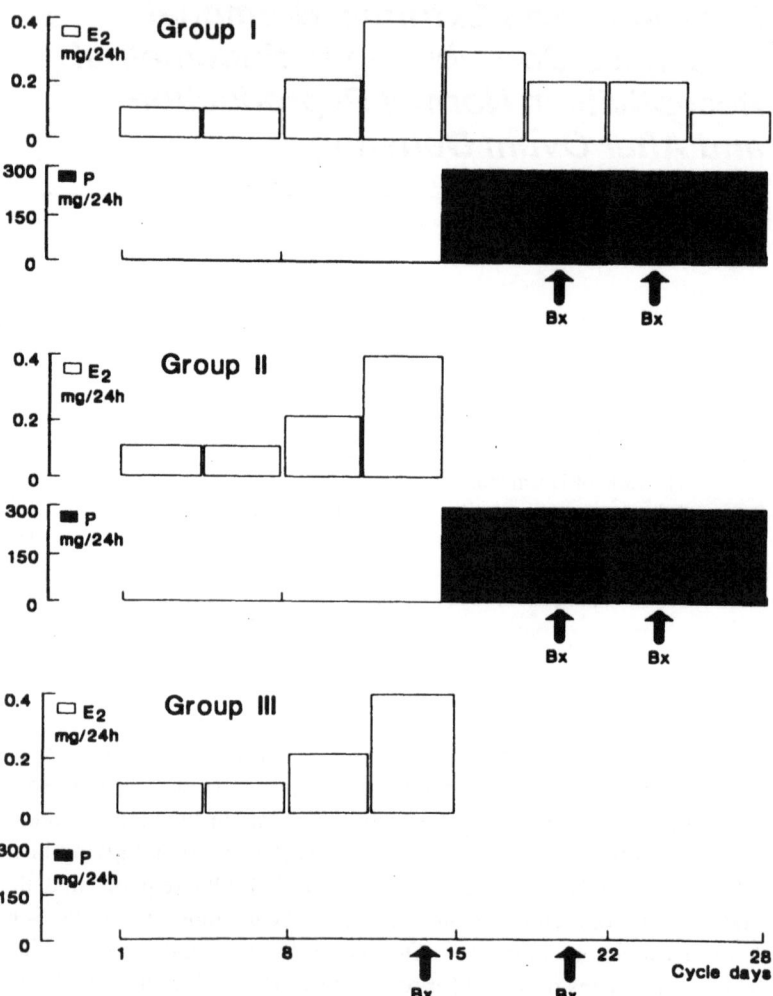

Fig. 1. Hormonal administration pattern

it was recognized that the hormonal requirements of IVF-OD are much more flexible than originally anticipated (De Ziegler 1995). Indeed, only two conditions have emerged as indispensable for the success of hormonal treatments for IVF-OD: (a) estradiol (E_2) priming should be sufficient with endometrial exposure to middle follicular phase levels lasting for at least 7 days but possibly, as long as 2 months (Navot et al. 1989, 1991). (b) The proper sequence of secretory changes in the endometrium must match the developmental stage of four to eight cell embryos (Rosenwaks 1987) or blastocysts (Lelaidier et al. 1995).

The simplicity of the necessary requirements for hormonal replacement regimens used to prime endometrial receptivity have substantially simplified the practical aspects of IVF-OD. However, this simplicity has hardly made the issue less interesting and has, rather, made hormonal substitution cycles designed for IVF-OD ideal experimental models for studying the respective roles of each hormonal factor in the control of endometrial receptivity.

The great predictability and reproducibility of endometrial effects triggered by progesterone irrespective of the woman's age contrasts with the prevailing concept that the uterus is the site of an aging process and progressively diminishes in its response to hormones. Contrary to this concept, IVF-OD data indicate that the endometrial response to nonoral E_2 and progesterone regimens show no adaptation of endometrial effects over time (Sauer et al. 1994). Some investigators have used hormonal replacement cycles designed for IVF-OD as study models to clarify the role played by the E_2/progesterone ratio on endometrial receptivity. First, it was determined that luteal E_2 is not necessary (De Ziegler et al. 1991a; Gosh and Sengupta 1994; Younis et al. 1994) and does not influence (De Ziegler and Bouchard 1993) the endometrial response to progesterone (Fig. 1). Contrasting, however, with the lack of influence that luteal E_2 has on endometrial effects of progesterone, luteal E_2 is an obligatory cofactor to the suppressing the effects of progesterone on gonadotropins (De Ziegler et al. 1992; Figs. 2,3).

As even extreme increases or decreases in plasma levels of luteal E_2 fail to affect the endometrial effects of progesterone, our interest has focused on the dose-response characteristics of progesterone effects. To clarify this issue, a clinical trial was designed to examine the effects induced by vaginal administration of progressively increasing doses of progesterone using a polycarbophil base sustained release preparation,

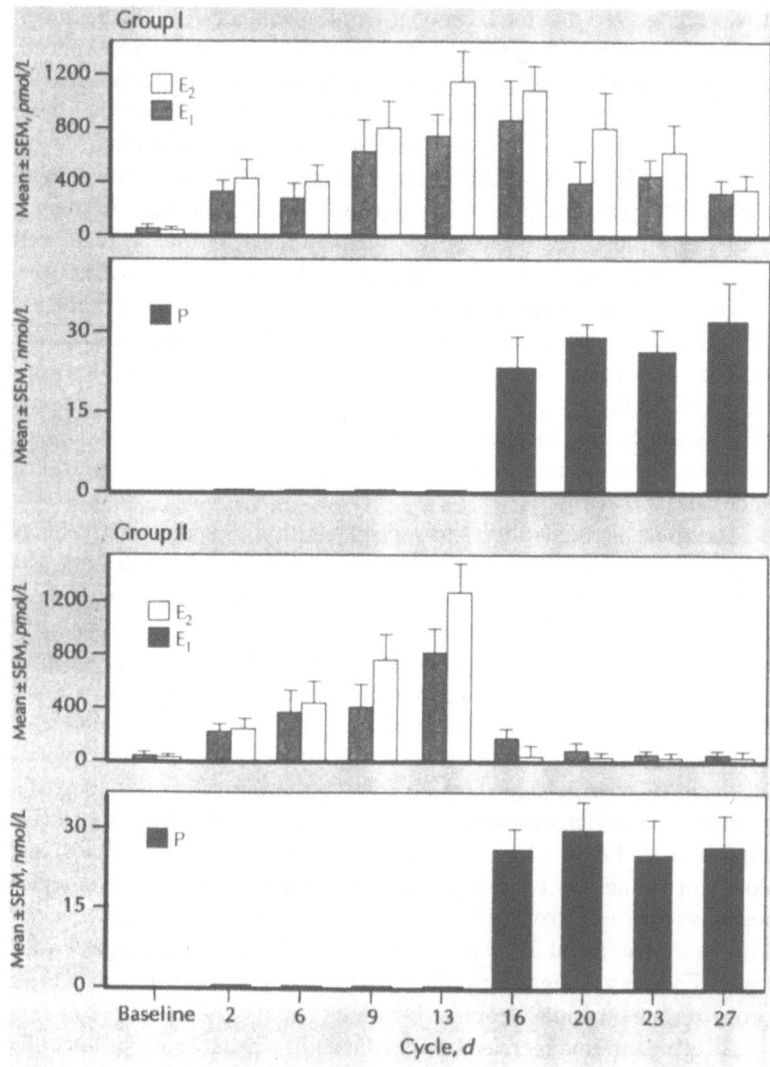

Fig. 2. Plasma E_2, E_1, and progesterone (P) levels. Group I women received E_2 and progesterone. Group II women did not receive E_2 during the luteal phase

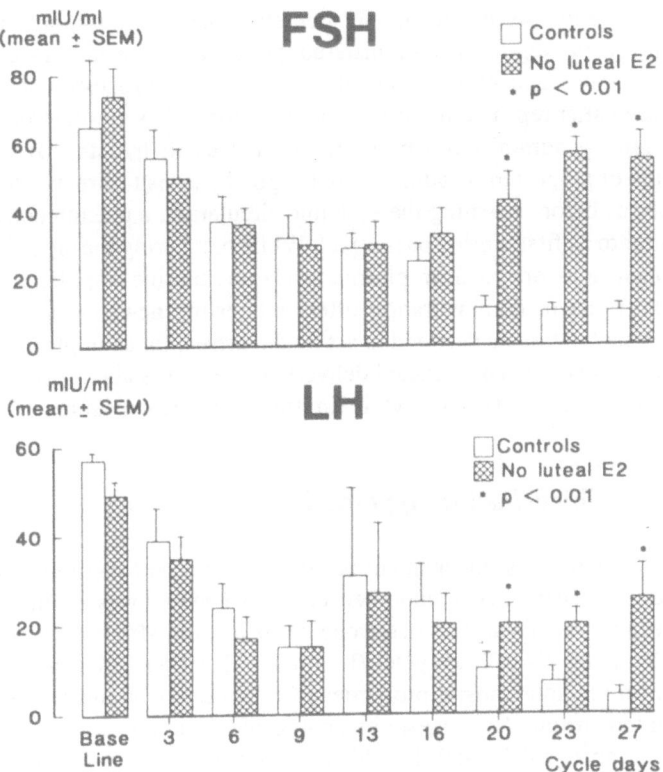

Fig. 3. Plasma follicle-stimulating hormone (*FSH*) and luteinizing hormone (*LH*) levels

Crinone-TVG (Fanchin et al. 1993). Unexpectedly, however, endometrial effects were similar at all doses of vaginal progesterone tested (45, 90, and 180 mg every 2nd day), which all mimicked the endometrial changes seen in the menstrual cycle despite markedly lower (subphysiological) plasma progesterone levels, particularly in the 45-mg dose group (Fanchin et al. 1993). The paradoxically strong effects on the endometrium of vaginally administered progesterone have been studied by Miles et al. (1994). Comparing plasma and uterine tissue levels of progesterone after vaginal or intramuscular administration, these investigators unequivocally demonstrated a remarkable uterine trophicity of vaginally administered progesterone which results in higher tissue concentrations despite lower plasma progesterone levels than seen after repeated intramuscular injections. This uterine trophicity of vaginally administered progesterone led us to hypothesize that a fraction of progesterone administered vaginally transits directly through the uterus before reaching the systemic circulation, a phenomenon that we refer to as first uterine pass effect. While hampering the significance of conclusions drawn from plasma levels, the uterine trophicity of the vaginal route of administration offers interesting new perspective for delivering treatments destined to act on the uterus, for example, uterorelaxant substances. The targeted delivery to the uterus allows maximalization of the desired effects while limiting systemic exposure.

9.2 The Third-Factor Hypothesis

As noted above, the mechanism originally proposed to account for the suboptimal receptivity of endometrium in IVF cycles was an imbalance between plasma E_2 and progesterone levels resulting from the markedly elevated E_2 levels of IVF cycles (Forman et al. 1988). This concept was based on the antagonistic properties that progesterone and E_2 have on the endometrium. As progesterone antagonizes the proliferative effects of E_2, it appeared logical that this antagonism was of the competitive mode. Hence our findings, later confirmed by others, on the lack of endometrial effects of even extreme changes in luteal E_2 levels came as a surprise. If alterations in plasma E_2 levels and the resulting changes in plasma E_2 to progesterone ratio were without impact on endometrial morphology and receptivity to embryos, what differences between IVF and menstrual cycles could hamper endometrial receptivity?

One consequence of controlled ovarian hyperstimulation (COH) cycles that may have been overlooked is the possible impact of an increase in production by the ovary of factors other than E_2 and progesterone brought by the gonadotropin treatment. That the ovaries could impact negatively on endometrial receptivity through substances other than E_2 and progesterone (hence, "third factor") was suggested from studies on uterine artery blood flow analyzed by pulsed Doppler. In women deprived of ovarian function either prematurely (De Ziegler et al. 1991b) or at the regular age (Bourne et al. 1990) uterine artery resistance is high in the absence of E_2 but lowers to minimal levels after only 2 weeks of exposure to early follicular phase levels of E_2. In this context the report that on the day of human chorionic gonadotropin administration a fair proportion of IVF candidates have high uterine artery resistance came as surprise. In women suffering from polycystic ovarian disease a similar paradox has been reported that disappears after suppression of ovarian function with a gonadotropin-releaseing hormone agonist and E_2 add-back therapy. The observation made in polycystic ovarian disease led us to hypothesize that also in COH the ovaries could impact negatively on uterine artery blood flow and receptivity to embryo implantation. According to this hypothesis, women whose uterine artery resistance tends to be too elevated during IVF cycles experience transitory effects resembling those of polycystic ovarian disease as a result of exogenous gonadotropins. To test this hypothesis we studied extensively the hormonal profile (E_2, progesterone, and androgens) seen after dministration of human menopausal gonadotropin (hMG) in IVF cycles. During the last day of hMG treatment in COH we observed a transitory increase in plasma androgens 12 h after hMG administration. Hence it is conceivable that in some women the ovarian production of androgens in response to hMG suffices to alter negatively uterine artery blood flow. An alternative hypothesis is that nonsteroid products of ovarian function are responsible for altering endometrial receptivity.

The practical consequence to be drawn from the third-factor hypothesis is that hMG doses should be decreased if possible after IVF cycles that show improper uterine blood flow.

9.3 Contractile Activity of the Nonpregnant Uterus: The Role of Hormones

Beyond their effects on the morphological characteristics of endometrial glands and stroma, ovarian hormones may also affect endometrial receptivity by altering uterine contractility. Earlier studies looking at patterns of intrauterine pressure recordings through open-ended fluid-filled catheters indicate that E_2 increases the frequency of uterine contractions while progesterone or progesterone and E_2 induce uterine relaxation through a decrease in frequency and an increase in amplitude of intrauterine pressure waves (Moawad and Bengtsson 1967). These authors have described "prelabor" and/or "labor" patterns of uterine contractions in the days preceding and during menses, with higher pressure amplitudes than at any other time during the menstrual cycle (Moawad and Bengtsson 1967). In an elegant work Martinez-Gaudio et al. (1973) recorded intrauterine pressure simultaneously from two or three different levels (lower, middle, and upper portions of the uterine cavity) using distinct fluid-filled catheters connected to individual pressure transducers. With this approach midcycle recordings revealed often different frequency of contractions at the three recording sites, suggesting poor propagation of contractions (Martinez-Gaudio et al. 1973) at this stage of the menstrual cycle. During the midsecretory phase a relative dyssynchrony prevailed between pressure recordings from the three different levels. During menstrual bleeding a tendency was noticed toward antegrade movement of the contractions that propagated from fundus to cervix with laborlike patterns of activity. However, numerous exceptions with nonpropagating contractions were also noted by these authors (Martinez-Gaudio et al. 1973). Taken together, these results indicate a tendency toward organized antegrade contractions during the menses and point also to the inappropriateness of the method used so far to record contractions in nonpregnant uterus (intrauterine pressure redording) in part because of its invasive nature.

The possible impact of uterine contractions on the outcome of embryo transfers (ET) after IVF has been studied by placing a drop of contrast medium in the uterine cavity on the occasion of pre-IVF mock cycles (Knutzen et al. 1992). Fluoroscopic recording and serial X-rays were used to study the possible displacements of the dye after mock transfers. Results were compared to the outcome of IVF cycles performed immediately after the mock cycle. All pregnancies (6/18) occurred in women in whom the dye remained in the uterine cavity after the mock transfer. In contrast, no women in whom the dye had been expelled toward the cervix and the vagina or the tube became pregnant in the following IVF cycle. These results are strongly supportive of the beneficial effects that uterine quiescence may exert on pregnancy rates following ET. Hence, a possible advantage may be gained from favoring uterine quiescence in women undergoing IVF-ET with timely use of specific uterorelaxants such as β-mimetics, NO donors such as nitroglycerin, or more simply, by supplementing uterine exposure to the most natural of all uterorelaxant substances, progesterone.

Originally, studies on uterine contractions were inherently limited by the invasive nature of the methodology available, requiring intrauterine pressure recording systems. Recently, however, the approach was dramatically changed when it became possible to assess uterine contractions from ultrasound recordings (Birnholz 1984; Abramovisc and Archer 1990; de Vries et al. 1990; Lyons et al. 1991; Chalubinski et al. 1993). The imprecision of the original transvesical scans (Birnholz 1984) has become a thing of the past with the availability of high-resolution transvaginal ultrasound systems (Abramovisc and Archer 1990; de Vries et al. 1990; Lyons et al. 1991; Chalubinski et al. 1993). However, the interpretation of uterine contractile activity from even the highest resolution scans raises questions about the validity of the conclusions drawn through naked-eye analysis of rapidly displayed scans. Does the contractile activity apparent on ultrasound truly correspond to efficient uterine contractions leading to intrauterine pressure elevations? To date no echographic-pressure correlation has been established. Hence, despite the great potential interests for evaluating uterine contractile activity through this high-tech noninvasive approach, transvaginal ultrasound assessment of uterine contractions must be validated against the existing reference, i.e., changes in intrauterine pressure, before it can lead to meaningful interpretations. In our preliminary work (Bulletti, Massonneau and de Ziegler, unpublished observation) we observed that all changes in uterine pressure are probably detectable by ultrasound scans. However, it is conceivable that the converse is not always true, and that all forms of uterine contractility detected on ultrasound do not translate into significant intrauterine pressure changes. Indeed, some myometrial activity may be functionally inadequate (pathologically or physiologically) because of lack or improper coordination of the myometrial contractile activity which results in various forms of uterine dyskinesia. Some contractions recorded on uterine scans have been interpreted as displaying highly sophisticated time-spatial organization resulting in true ante- or retrograde peristaltic movement (Salamanka and Beltran 1995). In particular, during menses a laborlike pattern of contractile activity results in powerful antegrade peristaltic contractions that play a physiological role in the proper external expulsion of menstrual blood.

Specific clinical issues which may be affected by uterine contraction include the incidence of ectopic pregnancies and endometriosis. Ectopic pregnancies occurring in women whose tubes are healthy have always raised puzzling questions about their etiology. Most intriguing has been the long-recognized increase risk of recurrence of ectopic pregnancy among women with normally appearing tubes whose first ectopic pregnancy had been treated by surgical removal of the affected tube. One factor compounding the complexity of this issue is the wide degree of difference in tubal contractions reported in different species that makes generalizations drawn from animal studies dubious. In ewes a discontinuous mode of progression has been described for the tube to uterus transport of the conceptus in which a prolonged arrest takes place at the level of the isthmic to ampullary junction. The arrest in the conceptus' progression results from retrograde tubal contractions that maintain the conceptus at the isthmotubal junction but its control appears most complex. Independent observations in nonhuman (Eddy et al. 1975, 1976) and human primates (Croxatto et al. 1978) concur in describing similar arrests in the progression of the conceptus at the isthmic-ampullary junction. In women the fertilized oocyte reaches the uterine cavity 4–5 days after the surge in luteinizing hormone (LH). On the other hand, a slow but nearly continuous transtubal transport of the conceptus is seen in rabbits in which the embryo reaches the uterine cavity 3–4 days after the LH surge. In women in the late follicular phase recordings of electrical activity at the tubal surface have revealed waves originating from both extremities that progress slowly at 1–3 mm/s and converge toward the isthmic-ampullary junction. During the luteal phase practically all tubal electrical activity consists of slow waves that progress toward the uterus (Maia and Coutinho 1970). Furthermore, in several areas spontaneous contractile activity of tubal muscle cells takes a pacemaker function. It is the relative importance of any given pacemaker activity over that of different areas that determines the ultimate direction of movement of the tubal contractions. In vitro studies support this theory by showing two types of tubal muscle cells. Some display spontaneous or pacemaker contractile activity while others more numerous are spontaneously inactive and contract only when exposed to the depolarized current of a nearby contracting cell.

9.4 Tubo-uterine Contractility and Embryo Placement

The hormonal control of the transtubal transport of the conceptus has not yet been completely elucidated. In most species progesterone administration at the time of ovulation slows the transtubal transit time of the conceptus. On the other hand, E_2 induces a prolonged blockade of oocyte development when administered at the time of ovulation. Supportive of distinctively different effects of hormones on tubal contractility are the findings of Nozaki and Ito (1987) who showed that E_2 hyperpolarizes longitudinal cells while progesterone exerts opposite effects (Fuentealba et al. 1987). Treatment with the competitive antiprogestin RU-486 exerts, however, paradoxical action in that it also accelerates (as progesterone) the transtubal transport of concepti. Furthermore, nerve endings producing vasoinhibitory peptide have been found in abundance in the isthmic-ampullary junction where they are probably involved in the transitory block the conceptus' transit observed in this area in women.

In the uterus the contractile activity is believed to participate in the proper placement of the conceptus in order to favor implantation while it must be recognized that the situation prevailing in humans in whom the uterus results from the fusion of two mullerian components may be dramatically different. Preliminary work in prematurely menopaused women speaks for a possible physiological role of these mechanisms in the control of embryo implantation in humans (De Ziegler et al. 1996). In women deprived of ovarian function receiving transdermal estradiol, progesterone administered transvaginally (Crinone-TVG 4% and 8%) triggered new patterns of uterine contraction that combined antegrade and retrograde activities that converged and stopped in the middle of the uterine cavity. Further work will determine whether some forms of uterine dyskinesia exist in women who present repeated implantation failures after IVF or early pregnancy losses. Pragmatic approaches aiming at decreasing uterine contractile activity after ET will also need to be tested to determine their true clinical value. Furthermore, the new emerging understanding of the possible role(s) of uterine contractions in human implantation forces top concider also that drugs affecting uterine contractility, for exemple, antiprogestins, may also affect endometrial receptivity by this mechanism.

9.5 Endometriosis

Endometriosis, a disorder known to take a significant toll on fertility, may also be influenced by uterine contractility. At the time of menses the laborlike pattern of peristalticlike uterine contractions is likely to play a significant role in the physiological process of external expulsion of menstrual blood. Conversely, it is conceivable that functional disturbances of menstrual flow expulsion augments the degree of retrograde menstruation (Halme et al. 1984) and favor the development of endometriaosis implants, following Sampson's (1927) theory. While menses that follow the demise of the corpus luteum and withdrawal of exogenous progesterone or progestin treatment are not inherently different, the subjective premenstrual contractile activity is. Indeed, it has long been established that premenstrual cramps that may be present in the menstrual cycle are classically alleviated in artificial cycles such as in women receiving oral contraception. This indicates that substances produced by the corpus luteum other than sex steroids are likely to play a role on uterine contractions, possibly influencing the functionality of menstrual blood expulsion. Future work will determine whether uterorelaxant therapies may diminish retrograde menstruation when deemed necessary and hence allievate dysmenorrhea and possibly prevent the development and/or the recurrence of endometriosis. Preliminary work reported by Salamanca and Beltran (1995) supports this hypothesis that endometriosis is linked to a form of uterine dyskinesia. These authors indicated that retrograde displacement of uterine contractions at the time of menstruation was found in women suffering from endometriosis.

9.6 Conclusion

Hormonal replacement cycles used in IVF-OD have succeeded in achieving excellent endometrial receptivity to embryo implantation. The absolute requirements have proven to be extremely simple: proper E_2 priming lasting from 7 to 28 days should be followed by progesterone treatment. The degree of embryo maturation must match that of secretory changes induced by progesterone on the endometrium. Vaginal administration of progesterone has been shown to result in a remarkable targeting toward the uterus. Further work will tell whether the uterorelaxing properties of progesterone exert significant benefit on embryo implantation.

References

Abramovisc J-S, Archer DF (1990) Uterine endometrial persistalsis: a transvaginal ultrasound study. Fertil Steril 54:451–454

Birnholz JC (1984) Ultrasonic visualization of endometrial movements. Fertil Steril 41:157–158

Bourne T, Hillard TC, Whitehead MI, Crook D, Campbell S (1967) Oestrogens, arterial status, and postmenopausal women. Lancet 335:1471

Chalubinski K, Deutinger J, Bernaschek G (1993) Vaginosonography for recording of cycle-related myometrial contractions. Fertil Steril 59:225–228

Croxatto HB, Ortiz ME, Diaz S, Hess R, Balamaceda J, Croxatto HD (1978) Studies on the duration of egg transport by the human oviduct. Ovum location at various intervals following LH peak. Am J Obstet Gynecol 132:629–634

de Vries K, Lyons EA, Ballard G, Levi CS, Lindsay DJ (1990) Contractions of the inner third of the myometrium. Am J Obstet Gynecol 162:679–682

de Ziegler D (1995) Hormonal strategies for preparing the human endometrium prior to oocyte donation. Semin Reprod Endocrinol 13:192–197

de Ziegler D, Bouchard P (1993) Understanding endometrial physiology and menstrual disorders in the 1990's. Curr Opin Obstet Gynecol 5:378–388

de Ziegler D, Cornel C, Bergeron C, Hazout A, Bouchard P, Frydman R (1991a) Controlled preparation of the endometrium with exogenous estradiol and progesterone in women having functioning ovaries. Fertil Steril 56:851–855

de Ziegler D, Bessis R, Frydman R (1991b) Vascular resistance of uterine arteries: physiological effects of estradiol and progesterone. Fertil Steril 55:775–779

de Ziegler D, Bergeron C, Cornel C et al (1992) Effects of luteal estradiol on the secretory transformation of human endometrium and plasma gonadotropins. J Clin Endocrinol Metab 74:322–331

de Ziegler D, Fanchin R, Bulletti C, Massonneau M (1996) Progesterone (P) decreases the frequency and alters the direction of peristaltic like contractions of the non pregnant uterus. Society of Gynecologic Investigation, Philadelphia

Eddy CA, Garcia RG, Kraemer DS, Pauerstein CJ (1975) Detailed time course of ovum transport in the rhesus monkey, Macaca mulatta. Biol Reprod 13:363–369

Eddy CA, Turner TG, Kraemer DS, Pauerstein CJ (1976) Pattern and duration of ovum transport in the baboon (Papio anubis). Obstet Gynecol 47:644–658

Fanchin R, Bergeron C, Leutr-Ksniusch H, Frydman R, Bouchard P, de Ziegler D (1993) Dose effect study of transvaginal progesterone (P) administration: discrepancy between plasma P and endometrial effects speaks for a first uterine pass. SGI

Forman R, Fries N, Testart J, Belaisch-Allart J, Hazout A, Frydman R (1988) Evidence for an adverse effect of elevated serum estradiol concentrations on embryo implantation. Fertil Steril 49:118–27

Fuentealba B, Nieto M, Croxatto HB (1987) Ovum transport in pregnant rats is little affected by RU 486 and exogenous progesterone as compared to cycling rats. Biol Reprod 37:768–774

Gosh D, Sengupta J (1994) Another look into the issue of peri-implantation oestrogen. Hum Reprod 10:1–7

Halme J, Hammond MG, Hulka JF, Raj SG, Talbert LM (1984) Retrograde menstruation in healthy women and in patients with endometriosis. J Am Coll Obstet Gynecol 64:151–154

Knutzen V, Stratton CJ, Sher G, McNamee PI, Huang TT, Soto-Albors C (1992) Mock embryo transfer in early luteal phase, the cycle before in vitro fertilization and embryo transfer: a descriptive Study. Fertil Steril 57:156–162

Lelaidier C, de Ziegler D, Freitas S, Olivennes F, Hazout A, Frydman R (1995) Endometrium preparation with exogeneous estradiol and progesterone for the transfer of cryopreserved blastocysts. Fertil Steril 63:919–921

Lutjen P, Traunson A, Leeton J, Findlay J, Wood C, Renow P (1984) The establishement and maintenance of pregnancy using in vitro fertilization and embryo donation in a patient with primary ovary failure. Nature 307:174–175

Lyons EA, Taylor PJ, Zheng XH, Ballard G, Levi CS, Kredentser JV (1991) Characterization of subendometrial myometrial contractions throughout the menstrual cycle in normal fertile women. Fertil Steril 55:771–774

Maia HS, Coutinho EM (1970) Peristalsis and antiperistalsis of the human fallopian tube during the menstrual cycle. Biol Reprod 2:305–314

Martinez-Gaudio M, Yoshida T, Bengtsson LP (1973) Propagated and non-propagated myometrial contractions in menstrual cycles. Am J Obstet Gynecol 115:107–111

Miles RA, Pauslon RJ, Lobo RA, Press MF, Dahmoush L, Sauer MV (1994) Pharmacokinetics and endometrial tissue levels of progesterone after administration by intramuscular and vaginal routes: a comparative study. Fertil Steril 62:485–490

Moawad AH, Bengtsson LP (1967) In vivo studies of the motility patterns of the nonpregnant human uterus. Am J Obstet Gynecol 98:1057–1064

Navot D, Laufer N, Kopolvic J et al (1984) Artificially induced endometrial cycles and establishement of pregnancies in the absence of ovaries. N Engl J Med 314:806–811

Navot D, Anderson TL, Doresch K, Scott RT, Kreiner D, Rosenwaks Z (1989) Hormonal manipulation of endometrial maturation. J Clin Endocrinol Metab 68:801–807

Navot D, Bergh PA, Williams M, Garrisi GJ, Guzman I, Sandler B, Fox J, Schreiner-Engel P, Hofman GE, Grunfeld L (1991) An insight into early reproductive process through the in vivo model of ovum donation. J Clin Endocrinol Metab 72:408–414

Nozaki M, Ito Y (1987) Changes in physiological properties of rabbit oviduct by ovarian steroids. Am J Physiol 252:R1059–1065

Rosenwaks Z (1987) Donor eggs: their application in modern reproductive technologies. Fertil Steril 47:895–909

Salamanka A, Beltran E (1995) Subendometrial contractility in menstrual phase visualized by transvaginal sonography in patients with endometriosis. Fertil Steril 64:193–195

Sampson JA (1927) Peritoneal endometriosis due to the menstrual dissemination of endometrial tissue into the peritoneal cavity. Am J Obstet Gynecol 14:422

Sauer MV, Pauson RJ, Ary BA, Lobo RA (1994) Three hundred cycles of oocyte donation at the University of Southern California: assessing the effect of age and infertility diagnosis on pregnancy and implantation rates. J Assist Reprod Genet 11:92–96

Younis JS, Ezra Y, Sherman Y, Simon A, Schenker JG, Laufer N (1994) The effect of estradiol depletion during the luteal phase on endometrial development. Fertil Steril 62:103–107

10 Clinical Significance of Integrin Cell Adhesion Molecules as Markers of Endometrial Receptivity

B.A. Lessey, A.J. Castelbaum, S.G. Somkuti, L. Yuan, and K. Chwalisz

10.1 Introduction

The advent of assisted reproductive technologies has focused attention on the endometrium as a critical component in the process of human reproduction. Despite the use of oocytes from young donors, in vitro fertilization success rates rarely exceed 40%. Unfortunately, our understanding of uterine receptivity has lagged behind other critical reproductive processes including oocyte and follicular maturation, fertilization, and tubal transport. A better understanding of the dynamic cascade culminating in implantation will lead to more targeted therapies for infertility, and possibly improved methods of contraception.

The histological criteria for evaluating luteal-phase endometrial maturation was noted by Noyes and colleagues nearly 50 years ago (Noyes et al. 1950). It remains a commonly used though crude index of uterine receptivity. Theoretically the endometrial biopsy is an in vivo assay of estrogen and progesterone effect. However, women with in-phase endometrium may exhibit significant variations in serum progesterone levels when measured singly or serially. In addition, many hormone-replacement regimes for donor oocyte embryos result in out-of-phase and yet receptive endometrium. The need for improved markers of uterine receptivity is apparent.

Integrins are a class of cell adhesion molecules in the uterus whose temporal and spatial expression makes them reliable markers of endometrial maturation and receptivity. Investigation of endometrial integrins has led to a more detailed understanding of uterine receptivity. Detailed examination of integrin expression during the midluteal phase has also suggested the existence of multiple types of defects in uterine receptivity in certain women with infertility (Lessey et al. 1992, 1994b, 1995a). Recent insights into the coregulation of endometrial integrins and progesterone receptors during the midluteal phase are provocative and may lead to better in vitro models for the study of implantation (Lessey et al. 1996a).

10.2 Integrins: A Family of Cell Adhesion Molecules

Integrins are a family of transmembrane glycoproteins, identified almost a decade ago, as the *integral* receptors for the extracellular matrix (ECM; Horwitz et al. 1985; Buck et al. 1986; Buck and Horwitz 1987; Hynes 1987; Ruoslahti and Pierschbacher 1987; Hemler et al. 1987; DeSimone et al. 1987). They are heterodimeric complexes of α- and β-subunits. To date, 15 α- and 8 β-subunits have been characterized, and their number is expected to grow (Ruoslahti et al. 1994). While the combinatorial potential of such a large number of subunits is staggering, the actual number of known integrins is more limited (presently numbering 20) because of constraints on subunit pairing. The integrins play substantive roles in such diverse processes as the immune response, wound healing, cellular development and differentiation, tumor metastasis, and mammalian fertilization (Hynes 1992) and perhaps are involved in the process of human implantation as well (Lessey et al. 1992; Tabibzadeh 1992).

The integrin receptor binding region for ECM requires amino acid sequences from both the α- and β-subunits. Different integrins recognize various ligands, and ligand preference for a given integrin may vary depending on the cell type involved (Elices and Hemler 1989; Elices et al. 1991; Languino et al. 1989) or the cells' membrane composition (Conforti et al. 1990). The cytoplasmic tail of the subunit may regulate extracellular conformation and ligand preference (Filardo and Cheresh 1994) and has functions in signal transduction (Chan et al. 1992). The β-subunit interacts with the actin filaments of the cytoskeleton through connections by the cytoplasmic tail with protein components such as talin and α-actinin (Hemler 1990) and may also play a role in both signal transduction (Akiyama et al. 1994) and the regulation of a migratory versus stationary phenotype (Pasqualini and Hemler 1994).

All cells express integrins on their surface (except red blood cells). Many different integrins are present on any given cell and a variety of cells often express the same integrin. The pattern of integrin expression ultimately forms the basis for certain characteristics of the cell, including its location within a tissue, cell shape and polarity, even its ability to respond to steroid hormones (Streuli et al. 1991). Epithelial cells, for example, maintain a repertoire of integrins distinct from that of stromal or vascular cells. In this way integrins appear to have a central role in cellular differentiation and offer a molecular paradigm for the relationship between cellular structure and function.

10.3 Regulation of Integrin Expression

The regulation of integrin expression is complex and cell type specific. While exceptions exist, the two central integrin subunits α_v and β_1, each pair with many other subunits and appear to be made in abundance (Heino et al. 1989; Sheppard et al. 1992). By tightly regulating the production of the other pairing subunits the cell controls expression of specific intact integrins, and thus cellular morphology.

Cells express only those integrins required to maintain function appropriate to that cell. A hallmark of malignant cells is a disordered pattern of integrin expression, contributing to an aberrant cellular phenotype (Ruoslahti 1992). Loss of a specific integrin ($\alpha_2\beta_1$) expression in endometrial adenocarcinoma cells was found to be associated with an increased incidence of nodal metastases (Lessey et al. 1995b). Similarly, altered integrin expression has been noted for metastatic melanoma (Albelda et al. 1990), breast (Koukoulis et al. 1991), and gastrointestinal tumors (Koretz et al. 1991).

Environmental stressors can rapidly change the integrin composition of normal cells. For example, when skin is injured, fibroblasts respond with an immediate alteration in genomic expression of specific integrins (Cheresh 1991). "Up regulation" of ECM production and stimulation of cell migration and/or proliferation is a critical part of the repair process, basic to our survival. An "adhesion cascade" directed at modulation of cell adhesion molecular expression contributes significantly to the inflammation process (Albelda et al. 1994).

Growth factors and cytokines are important regulators of integrins. Endothelial cells increase their expression of $\alpha_2\beta_1$, $\alpha_3\beta_1$, $\alpha_5\beta_1$, $\alpha_6\beta_1$, $\alpha_6\beta_4$, and $\alpha_v\beta_5$ in response to basic fibroblast growth factor (bFGF) and simultaneously "downregulate" $\alpha_1\beta_1$ and $\alpha_v\beta_3$ (Boll et al. 1991). Conversely, the inflammatory cytokines interleukin-1 and tumor necrosis factor-α cause a decline in $\alpha_6\beta_1$ (Defilippi et al. 1992), and an increase in $\alpha_v\beta_3$ on endothelial cells (Leslie et al. 1990) and endometrial stromal cells (Grosskinsky et al. 1996) in vitro. These cytokines also increase $\alpha_1\beta_1$ expression on fibroblasts (Santala and Heino 1991). The paracrine and autocrine cross-talk between cytokines and integrins is an exciting and evolving area of cellular biology, with wide implications for human health and disease states.

Transforming growth factor-β appears to be an important growth factor in the modulation of integrins and the ECM in general. It has known roles in cell proliferation and differentiation (D'Souza et al. 1990; Sporn et al. 1987), tissue remodeling, and repair (Mustoe et al. 1987) and appears to promote the synthesis and secretion of several ECM components, including fibronectin, osteopontin, and proteoglycans (Ignotz and Massagué 1986; Bassols and Massagué 1988; Noda et al. 1988; Pearson et al. 1988). This growth factor also appears to inhibit ECM degradation (Laiho et al. 1986) and alter specific integrin expression in many cell types (Milazzo et al. 1992; Ignotz and Massague 1987; Sheppard et al. 1992; Ignotz et al. 1989; Heino and Massague 1989; Santala and Heino 1991). The changing patterns of transforming growth factor-β in human endometrium during the menstrual cycle is likely involved in regulating the dynamic patterns of integrin expression noted there (Chegini et al. 1994).

10.4 Integrins in the Endometrium

We and others have previously described the temporal and spatial distribution of endometrial integrins throughout the menstrual cycle and early pregnancy (Lessey et al. 1992; Tabibzadeh 1992; Van der Linden et al. 1995; Klentzeris et al. 1993; Ruck et al. 1994; Bridges et al. 1994). The endometrial epithelium expresses those integrins that recognize basement membrane components (laminin and collagen), while mesenchyme (stromal cells) express receptors for fibronectin. As shown in Fig. 1, a photomicrograph of immunostaining for various integrin subunits, epithelial cells express $\alpha_2\beta_1$ (A), $\alpha_3\beta_1$ (B), $\alpha_6\beta_1$, and $\alpha_6\beta_4$ (C and D). The stromal cells express primarily $\alpha_5\beta_1$, the classic fibronectin receptor (F).

While most endometrial integrins are constitutively expressed, several integrins are coexpressed only during cycle day 20–24, thought to correspond to a *window* of implantation (Bergh et al. 1992), and therefore have been intensively examined as candidate markers of uterine receptivity (Lessey et al. 1992; Tabibzadeh 1992; Lessey et al. 1994a). Trophoblast invasion and degradation of the ECM are critical to early placentation. Interestingly, the pattern of integrin expression in the decidual tissue of early pregnancy differs significantly from that seen in the luteal phase (Lessey et al. 1994a; Ruck et al. 1994). Hormonal and growth factor signals may be an important regulatory components of the transformation of secretory endometrium into decidua.

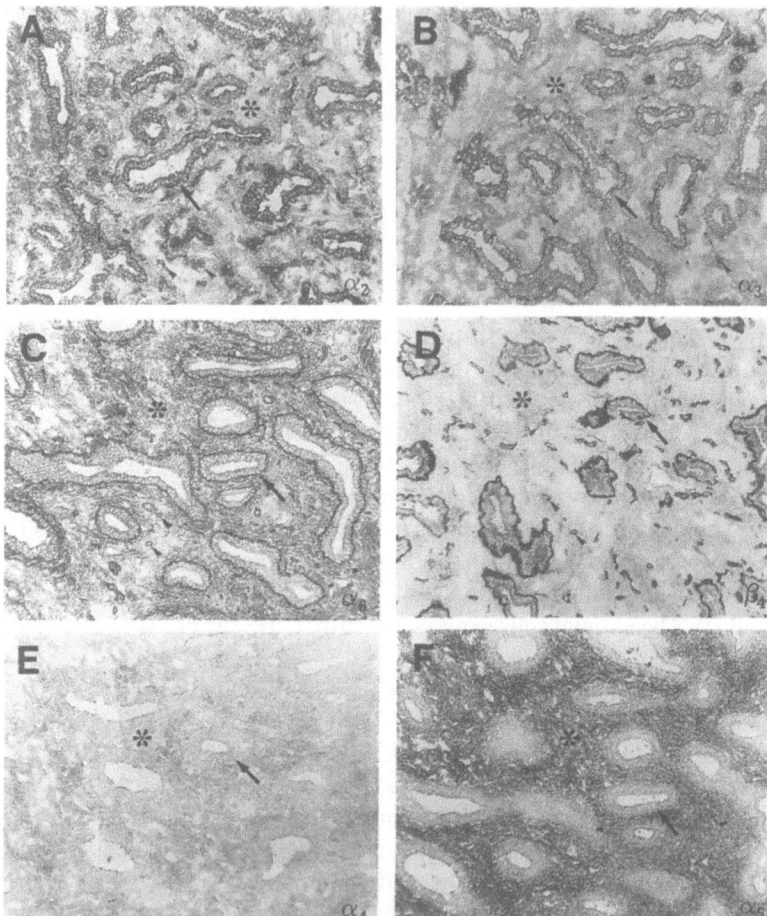

Fig. 1A–F. The profile of integrins in normal endometrium in frozen sections. Immunohistochemical staining of the collagen/laminin receptor subunits: α_2 (**A**), α_3 (**B**), α_6 (**C**), and β_4 (**D**) shows prominent staining of epithelium (*arrows*) and microvessels (*arrowheads*) without significant stromal staining (*asterisks*) for α_2, α_3, and β_4. Note basolateral staining α_3 and α_6, and basal staining for β_4. The immunoreactions (*dark staining*) were developed by the avidin-biotin-peroxidase complex using diaminobenzidine as a chromagen. For greater sensitivity, no counterstain was applied. ×125. (Lessey et al. 1992, with permission from Rockefeller Press, New York)

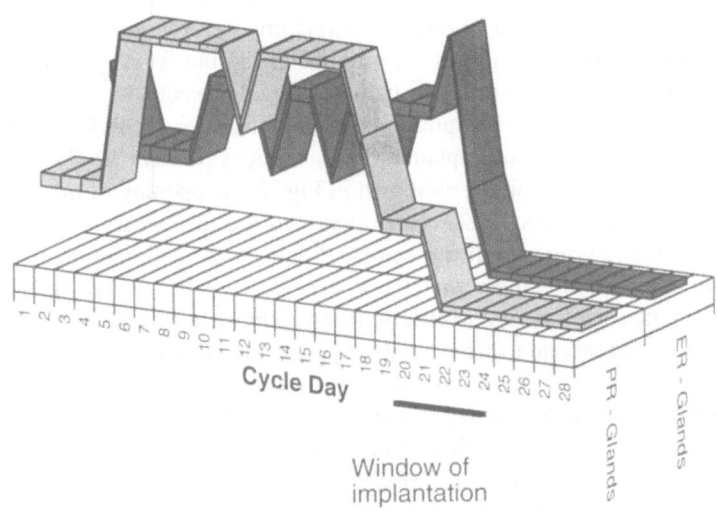

Fig. 2. Relative immunohistochemical staining intensities for estrogen and progesterone receptors during the normal menstrual cycle. (Adapted from Garcia et al. 1988)

10.4.1 Steroid Hormones and the Establishment of Uterine Receptivity

It has long been suspected that the endometrium undergoes a defined period of receptivity (for review, see Rogers and Murphy 1989; Stallmach et al. 1992; Anderson and Hodgen 1989). Using the rabbit model, Chung (1950) demonstrated the ability to transfer embryos from a hyperstimualted donor animal to a recipient uterus and successfully achieve pregnancy. A "window of implantation" may have been first suggested by Finn (1977) but has been demonstrated in various animal models (Beier 1974; Hodgen 1983; Psychoyos 1986). Only recently has the demonstration of a temporal window been systematically described in the human (Navot et al. 1986, 1991a,b) using the model of donor embryos into hormonally prepared recipients. The timing of embryo attachment in the human was initially suggested by the work of Hertig et al. (1956), who evaluated luteal-phase hysterectomy specimens for the presence of early gestations. All free-floating embryos were found in the uteri of women undergoing hysterectomy before cycle day 19–20, whereas implanted embryos were uniformly found from cycle day 21 onward. More recent studies utilizing extremely sensitive β-hCG serum measurements during cryopreserved embryo transfer cycles has defined a presumed window of implantation spanning cycle days 20–24 (Bergh et al. 1992). Interestingly, as shown in Fig. 2, the opening of this "window" on cycle days 19–20, corresponds to the disappearance of both estrogen and progesterone receptors (PR) from the endometrial epithelium. This would imply that these steroids may have dual functions within the secretory endometrium: first to stimulate synthesis of certain proteins and second to temporarily suppress the production of others. A receptor-mediated paradigm for embryo attachment and invasion has been postulated (Yoshinaga 1989) as has the establishment of blocking proteins such as mucins (Surveyor 1993). The timely disappearance of epithelial PR creates a *functional* loss of progesterone, despite rising serum levels of these hormone in the midsecretory phase and may explain some of the shifts in protein expression that have been described during the time of maximal uterine receptivity.

10.4.2 Integrin Expression and Endometrial Receptivity

The hallmark of endometrial integrins appears to be their complex pattern of temporal and spatial changes during the menstrual cycle and in early pregnancy. As outlined above, growth factors and cytokines are actively involved in the regulation of integrin expression. The endometrium is the first example of steroid hormone regulation of integrin expression (Lessey et al. 1992; 1994a; Tabibzadeh 1992). Surveillance of endometrial integrins may offer insights into the complex and dynamic processes of endometrial receptivity and implantation. As shown in the scattergram (Fig. 3) and photomicrographs (Fig. 4), three integrins appear to undergo orchestrated changes on endometrial epithelium during the menstrual cycle. Each of the three, $\alpha_1\beta_1$ (a collagen-laminin receptor), $\alpha_4\beta_1$ (a fibronectin receptor), and $\alpha_v\beta_3$ (the vitronectin receptor), exhibit increased immunostaining during the secretory phase of the menstrual cycle. There is coexpression of the $\alpha_4\beta_1$ and $\alpha_v\beta_3$ integrins

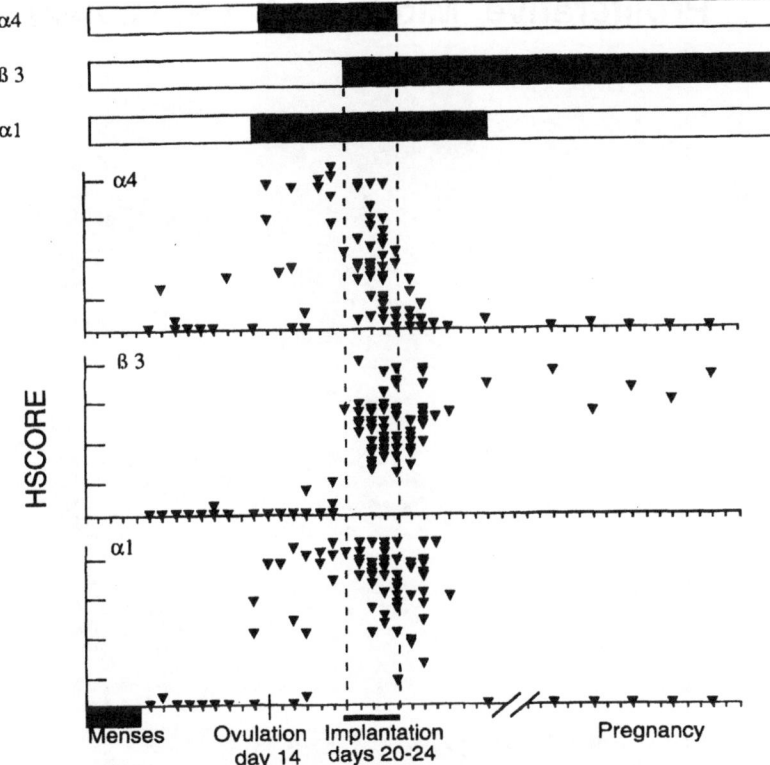

Fig. 3. Relative intensity of staining for the epithelial α_4, β_3, and α_1 integrin subunits throughout the menstrual cycle and in early pregnancy. Immunohisto-chemical staining was assessed by a blinded observer using the semi-quantita-tive HSCORE (ranging from 0 to 4), as previously described (Lessey et al. 1994a), and correlation to the estimate of histological dating based on patho-logical criteria or by last menstrual period in patients undergoing therapeutic pregnancy termination. The negative staining (*open bars*) was shown for im-munostaining of an average HSCORE ≤ 0.7, for each of the three integrin subunits. Positive staining for all three integrin subunits was seen only during a 4-day interval corresponding to cycle days 20–24, based on histological dating criteria. This interval of integrin coexpression corresponds to the putative win-dow of implantation. Of the three only the $\alpha_v\beta_3$ integrin was seen in the epi-thelium of pregnant endometrium. (From Lessey et al. 1994a, reproduced with permission of the American Fertility Society)

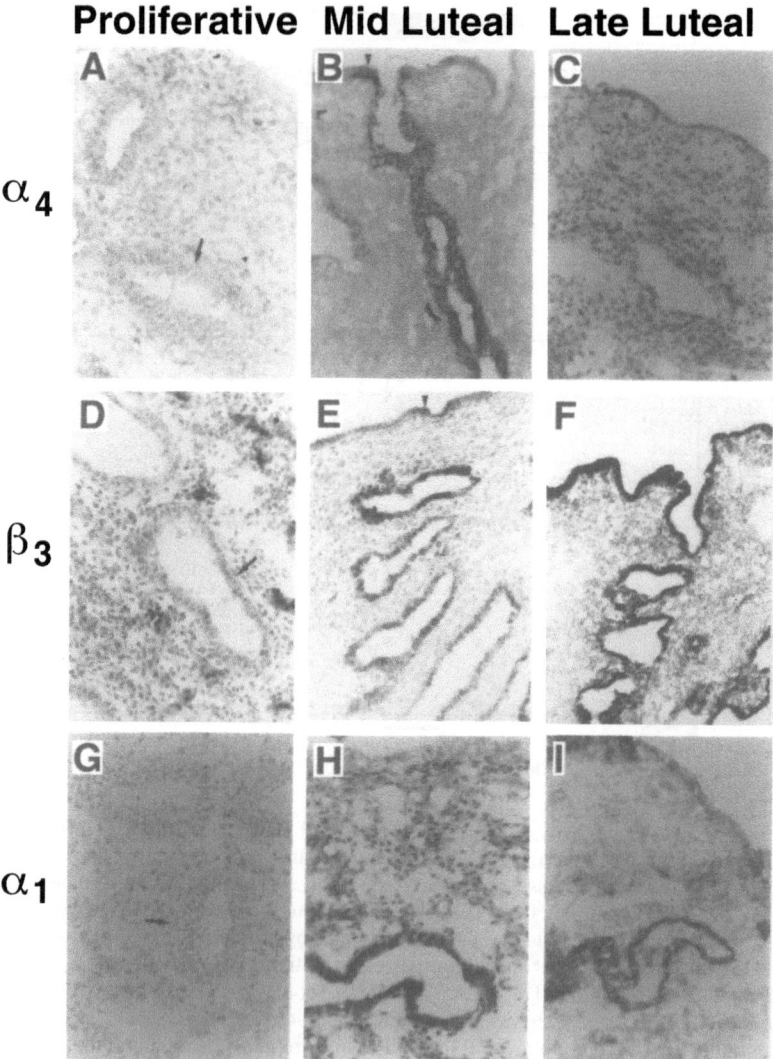

Proliferative   Mid Luteal   Late Luteal

α_4

β_3

α_1

Fig. 4. Legend see p. 203

during the putative window of implantation. These integrins serve as markers of normal endometrial maturation and endometrial receptivity. These particular integrins are of interest, since each of them bind ligands associated with the embryo, and therefore may be actively involved in the process of implantation. The $\alpha_4\beta_1$ integrin binds the alternatively spliced form of fibronectin (oncofetal fibronectin). The $\alpha_v\beta_3$ vitronectin receptor recognizes multiple Arg-Gly-Asp (RGD) containing ligands and may confer the ability of a cell with this integrin to interact with other cells which possess $\alpha_v\beta_3$. It is now known that the embryo expresses fetal fibronectin (Feinberg et al. 1991), and both mouse (Sutherland et al. 1993) and human embryos (Campbell et al. 1995) possess the $\alpha_v\beta_3$ vitronectin receptors on the outer apical cell surfaces. A candidate bridging molecules which contain the RGD sequence (osteopontin) have also been identified in the human endometrium (Young et al. 1990) and proposed to be involved in implantation (Coutifaris and Lessey 1993).

We (Lessey et al. 1992, 1994b, 1995a) and others (Klentzeris et al. 1993) have noted aberrant expression of integrin in certain infertility states (see below). Hormonal deficiency (Lessey et al. 1992) or disruption of normal paracrine cross-talk (Lessey et al. 1994b) may predispose to these observed defects in integrin expression and potential alterations

---

◀ **Fig. 4A–I.** Immunostaining of α_4, β_3, and α_1 integrin subunits in proliferative phase vs. middle and late secretory phase endometrium. The staining intensity of α_4, β_3, and α_1 in the proliferative phase (**A,D,G**, respectively), middle (**B,E,H**, respectively) and late luteal-phase (**C,F,I**, respectively) endometrium. Epithelial staining was judged as "0" HSCORE for all three integrin subunits in the proliferative epithelial cells (*arrowheads*; **A,D,G**). Immunostaining for α_4 in day 22 endometrium (**B**; example of an HSCORE of 2.5), β_3 (**E**) and α_1 (**H**) demonstrates a significant increase in glandular staining. All three integrin subunits were expressed on glandular epithelial cells of the midluteal phase (**B,E,H**). Note the increase in luminal β_3 staining (corresponding to an HSCORE of 3.5) in late luteal phase (**E**), whereas α_4 and α_1 failed to be expressed on luminal epithelium at any time during the menstrual cycle, though extension of staining to include the luminal epithelium around the glandular orifice was often seen (**B,E**). The α_4 immunostaining was absent on glandular epithelium after day 24 (**C**), while both α_1 and β_3 continued to be expressed (F and I, respectively). ×100–200. (From Lessey1994a, reproduced with permission by theAmerican Fertility Society)

in uterine receptivity. Insights into the regulation of endometrial integrins among fertile and infertile women will be important in developing better diagnostic and treatment strategies for infertile couples and towards the development of improved contraceptive techniques.

10.5 Significance of Integrins for Infertility and Contraception

In the context of a book on targeting the endometrium for contraception it is useful to examine defects in uterine receptivity found in varied infertility states. Infertility affects up to 2.5 million couples in the United States (Marchbanks et al. 1989) and this number is expected to grow with the aging of the "baby boom" generation. Luteal-phase deficiency and endometriosis are two disorders that we feel manifest infertility on the basis of defects in endometrial function. Luteal-phase deficiency may account for up to 20% of all cases of infertility (Li and Cooke 1991). Endometriosis affects only 5% of the general population but is found in up to 40% of women with infertility (Verkauf 1987; Mahmood and Templeton 1991). A high percentage of women with unexplained infertility may also have abnormal endometrium (Lessey et al. 1994a; Li and Cooke 1992).

We have postulated two distinct types of uterine receptivity defects (Lessey et al. 1994a). In the first, designated "type I" defects, the endometrium is histologically delayed, presumably due to inadequate progesterone secretion or action. In 1992 we demonstrated that women with "out-of-phase" endometrium also have a delayed appearance of the $\alpha_v\beta_3$ integrin. The $\alpha_v\beta_3$ integrin is usually expressed by cycle day 20 (Lessey et al. 1992), coincident with the opening of the window of implantation. In a second putative pathway, designated "type II" defects, the endometrium appears histologically in phase, no $\alpha_v\beta_3$ is expressed (Lessey et al. 1994b). These type II defects are occult since conventional histology as judged by Noyes criteria is found to be normal. This newly designated defect is seen primarily in women with minimal and mild endometriosis, but was also seen in women with hydrosalpinges (Lessey et al. 1994) and endometritis (unpublished data). Evaluating the endometrium with markers of uterine receptivity may allow identification of occult uterine receptivity defects analogous to the clomid challenge test in uncovering occult diminished ovarian reserve.

That mild or minimal endometriosis is associated with infertility has been suggested by numerous investigators (see review see Bancroft et al. 1989) and by at least two prospective controlled laparoscopic studies (Verkauf 1987; Mahmood and Templeton 1991). The mechanism by which minimal endometriosis causes infertility, however, remains uncertain and controversial (Bancroft et al. 1989). Adverse effects on folliculogenesis (Doody et al. 1988; Lentz et al. 1990), ovulation (Schenken et al. 1984; Brosens et al. 1978), luteal-phase function (Grant 1966; Cheesman et al. 1982; Ayers et al. 1987), ovum transport (Drake et al. 1981; Suginami et al. 1990), sperm quality (Soldati et al. 1989) and function (Klein et al. 1990), fertilization (Sueldo et al. 1987), and embryo quality (Morcos et al. 1985; Damewood et al. 1990) have all been postulated to contribute to the infertility seen in these patients. Peritoneal fluid factors and/or the activation of peritoneal macrophages (Haney et al. 1981; Halme et al. 1983), and alterations in immune function (Dmowski et al. 1981; Oosterlynck et al. 1991) have been implicated in these effects. Few researchers that have suggested that uterine receptivity is adversely affected by the presence of endometriosis (Muscato et al. 1982; Yovich et al. 1988; Lessey et al. 1994b), yet limited data from surgically induced endometriosis in animal models support this hypothesis (Hahn et al. 1986). Structural and biochemical abnormalities of the native endometrium have been described as well, in women with endometriosis when compared to that of normal fertile controls (Fedele et al. 1990).

10.6 Progesterone and Defects in Endometrial Receptivity

To study the role of progesterone in these potential uterine receptivity defects we have previously employed in vivo and in vitro models. Endometrial integrins, as demonstrated above, appear to be hormonally regulated. Using the well-differentiated adenocarcinoma cell line, the Ishikawa cells, we have examined the role of the sex steroids in the expression of two of these cycle-dependent integrins, $\alpha_1\beta_1$ and $\alpha_v\beta_3$. These cells maintain functional estrogen and progesterone receptors (Lessey et al. 1996a) and express integrins similar to normal en-

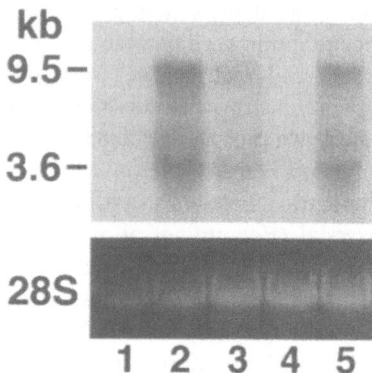

Fig. 5. Northern blot of total RNA from Ishikawa cells treated with estradiol, progesterone, and antiprogestin, onapristone. Equal amounts of total RNA were loaded (see the 28S ribosomal subunit, *bottom lane*) from Ishikawa endometrial adenocarcinoma cells treated with no steroids (lane 1), estradiol (10–8 *M*), estradiol plus progesterone (10–6 *M*), progesterone alone, or estradiol plus progesterone plus the antiprogestin onapristone (ZK-98299). There was an increased induction of progesterone receptor transcripts in the estradiol treated group, blocked by the addition of progesterone. The inhibitory effect of progesterone on PR was reversed by the addition of the antiprogestin onapristone

dometrial epithelium (Castelbaum et al. 1995). As with endometrial epithelium (Lessey et al. 1992; Tabibzadeh 1992), Ishikawa cells express the α_1 subunit in response to progesterone, and this increase is blocked by the antiprogestin, ZK-98299 (Onapristone). As shown in the northern blot (Fig. 5), PR is increased by the action of estradiol (lane 2) but downregulated by the presence of estradiol plus progesterone (lane 3) or progesterone alone (lane 4). The effect of progesterone is reversed by the addition of equimolar Onapristone (lane 5). The α_1 subunit is also specifically increased by estradiol plus progesterone in these cells (Lessey et al. 1996a) and this effect is blocked by antiprogestin treatment. These cells also express the $\alpha_v\beta_3$ integrin. The availability of a cell line that maintains functional ER and PR will likely increase our ability to directly study the regulation of hormonally regulated integrins in endometrial epithelium.

To examine the relationship between progesterone action and integrins as markers of endometrial receptivity, immunohistochemistry was employed on endometrial biopsies from women with infertility and suspected defects in endometrial receptivity (Lessey et al. 1996b). The results of immunohistochemistry for PR was significantly different in women with luteal-phase defect (LPD, type I defects) compared to those with suspected "type II" defects and endometriosis, those with LPD who were medically treated and compared to fertile and infertile controls ($p \leq .001$). In cases of histologic delay there was a greater expression of epithelial PR, normally downregulated by cycle days 20–24.

The integrin profile between groups was not different for epithelial $\alpha_1\beta_1$ or $\alpha_4\beta_1$ between groups (data not shown). In contrast, the $\alpha_v\beta_3$ integrin was significantly reduced in the epithelial cells of endometrial biopsies from women with LPD and in women with type II defects, but present in the patients with corrected LPD and the fertile and infertile controls. These data are summarized in Fig. 6.

While it is possible that integrins play a direct role in the cascade of molecular events leading to implantation, there is little doubt that circulating progesterone and the endometrial PR are critical to nidation (Baulieu 1989). Based on this study, epithelial PRs are downregulated in normal, in-phase endometrium at the time of implantation. Progesterone receptors persist, however, in women with histological delay consistent with LPD. Using the $\alpha_v\beta_3$ integrin as markers of receptivity, it was shown that women with LPD and persistence of PR have aberrant (low) $\alpha_v\beta_3$ expression that corrected following medical treatment. Women with type II defects and in-phase endometrium were also missing the $\alpha_v\beta_3$ integrin but had normal downregulation of PR and in-phase endometrium.

It is likely that paracrine mediators also play a role in the regulation and dysregulation of endometrial function. As demonstrated by these data, progesterone and its receptor act in concert to regulate at least two of the cycle-dependent integrins in the human endometrium. In the case of $\alpha_1\beta_1$ progesterone is clearly stimulatory. For $\alpha_v\beta_3$ progesterone in estrogen-primed endometrial epithelium appears to be inhibitory. While the action of progesterone can be understood in the context of LPD (the lack of PR disappearance results in continued suppression of the $\alpha_v\beta_3$ integrin), it cannot explain the lack of this marker in women with type II defects and endometriosis. As previously postulated, paracrine or in-

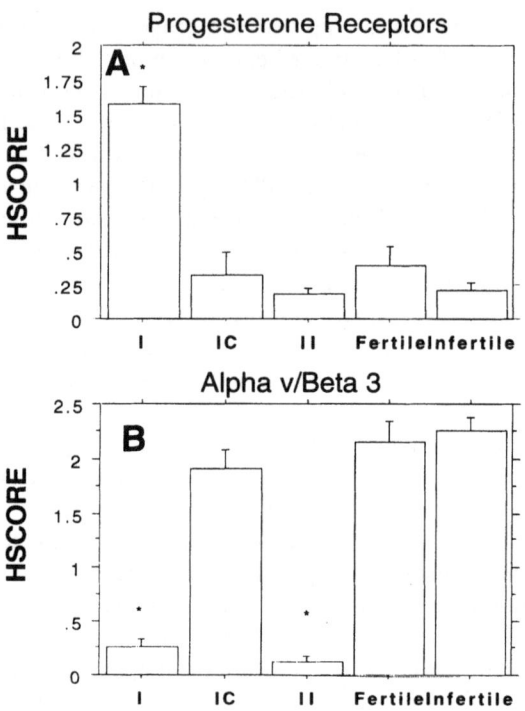

Fig. 6A,B. Relative intensity of staining for the epithelial β3 integrin subunit and progesterone receptor in endometrial biopsies from fertile and infertile women. **A** Immunostaining was compared for PR in epithelial cells in women with out-of-phase histology before (*OOP*; type I defects; $n=80$) and after successful medical treatment (*IC*; $n=16$), women with in-phase endometrium, endometriosis and aberrant β3 expression (type II defects; $n=21$), and fertile ($n=26$) and infertile ($n=38$) controls. **B** Similar comparisons were made for the $\alpha_v\beta_3$. Intensity and distribution of staining was quantified using the semiquantitative HSCORE as previously reported (Lessey et al. 1994a). A significant elevation in PR was seen only in OOP endometrial biopsies, in epithelial cells. The elevation of PR may account for the loss of β3 expression found in women with OOP biopsies but cannot account for the loss of this integrin in type II defects, since PR was normally suppressed in these women. *Asterisks*, significant differences, using analysis of variance with Scheffe's correction. (Adapted from Lessey et al. 1995c)

flammatory cytokine mediated changes may prevent the timely expression of this integrin in such cases (Lessey et al. 1994b).

10.7 Pharmacological Strategies
to Target the Endometrium for Contraception

The importance of progesterone on the events of implantation have led researchers to develop strategies to disrupt the window of implantation by pharmacological methods. Synthetic antiprogestins such as ZK 98.734 (Schering, Berlin, Germany) and RU 486 (Roussel-Uclaf, Romainville, France) are potent inhibitors of progesterone action and have been shown by Beier and co-workers to delay key protein markers of uterine receptivity in the rabbit (Hegele-Hartung and Beier 1986; Beier et al. 1987). These data have been extended and demonstrate indirect effects on corpus luteum function as well (Beier et al. 1991; Hegele-Hartung et al. 1992) and have set the stage for the use of antiprogestins in humans (Beier et al. 1994).

Based on the data presented above, one of the primary effects of progesterone in the uterus is the timely demise of its own receptor in endometrial epithelium. The onset of uterine receptivity may be determined not only by the timely expression of progesterone-induced proteins, but also perhaps the release of progesterone suppressed factors. The integrins are reliable and dynamically expressed marker proteins of the window of implantation in humans. As such, we propose that they may be useful to study the hormonal and paracrine factors that influence the onset of receptivity in women. The lack of $\alpha_v\beta_3$ expression is associated with infertility and an insufficiency in circulating progesterone (Lessey et al. 1992). Alternatively, aberrant expression of $\alpha_v\beta_3$ is seen in endometriosis, in which we postulate the presence of an altered paracrine milieu in or around the endometrium (Lessey et al. 1994b). The former condition (LPD) is characterized by abnormalities in the distribution of the epithelial PR; the causative agent in the latter remains undefined.

Targeting the endometrium for purposes of contraception might involve either paracrine or endocrine manipulation. Analogous to the effect on uteroglobin (Hegele-Hartung and Beier 1986), antiprogestins administered in the proliferative or early secretory phase could delay the action of progesterone in downregulation of its own receptor. As illustrated above in both in vitro and in vivo studies, this would be expected to result in disturbances in the expression of $\alpha_v\beta_3$ and probably other peptides involved in implantation. It is likely that appropriately designed treatment would have few side effects other than slight alterations in cycle length. We recently demonstrated that pharmacological intervention in the form of oral contraceptives results in endometrial integrin profiles that are representative of "nonreceptive" endometrium (Somkuti et al. 1996). Postcoital contraception with antiprogestins such as RU-486 and high dose oral contraceptive are both highly efficacious, presumably through alterations in the establishment of endometrial receptivity. A preliminary study of late luteal biopsy specimens from women using the Yuzpe postcoital regime demonstrated no alteration in integrin expression (Taskin et al. 1994), though the methods used did not specifically examine the window of implantation (Lessey 1994).

Infertility patients with minimal or mild endometriosis are frequently asymptomatic. Lessons learned from the infertility associated with this disorder might one day allow a form of contraception based on paracrinology designed to prevent the expression of essential peptides involved in the cascade of molecular events leading to successful implantation. Factors present in the peritoneal fluid may hold the key to this pursuit. As previously demonstrated, transfer of peritoneal fluid from rabbits with surgically induced endometriosis into healthy rabbits is sufficient to recreate the defect in implantation noted in the animals with this disease (Hahn et al. 1986). Similar studies may be possible using in vitro models with peritoneal fluid from women with endometriosis and aberrant $\alpha_v\beta_3$ expression (Illera et al. 1995).

Fig. 7A–D. Schematic of possible mechanisms of contraception based on targeting endometrial receptivity. **A** Normally a period of receptivity defined the time of embryo attachment and invasion. **B** In LPD or after pharmacological intervention with antiprogestins this window may be shifted. **C** In endometriosis or through paracrine mediators the critical biochemical events of receptivity might be effectively blocked. **D** If integrins on embryo or endometrium are critical to inttial implantation events, competitive blockade of binding sites with specific amino acid sequences might effect a contraceptive outcome

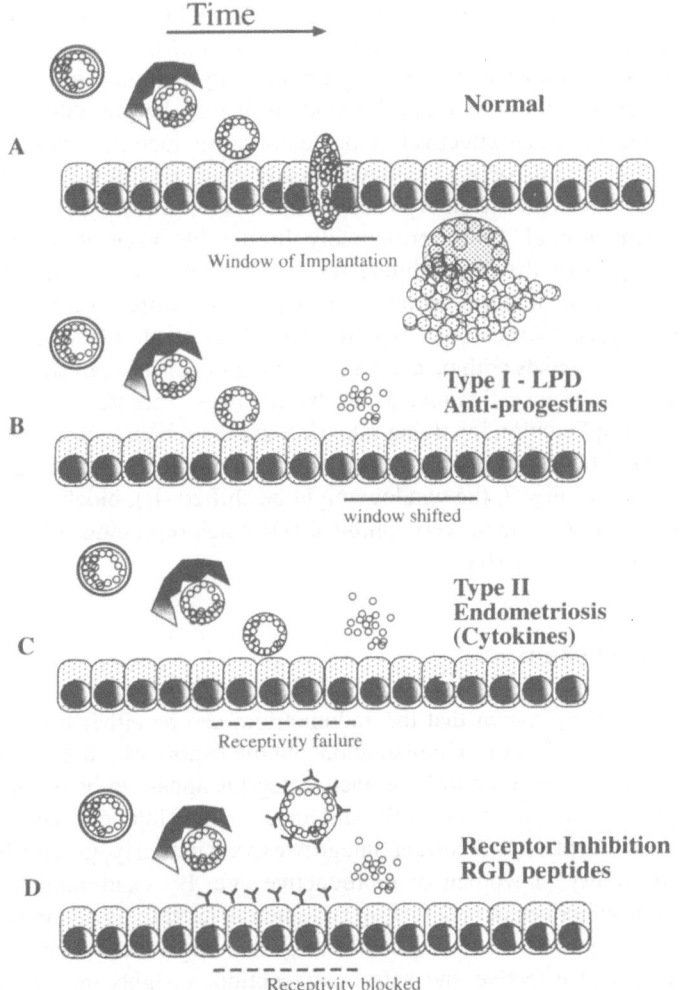

Fig. 7. Legend see p. 210

Finally, the function of integrins as cell adhesion molecules suggests that integrins themselves may be directly involved in embryo attachment to the endometrial lining. As each integrin maintins short amino acid target sequences required for binding, it may be possible to discover sequences that effectively block embryo interaction with the endometrium. Extensive studies have already been performed showing that RGD blocks mouse embryo attachment and outgrowth (Yelian et al. 1993; Armant et al. 1986), presumably through blockade of either the $\alpha_v\beta_3$ integrin or the $\alpha_5\beta_1$ fibronectin receptor. Recent evidence also suggests that α_4 integrin subunit is essential for normal placentation, based on gene "knock-out" experiments (Yang et al. 1995). As the endometrium makes both α_4 and β_3 containing integrins, both strategies warrant further investigation. Thus, based on a "receptor-mediated" model of implantation involving integrins and the window of implantation, three different strategies for contraception might be envisioned. As summarized in Fig. 7, the window might be shifted (B), biochemically inhibited (C) or competitively inhibited (D). Each represents a testable hypothesis for future studies.

10.8 Conclusions

It has long been known that the endometrium can be either hostile or receptive towards embryo implantation, but the factors which determine this dichotomy remain poorly defined. Integrins appear to be excellent cycle-specific markers of both endometrial development and endometrial receptivity. Aberrant integrin expression may predict low cycle fecundity in women of reproductive age. By examining those conditions which result in defects in endometrial receptivity and infertility it may be possible to devise new strategies to target the endometrium as a means of effective and safe contraception. Insights into uterine receptivity, using integrins as markers of implantation, may lead to rapid advances from benchtop investigation into practical therapies for infertility and family planning.

References

Akiyama SK, Yamada SS, Yamada KM, LaFlamme SE (1994) Transmembrane signal transduction by integrin cytoplasmic domains expressed in single-subunit chimeras. J Biol Chem 269:15961–15964

Albelda SM, Mette SA, Elder DE et al (1990) Integrin distribution in malignant melanoma: association of the beta 3 subunit with tumor progression. Cancer Res 50:6757–6764

Albelda SM, Smith CW, Ward PA (1994) Adhesion molecules and inflammatory injury. FASEB J 8:504–512

Anderson TL, Hodgen GD (1989) Uterine receptivity in the primate. Prog Clin Biol Res 294:389–399

Armant DR, Kaplan HA, Mover H, Lennarz WJ (1986) The effect of hexapeptides on attachment and outgrowth of mouse blastocysts cultured in vitro: evidence for the involvement of the cell recognition tripeptide Arg-Gly-Asp. Proc Natl Acad Sci U S A 83:6751–6755

Ayers JW, Birenbaum DL, Menon KM (1987) Luteal phase dysfunction in endometriosis: elevated progesterone levels in peripheral and ovarian veins during the follicular phase. Fertil Steril 47:925–929

Bancroft K, Vaughan Williams CA, Elstein M (1989) Minimal/mild endometriosis and infertility. A review. Br J Obstet Gynaecol 96:454–460

Bassols A, Massagué J (1988) Transforming growth factor b regulates the expression and structure of extracellular matrix chondroitin/dermatan sulfate proteoglycans. J Biol Chem 263:3039–3045

Baulieu EE (1989) Contragestion and other clinical applications of RU-486, an antiprogesterone at the receptor. Science 245:1351–1357

Beier HM, Elger W, Hegele-Hartung C (1987) Effects of antiprogestins on the endometrium during the luteal phase after postovulatory treatment. In: Naftolin F, DeCherney A (eds) The control of follicular development, ovulation and luteal function. Lessons from in vitro fertilization. Raven, New York, pp 331–343 (Serono symposia publications, vol 35)

Beier HM, Elger W, Hegele-Hartung C, Mootz U, Beier-Hellwig K (1992) Dissociation of corpus luteum, endometrium and blastocyst in human implantation research. J Reprod Fertil 92:511–523

Beier HM, Hegele-Hartung C, Mootz U, Beier-Hellwig K (1994) Modification of endometrial cell biology using progesterone antagonists to manipulate the implantation window. Hum Reprod 9 [Suppl 1]:98–115

Bergh PA, Navot D (1992) The impact of embryonic development and endometrial maturity on the timing of implantation. Fertil Steril 58:537–542

Boll W, Partin JS, Katz AI, Caplan MJ, Jamieson JD (1991) Distinct pathways for basolateral targeting of membrane and secretory proteins in polarized epithelial cells. Proc Natl Acad Sci U S A 88:8592–8596

Bridges JE, Prentice A, Roche W, Englefield P, Thomas EJ (1994) Expression of integrin adhesion molecules in endometrium and endometriosis. Br J Obstet Gynaecol 101:696–700

Brosens IA, Koninckx PR, Corveleyn PA (1978) A study of plasma progesterone, oestradiol-17β, prolactin and LH levels, and of the luteal phase appearance of the ovaries in patients with endometriosis and infertility. Br J Obstet Gynaecol 85:246–250

Buck CA, Shea E, Duggan K, Horwitz AF (1986) Integrin (the CSAT antigen):Functionality requires oligomeric integrity. J Cell Biol 103:2421–2428

Buck CA, Horwitz AF (1987) Integrin, a transmembrane glycoprotein complex mediating cell-substratum adhesion. J Cell Sci Suppl 8:231–250

Campbell S, Swann HR, Seif MW, Kimber SJ, Aplin JD (1995) Cell adhesion molecules on the oocyte and preimplantation human embryo. Hum Reprod 10:1571–1578

Castelbaum AJ, Somkuti SG, Ying L et al (1996) Characterization of integrin expression in a well-differentiated endometrial cancer cell line (Ishikawa). J Clin Endocrinol Metab (submitted)

Chan BM, Kassner PD, Schiro JA, Byers HR, Kupper TS, Hemler ME (1992) Distinct cellular functions mediated by different VLA integrin alpha subunit cytoplasmic domains. Cell 68:1051–1060

Cheesman KL, Ben-Nun I, Chatterton RT Jr, Cohen MR (1982) Relationship of luteinizing homrone, pregnanediol-3-glucoronide and estriol-16-glucuronide in urine of infertile women with endometriosis. Fertil Steril 38:542–548

Chegini N, Zhao Y, Williams RS, Flanders KC (1994) Human uterine tissue throughout the menstrual cycle expresses transforming growth factor-b1 (TGFb1), TGFb2, TGFb3, and TGFb type II receptor messenger ribonucleic acid and protein and contains [125I]TGFb1-binding sites. Endocrinology 135:439–449

Cheresh DA (1991) Integrins in thrombosis, wound healing and cancer. Biochem Soc Trans 19:835–838

Conforti G, Zanetti A, Pasquali-Ronchetti I, Quaglino D,Jr., Neyroz P, Dejana E (1990) Modulation of vitronectin receptor binding by membrane lipid composition. J Biol Chem 265:4011–4019

Coutifaris C, Lessey BA (1993) Co-expression of endometrial osteopontin and its receptor, the avb3 integrin, define the window of human receptivity to embryo implantation. Soc Gynecol Invest Toronto: S135

Damewood MD, Hesla JS, Schlaff WD, Hubbard M, Gearhart JD, Rock JA (1990) Effect of serum from patients with minimal to mild endometriosis on mouse embryo development in vitro. Fertil Steril 54:917–920

Defilippi P, Silengo L, Tarone G (1992) a6b1 integrin (laminin Receptor) is down-regulated by tumor necrosis factor a and interleukin-1 b in human endothelial cells. J Biol Chem 267:18303–18307

DeSimone DW, Stepp MA, Patel RS, Hynes RO (1987) The integrin family of cell surface receptors. Biochem Soc Trans 15:789–791

Dmowski WP, Steele RW, Baker GF (1981) Deficient cellular immunity in endometriosis. Am J Obstet Gynecol 141:377–383

Doody MC, Gibbons WE, Buttram VC,Jr. (1988) Linear regression analysis of ultrasound follicular growth series: evidence for an abnormality of follicular growth in endometriosis patients. Fertil Steril 49:47–51

Drake TS, O'Brien WF, Ramwell PW, Metz SA (1981) Peritoneal fluid thromboxane B2 and 6-keto-prostaglandin F2 alpha in endometriosis. Am J Obstet Gynecol 140:401–404

D'Souza SE, Ginsberg MH, Burke TA, Plow EF (1990) The ligand binding site of the platelet integrin receptor GPIIb-IIIa is proximal to the second calcium binding domain of its alpha subunit. J Biol Chem 265:3440–3446

Elices MJ, Hemler ME (1989) The human integrin VLA-2 is a collagen receptor on some cells and a collagen/laminin receptor on others. Proc Natl Acad Sci U S A 86:9906–9910

Elices MJ, Urry LA, Hemler ME (1991) Receptor functions for the integrin VLA-3: fibronectin, collagen, and laminin binding are differentially influenced by Arg-Gly-Asp peptide and by divalent cations. J Cell Biol 112:169–181

Fedele L, Marchini M, Bianchi S, Dorta M, Arcaini L, Fontana PE (1990) Structural and ultrastructural defects in preovulatory endometrium of normo-ovulating infertile women with minimal or mild endometriosis. Fertil Steril 53:989–993

Feinberg RF, Kliman HJ, Lockwood CJ (1991) Is oncofetal fibronectin a trophoblast glue for human implantation? Am J Pathol 138:537–543

Filardo EJ, Cheresh DA (1994) A β turn in the cytoplasmic tail of the integrin av subunit influences conformation and ligand binding of avb3. J Biol Chem 269:4641–4647

Finn CA (1977)The implantation reaction. In: Wynn RM (ed) Biology of the uterus. Plenum, New York, p 245

Grant A (1966) Additional sterility factors in endometriosis. Fertil Steril 17:514–519

Garcia E, Bouchard P, De Brux J, Berdah J, Frydman R, Schaison G et al (1988) Use of immunoctyochemistry of progesterone and estrogen receptors for endometrial dating. J Clin Endocrinol Metab 67:80–87

Grosskinsky CM, Yowell CW, Sun J, Parise L, Lessey BA (1996) Modulation of integrin expression in endometrial stromal cells in vitro. J Clin Endocrinol Metab 81:2047–2054

Hahn DW, Carraher RP, Foldesy RG, McGuire JL (1986) Experimental evidence for failure to implant as a mechanism of infertility associated with endometriosis. Am J Obstet Gynecol 155:1109–1113

Halme J, Becker S, Hammond MG, Raj MHG, Raj S (1983) Increased activation of pelvic macrohages in infertile women with mild endometriosis. Am J Obstet Gynecol 145:333–337

Haney AF, Muscata JJ, Weinberg JB (1981) Peritoneal fluid cell populations in infertility patients. Fertil Steril 35:696–698

Hegele-Hartung C, Beier HM (1986) Distribution of uteroglobin in the rabbit endometrium after treatment with an anti-progesterone (ZK 98.734): an immunohistochemical study. Hum Reprod 1:497–505

Hegele-Hartung C, Mootz U, Beier HM (1992) Luteal control of endometrial receptivity and its modification by progesterone antagonists. Endocrinology 131:2446–2460

Heino J, Ignotz RA, Hemler ME, Crouse C, Massague J (1989) Regulation of cell adhesion receptors by transforming growth factor-beta. Concomitant regulation of integrins that share a common beta 1 subunit. J Biol Chem 264:380–388

Heino J, Massague J (1989) Transforming growth factor-beta switches the pattern of integrins expressed in MG-63 human osteosarcoma cells and causes a selective loss of cell adhesion to laminin. J Biol Chem 264:21806–21811

Hemler ME, Huang C, Takada Y, Schwarz L, Strominger JL, Clabby ML (1987) Characterization of the cell surface heterodimer VLA-4 and related peptides. J Biol Chem 262:11478–11485

Hemler ME (1990) VLA proteins in the integrin family: structures, functions, and their role on leukocytes. Annu Rev Immunol 8:365–400

Hertig AT, Rock J, Adams EC (1956) A description of 34 human ova within the first 17 days of development. Am J Anat 98:435–493

Hodgen GD (1983) Surrogate embryo transfer combined with estrogen-progesterone therapy in monkeys: implantation, gestation, and delivery without ovaries. JAMA 250:2167–2171

Horwitz A, Duggan K, Greggs R, Decker C, Buck C (1985) The cell substrate attachment (CSAT) antigen has properties of a receptor for laminin and fibronectin. J Cell Biol 101:2134–2144

Hynes RO (1987) Integrins: a family of cell surface receptors. Cell 48:549–554

Hynes RO (1992) Integrins: versatility,modulation,and signaling in cell adhesion. Cell 69:11–25

Ignotz RA, Massagué J (1986) Transforming growth factor-b stimulates the expression of fibronectin and collagen and their incorporation into the extracellular matrix. J Cell Biol 261:4337–4345

Ignotz RA, Massague J (1987) Cell adhesion protein receptors as targets for transforming growth factor-beta action. Cell 51:189–197

Ignotz RA, Heino J, Massague J (1989) Regulation of cell adhesion receptors by transforming growth factor-beta. Regulation of vitronectin receptor and LFA-1. J Biol Chem 264:389–392

Illera MJ, Rumen J, Yuan LW, Lessey BA (1995) Peritoneal fluid from infertile women with endometriosis and aberrant endometrial integrin expression blocks embryo implantation in a mouse model. The Endocrine Society 77th Annual Meeting P2-98:315 (abstract)

Klein CE, Steinmayer T, Mattes JM, Kaufmann R, Weber L (1990) Integrins of normal human epidermis: differential expression, synthesis and molecular structure. Br J Dermatol 123:171–178

Klentzeris LD, Bulmer JN, Trejdosiewicz LK, Morrison L, Cooke ID (1993) Beta-1 integrin cell adhesion molecules in the endometrium of fertile and infertile women. Hum Reprod 8:1223–1230

Koretz K, Schlag P, Boumsell L, Moller P (1991) Expression of VLA-alpha 2, VLA-alpha 6, and VLA-beta 1 chains in normal mucosa and adenomas of the colon, and in colon carcinomas and their liver metastases. Am J Pathol 138:741–750

Koukoulis GK, Virtanen I, Korhonen M, Laitinen L, Quaranta V, Gould VE (1991) Immunohistochemical localization of integrins in the normal, hyperplastic, and neoplastic breast. Correlations with their functions as receptors and cell adhesion molecules. Am J Pathol 139:787–799

Laiho M, Saksela O, Andreasen PA, Keski-Oja J (1986) Enhanced production and extracellular matrix deposition of the endothelial-type plasminogen activator inhibitor in cultured human lung fibroblasts by transforming growth factor-b. J Cell Biol 103:2403–2410

Languino LR, Gehlsen KR, Wayner E, Carter WG, Engvall E, Ruoslahti E (1989) Endothelial cells use alpha 2 beta 1 integrin as a laminin receptor. J Cell Biol 109:2455–2462

Lentz SS, Kovach JS, McKean DJ, Wieand HS, Podratz KC (1990) Effector function of lymphokine-activated killer cells and cytotoxic T lymphocytes in ovarian epithelial carcinoma. Gynecol Oncol 38:191–196

Leslie KK, Watanabe S, Lei KJ et al (1990) Linkage of two human pregnancy-specific b1-glycoprotein genes: One is associated with hydatidiform mole. Proc Natl Acad Sci U S A 87:5822–5826

Lessey BA (1994) The use of integrins for the assessment of uterine receptivity. Fertil Steril 61:812–814

Lessey BA, Damjanovich L, Coutifaris C, Castelbaum A, Albelda SM, Buck CA (1992) Integrin adhesion molecules in the human endometrium. Correlation with the normal and abnormal menstrual cycle. J Clin Invest 90:188–195

Lessey BA, Castelbaum AJ, Buck CA, Lei Y, Yowell CW, Sun J (1994a) Further characterization of endometrial integrins during the menstrual cycle and in pregnancy. Fertil Steril 62:497–506

Lessey BA, Castelbaum AJ, Sawin SJ et al (1994b) Aberrant integrin expression in the endometrium of women with endometriosis. J Clin Endocrinol Metab 79:643–649

Lessey BA, Castelbaum AJ, Riben M, Howarth J, Tureck R, Meyer WR (1994c) Effect of hydrosalpinges on markers of uterine receptivity and success in IVF. Annual Meeting of the American Fertility Society (Abstract O-091:S45

Lessey BA, Castelbaum AJ, Sawin SJ, Sun J (1995a) Integrins as markers of uterine receptivity in women with primary unexplained infertility. Fertil Steril 63:535—542

Lessey BA, Albelda S, Buck CA, Castelbaum AJ, Yeh I, Kohler M, Berchuck A (1995b) Distribution of integrin cell adhesion molecules in endometrial cancer. Am J Pathol 146:717–726

Lessey BA, Ilesanmi A, Castelbaum AJ, Yuan L-W, Somkuti S, Chwalisz K (1996a) Characterization of a functional progesterone receptor in a well-differentiated endometrial adenocarcinoma cell line (Ishikawa). J Steroid Biochem Mol Biol (in press)

Lessey BA, Yeh I-T, Castelbaum AJ, Korzeniowski P, Sun J, Chwalisz K (1996b) Endometrial progesterone receptors and markers of uterine receptivity in the window of implantation. Fertil Steril 65:477–483

Li TC, Cooke ID (1991) Evaluation of the luteal phase. Hum Reprod 6:484–499

Li TC, Cooke ID (1992) Uterine factors in infertility. Curr Opin Obstet Gynecol 4:212–219

Mahmood TA, Templeton A (1991) Prevalence and genesis of endometriosis. Hum Reprod 6:544–549

Marchbanks PA, Peterson HB, Rubin GL, Wingo PA (1989) Research on infertility: definition makes a difference. The Cancer and Steroid Hormone Study Group. Am J Epidemiol 130:259–267

McLaren A (1985) The control of implantation. In: Thompson W, Joyce DN, Newton JR (eds) In vitro fertilization and donor insemination. Royal College of Obstetricians and Gynaecologists, London, p 13

Milazzo G, Yip CC, Maddux BA, Vigneri R, Goldfine ID (1992) High-affinity insulin binding to an atypical insulin-like growth factor-I receptor in human breast cancer cells. J Clin Invest 89:899–908

Morcos RN, Gibbons WE, Findley WE (1985) Effect of peritoneal fluid on in vitro cleavage of 2-cell mouse embryos: possible role in infertility associated with endometriosis. Fertil Steril 44:678–683

Muscato JJ, Haney AF, Weinberg JB (1982) Sperm phagocytosis by human peritoneal macrophages: a possible cause of infertility in endometriosis. Am J Obstet Gynecol 144:503–510

Mustoe TA, Pierce GF, Thomason A, Gramates P, Sporn MB, Deuel TF (1987) Accelerated healing of incisional wounds in rats induced by transforming growth factor-b. Science 237:1333–1336

Navot D, Bergh PA, Williams M et al (1991a) An insight into early reproductive processes through the in vivo model of ovum donation. J Clin Endocrinol Metab 72:408–414

Navot D, Scott RT, Droesch K, Veeck LL, Liu H-C, Rosenwaks Z (1991b) The window of embryonic transfer and the efficiency of human conception in vitro. Fertil Steril 55:114

Noda M, Yoon K, Prince CW, Butler WT, Rodan GA (1988) Transcriptional regulation of osteopontin production in rat osteosarcoma cells by type B transforming growth factor. J Biol Chem 263:13916–13921

Noyes RW, Hertig AI, Rock J (1950) Dating the endometrial biopsy. Fertil Steril 1:3–25

Oosterlynck DJ, Cornillie FJ, Waer M, Vandeputte M, Koninckx PR (1991) Women with endometriosis show a defect in natural killer activity resulting in a decreased cytotoxicity to autologous endometrium. Fertil Steril 56:45–51

Pasqualini R, Hemler ME (1994) Contrasting roles for integrin b1 and b5 cytoplasmic domains in subcellular localization, cell proliferation, and cell migration. J Cell Biol 125:447–460

Pearson CA, Pearson D, Shibahara S, Hofsteenge J, Chiquet-Ehrismann R (1988) Tenascin: cDNA cloning and induction by TGF-beta. EMBO J 7:2977–2982

Psychoyos A (1986) Uterine receptivity for nidation. Ann N Y Acad Sci 476:36–42

Rogers PAW, Murphy CR (1989)Uterine receptivity for implantation: human studies. In: Yoshinaga K (ed) Blastocyst implantation. Adams Publishing Group, Boston, p 231

Ruck P, Marzusch K, Kaiserling E et al (1994) Distribution of cell adhesion molecules in decidua of early human pregnancy: an immunohistochemical study. Lab Invest 71:94–101

Ruoslahti E, Pierschbacher MD (1987) New perspectives in cell adhesion: RGD and integrins. Science 238:491–497

Ruoslahti E (1992) Control of cell motility and tumour invasion by extracellular matrix interactions. Br J Cancer 66:239–242

Ruoslahti E, Noble NA, Kagami S, Border WA (1994) Integrins. Kidney Int 45 [Suppl 44]: S17–22

Santala P, Heino J (1991) Regulation of integrin-type cell adhesion receptors by cytokines. J Biol Chem 266:23505–23509

Schenken RS, Asch RH, Williams RF, Hodgen GD (1984) Etiology of infertility in monkeys with endometriosis: luteinized unruptured follicles, luteal phase defects, pelvic adhesions, and spontaneous abortions. Fertil Steril 41:122–130

Sheppard D, Cohen DS, Wang A, Busk M (1992) Transforming growth factor b differentially regulates expression of integrin subunits in guinea pigs airway epithelial cells. J Biol Chem 267:17409–17414

Soldati G, Piffaretti-Yanez A, Campana A, Marchini M, Luerti M, Balerna M (1989) Effect of peritoneal fluid on sperm motility and velocity distribution using objective measurements. Fertil Steril 52:113–119

Somkuti SG, Yowell CW, Fritz MA, Lessey BA (1995) The effect of oral contraceptive pills on markers of endometrial receptivity. Fertil Steril 65:484–488

Sporn MB, Roberts AB, Wakefield LM, de Crombrugghe B (1987) Some recent advances in the chemistry and biology of transforming growth factor-beta. J Cell Biol 105:1039–1045

Stallmach A, Rosewicz S, Kaiser A, Matthes H, Schuppan D, Riecken EO (1992) Laminin binding in membranes of a rat pancreatic acinar cell line are targets for glucocorticoids. Gastroenterology 102:237–247

Streuli CH, Bailey N, Bissell MJ (1991) Control of mammary epithelial differentiation: basement membrane induces tissue-specific gene expression in the absence of cell-cell interaction and morphological polarity. J Cell Biol 115:1383–1395

Sueldo CE, Lambert H, Steinleitner A, Rathwick G, Swanson J (1987) The effect of peritoneal fluid from patients with endometriosis on murine sperm-oocyte interaction. Fertil Steril 48:697–699

Suginami H, Yano K, Nakahashi N, Takeda Y (1990) Fallopian tube and fimbrial function in endometriosis: with a special reference to an ovum capture inhibitor. Prog Clin Biol Res 323:81–97

Surveyor GA, Gendler SJ, Pemberton L, Spicer AP, Carson DD (1993) Differential expression of Muc-1 at the apical cell surface of mouse uterine epithelial cells. FASEB J 7:1151

Sutherland AE, Calarco PG, Damsky CH (1993) Developmental regulation of integrin expression at the time of implantation in the mouse embryo. Development 119:1175–1186

Tabibzadeh S (1992) Patterns of expression of integrin molecules in human endometrium throughout the menstrual cycle. Hum Reprod 7:876–882

Tabibzadeh SS, Santhanam U, Sehgal PB, May LT (1989) Cytokine-induced production of IFN-beta 2/IL-6 by freshly explanted human endometrial stromal cells. Modulation by estradiol-17 beta. J Immunol 142:3134–3139

Taskin O, Brown RW, Young DC, Poindexter AN, Wiehle RD (1994) High doses of oral contraceptives do not alter endometrial a1 and avb3 integrins in the late implantation window. Fertil Steril 61:850–855

Van der Linden PJQ, De Goeij AFPM, Dunselman GAJ, Erkens HWH, Evers JLH (1995) Expression of cadherins and integrins in human endometrium throughout the menstrual cycle. Fertil Steril 63:1210–1216

Verkauf BS (1987) Incidence, symptoms, and signs of endometriosis in fertile and infertile women. J Fla Med Assoc 74:671–675

Yang JT, Rayburn H, Hynes RO (1995) Cell adhesion events mediated by a4 integrins are essential in placental and cardiac development. Development 121:549–560

Yelian FD, Edgeworth NA, Dong LJ, Chung AE, Armant DR (1993) Recombinant entactin promotes mouse primary trophoblast cell adhesion and migration through the Arg-Gly-Asp (RGD) recognition sequence [published erratum appears in J Cell Biol 1993 122(1):279]. J Cell Biol 121:923–929

Yoshinaga, K. (1989) Receptor concept in implantation research. In: Yoshinaga K, Mori T (eds) Development of preimplantation embryos and their environment. Alan, New York, p 379

Young MF, Kerr JM, Termine JD et al (1990) cDNA cloning, mRNA distribution and heterogeneity, chromosomal location, and RFLP analysis of human osteopontin (OPN). Genomics 7:491–502

Yovich JL, Matson PL, Richardson PA, Hilliard C (1988) Hormonal profiles and embryo quality in women with severe endometriosis treated by in vitro fertilization and embryo transfer. Fertil Steril 50:308–313

11 Endometrial Contraception with Progesterone Antagonists: An Experimental Approach

K. Chwalisz, I. Gemperlein †, C.P. Puri, S. Shao-Qing, and R. Knauthe

11.1 Introduction

Progesterone plays a pivotal role in female reproduction in mammals during almost all stages of the ovarian cycle and pregnancy. It is involved in the control of ovulation, prepares the endometrium for implantation, regulates the entire implantation process, and in later stages of pregnancy is responsible for its maintenance by suppressing uterine contractility. The sudden withdrawal of progesterone action at the end of the nonfertile cycle leads to the constriction of spiral arteries and in turn to menstruation in humans and nonhuman primates. The decrease in serum progesterone concentrations (e.g., in rabbits, rats and sheep) or its functional withdrawal in the myometrium and decidua (primates, guinea pigs) is the most important event during parturition in mammals (for review see Chwalisz 1993).

The presence of progesterone during the periovulatory stage of the ovarian cycle is essential for ovulation. Progesterone acts synergistically with estradiol in inducing the surge in luteinizing hormone (LH) prior to ovulation at the hypothalamus/hypophysis level (Hoff 1983) and most likely plays an important role during folliculogenesis and ovulation, acting directly on the ovary.

In the uterus progesterone controls the growth and differentiation of endometrial and myometrial cells and regulates a variety of cell functions directly by either stimulating or inhibiting structural and functional proteins but also indirectly by functionally opposing estradiol (E_2) action. In the nonpregnant uterus there are different progesterone effects on uterine cell proliferation which vary among the different species. In primates during the luteal phase progesterone inhibits the estrogen-induced mitotic activity in the functional zones of the endometrium but shows a stimulatory effect on the proliferation of endometrial stem cells which are responsible for endometrial regeneration after menstruation in the basalis (Padykula 1991). These differential effects of progesterone may explain to some extent the antiproliferative activity of antiprogestins on the primate endometrium.

In the fertile cycle progesterone, synergistically with estrogen, regulates the transport of the embryo through the oviduct and induces secretory changes required for implantation in the endometrium. In the primate endometrium during the period between ovulation and implantation there are remarkable morphological and biochemical changes in the luminal and glandular epithelial cells under the influence of rising progesterone levels. These changes include the appearance of glycogen deposits in the basal cytoplasm, an increasingly abundant golgi apparatus in the appical cytoplasm, and a continuous increase in secretory vesicles. The maximum secretory capacity of the glandular epithelium is reached approximately 6 days after the LH peak (i.e., around implantation) and remains high for several days thereafter. The secretory endometrial proteins produced by endometrial glands and cell surface proteins such as integrins and proteoglycans, and probably other cellular and extracellular components, most likely determine the endometrial receptivity for blastocyst implantation. These changes are totally dependent on progesterone action after estrogen priming. Therefore, the luteal-phase endometrium, in particular during the perimplantation period, may be a very sensitive target for contraception especially with antiprogesterone agents. However, it is now evident that the progesterone effects are further modulated by peptide hormones, growth factors, and cytokines secreted by a variety of cell types within the endometrium, including immunocompetent cells (Tabibzadeh and Babaknia 1995; Loke and King 1995).

During the past decade several possibilities for using antiprogestins in fertility regulation have been suggested, based either on the inhibition of ovulation or the prevention of implantation after postcoital or early luteal-phase treatment (see Puri 1995 for review). However, only postcoital treatment with mifepristone (Glasier et al. 1992) and its early luteal-phase administration on LH+2 (Gemzell-Danielsson et al. 1993) have as yet been proven to be effective in women. The contraceptive effects of mifepristone in these approaches are most likely due to its effects on the endometrium. The postcoital treatment with mifepristone can be used only occasionally, otherwise it interferes with ovulation and induces amenorrhea. The use of mifepristone on LH+2 is rather inconvenient since the LH surge must be identified in every cycle.

An alternative approach is to administer an antiprogestin in a dose which closes the "implantation window" by acting selectively on the endometrium, but does not affect the ovarian and menstrual cyclicity. This approach, (i.e., inhibition of endometrial receptivity) is based on the observation made in laboratory animals and nonhuman primates that the endometrium is much more sensitive to antiprogestins than the hypophyseo-hypothalamo-ovarian axis. This chapter summarizes the evidence from animal studies supporting this concept.

11.2 Progesterone and the Uterine Receptivity for Blastocyst Implantation

Successful blastocyst implantation is strictly dependent on the synchrony between the developmental program of the embryo itself and the cascade of cellular and molecular events that occur in the endometrium during the peri-implantation period of the fertile cycle. In all mammals the endometrium is receptive to blastocyst implantation only during a specific period after ovulation. This stage of the luteal phase is called "implantation window." This concept was first proposed by M.C. Chang (1950) in rabbits, but the term "implantation window" was established by Psychoyos (1973) in rats and then extended to mice (McLaren 1973; Finn and Martin 1974). In rodents uterine receptivity is functionally divided into prereceptive, receptive, and nonreceptive (refractory) phases (Psychoyos 1973). In mice and rats uterine receptivity occurs only for a limited period during pregnancy or pseudopregnancy. The prereceptive uterus on day 3 becomes receptive on day 4 (day of implantation) and is refractory from day 5 onwards. In rodents the phases of uterine sensitivity with respect to implantation are strictly dependent on changes in ovarian steroid secretion. The prereceptive (neutral) phase, which is determined by progesterone exposure (after estradiol priming), becomes receptive for a short period of time (approx. 24 h) if exposed to ovarian estrogen peak. The endometrium then proceeds to the nonreceptive (refractory) phase as long as it is being exposed to progesterone (Psychoyos 1973).

Similar phases of endometrial receptivity can be defined in primates, despite differences in the role of ovarian estrogen. The results of embryo transfer studies indicate that the implantation window (transfer window) also exists in humans. In women the successful implantation may only take place between days 20–24 of a histologically defined 28-day cycle, i.e., during the period of highest progesterone levels (Navot et al. 1991). The optimum condition for nidation is estimated to be on days 20–22 of the normal cycle, i.e., 7 days after the LH surge (Bergh et al. 1992). There are data indicating that under certain clinical conditions (e.g., endometriosis) receptivity can be impaired which can lead to infertility despite a normal ovarian and menstrual cycle and the presence of normal endometrial histology (Lessey et al. 1994). In such clinical situations the implantation window appears to be "closed" due to a yet unidentified mechanism. This observation also suggests that the implantation window is not exclusively regulated by sex steroids, since both progesterone and estradiol levels were normal.

There are few morphological examples for early human implantation stages. However, considerable information can be inferred from nonhuman primates (Enders 1993). In primates the morphological changes associated with the implantation process can be divided into the following stages: (a) apposition of the trophoblast and uterine epithelium, (b) adhesion of the blastocyst to the apical surface of the epithelium, which involves the formation of junctional complexes between the two cell types, and (c) epithelial penetration, which includes the trophoblast invasion of the endometrium, formation of the trophoblastic plate, lacunar stage, and finally placental formation (Enders and Schlafke 1989).

11.2.1 Hormonal Regulation of Endometrial Receptivity

It is becoming increasingly clear that the opening of the implantation window is strictly but not solely dependent on the steroid hormones progesterone and estradiol. However, the necessary steroid hormonal requirements for endometrial receptivity, in particular concerning the role of estrogen, are species specific. In rodents, which belong to the category of species with "facultative delayed implantation," the ovarian estrogen is essential for implantation, and a blastocyst does not implant in ovariectomized pregnant or pseudopregnant rats or mice which are supplemented with progesterone alone (Psychoyos 1986). In this situation the blastocyst enters a state of diapause which can be terminated by the additional administration of a small amount of estrogen. In eutherian species, not exhibiting embryonic diapause, ovarian estrogen is not required for implantation. In guinea pigs, rabbits, and primates ovarian estrogen is not essential for implantation, and ovariectomy during the first day of pregnancy does not inhibit implantation, provided exogenous progesterone is supplied continuously.

Blastocyst-transfer experiments in delayed-implanting mice suggest that endometrial receptivity is also regulated by the blastocyst's state of activity (Paria et al. 1993). The window of implantation in the receptive uterus remain operative for a shorter period for dormant blastocysts than for normal or E$_2$-activated dormant blastocysts. Therefore, both the ovarian sex steroids and the embryonic signals play an important role in receptivity. These studies also suggest that the blastocyst is also a target for steroid hormones and perhaps antihormones.

Uterine stromal cell differentiation is essential for the successful establishment of pregnancy in mammals. It is characterized by a substantial increase in the size of the stromal cell compartment through both cell proliferation and cell growth. Decidualization is a feature unique to species exhibiting invasive hemochorial placentation, whereby the decidua most likely controls the trophoblastic invasion (Loke and King 1995). In rodents decidualization is localized to areas of embryo attachment and can be induced by physical stimuli, whereas in primates it is induced by luteal-phase progesterone. However, the presence of progesterone is essential for decidualization in both rodents and primates.

Although the precise mechanisms involved in the regulation of the "implantation cascade" remain unknown, it is clear that several adhesion molecules, growth factors, cytokines, and matrix metalloproteinases play a role in this process. However, the studies with progesterone antagonists reviewed in brief below strongly indicate that progesterone exerts an overall control on uterine receptivity and most likely on all implantation stages, since treatment with progesterone antagonists inhibits endometrial receptivity and interrupts early pregnancy in all species investigated to date. Interestingly, an acute antiprogestin treatment during the prereceptive phase can delay the endometrial protein secretion and shift (transpose) the implantation window, as demonstrated by embryo transfer experiments in rabbits (Hegele-Hartung et al. 1992; Beier et al. 1994). These results indicate that the antiprogestin effects on the endometrium are reversible. Therefore, depending on the timing, dose, and treatment duration the implantation window can be either manipulated or closed by antiprogestins.

11.2.2 Steroid Hormone Receptors and the Implantation Window

The cellular distribution of estrogen receptors (ER) and progesterone receptors (PR) in the human endometrium, as assessed by immunohistology, show a cyclic pattern during the menstrual cycle. Both glandular and stromal cell expression of ER increases during the proliferative phase and then gradually declines to undetectable levels during the midluteal phase, approximately on days 19–20 of the cycle, which closely corresponds to the opening of the implantation window. A similar pattern is shown for the PR expression in the endometrial epithelium (gradual increase during proliferative phase, rapid decline on day 19–22), but PR is maintained in the stroma throughout the luteal phase although at slightly lower levels (Lessey et al. 1988).

These changes reflect an increase in serum progesterone concentrations, since it is well established that progesterone downregulates the expression of both ER and PR at the genomic level. The differential expression in PR in the endometrial epithelium and stroma indicate that there are differences in progesterone sensitivity to different cell types, the endometrial epithelial cells being much more sensitive to progesterone downregulation than the endometrial stroma. Interestingly, the PR expression in the endometrial epithelium is upregulated in infertile women with a luteal-phase defect (Lessey et al. 1995). Failure of PR downregulation is associated with aberrant $\alpha_v\beta_3$ integrin expression, a marker of uterine receptivity, in women with luteal-phase defect. This observation suggests that the establishment of normal endometrial receptivity in humans is closely associated with the downregulation of epithelial PR.

The PR consists of two isoforms: an A receptor (hPR-a), which contains 933 amino acids, and a B receptor (hPR-b), which lacks the N-terminal 164 amino acids (Horwitz and Alexander 1993). The B receptor functions as a hormone-dependent positive regulator of specific progesterone-induced genes, whereas hPR-a can inhibit the activity of B receptors (Sartorius et al. 1993; Vegato et al. 1993) and other members of the steroid receptor family, including ER. The ratio of B to A receptors in the progesterone target tissue may therefore determine its response to progestational and antiprogestational agents. The expression of PR isoforms changes during the human menstrual cycle (Feil et al. 1988); however, very little is known about their role in implantation to date.

11.2.3 Progesterone and the Molecular Aspects of Implantation

The first step of the implantation process is characterized by the adhesion of the blastocyst's trophectoderm to the uterine surface epithelium. This initial embryo-endometrial contact (apposition) seems to represent a crucial step in the implantation process. At the time of implantation changes in the surface epithelium must occur to allow attachment and subsequently implantation. The uterine epithelium plays a crucial role in receptivity, since after its removal implantation can occur independently of hormonal control (Cowell 1969).

There have been numerous attempts to identifiy the biochemical markers of endometrial receptivity or other specific mechanisms required for blastocyst implantation. Recently two different concepts of the mechanism of receptivity have been proposed. According to the first concept, the receptivity stage is determined by the appearance of "essential" factors which, acting as receptors, allow the initial embryo-endometrial contact, or are of pivotal importance during more advanced stages of the implantation process.

According to the second concept, receptivity is rather determined by the release of a factors(s) which prevents endometrial receptivity during the nonreceptive phase (McLaren 1973; Surveyor et al. 1995). The human blastocyst can readily adhere to other tissues, including the oviducts, which do not show cyclical changes typical for the endometrium. These observations indicate that the uterus is normally very hostile to implantation and becomes receptive only during a specific period subject to appropriate hormonal stimulation. Numerous experimental and clinical studies indicate that under estrogen dominance the uterine enviroment is hostile to implantation, and under progesterone dominance (after estrogen priming) the endometrial epithelium becoms receptive to the blastocyst. However, pregnancy and blastocyst signals most likely modulate this response.

In summary, the implantation window can be determined by both the upregulation of the "essential implantation factors" (receptivity markers) and the downregulation of factors which prevent implantation (e.g., MUC-1 in mice). Progesterone is very likely to be the most important factor regulating these events (Fig. 1).

Non-receptive Uterus:
Estrogen Dominance

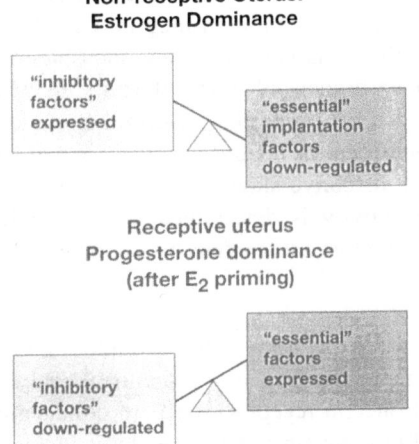

Receptive uterus
Progesterone dominance
(after E_2 priming)

Fig. 1. Hypothetical mechanisms involved in the regulation of the "implantation window"

11.2.3.1 *"Essential" Implantation Factors (Receptivity Markers)*
Several genes are switched on during the luteal phase, including those encoding the adhesion molecules (integrins), growth factors, and cytokines (for review see Tabibzadeh and Babaknia 1995; Edwards 1995). It is likely that progesterone, directly or indirectly, regulates the expression of the receptivity markers. Progesterone can stimulate gene expression via its receptor. However, only a few genes have been shown to be directly regulated by progesterone, including uteroglobin in the rabbit uterus (Beier 1975), c-*myc* in the rodent uterus (Huet-Hudson et al. 1989), uteroferrin in the pig uterus (Fliss et al. 1991), insulin-like growth factor (IGF) binding protein 1 in the primate uterus (Fazleabas and Verhage 1994), heparin-binding epidermal growth factor (HB-EGF) in the rodent uterus (Zhang et al. 1995), calcitonin in glandular epithelial cells of rat uterus (Ding et al. 1994), amphiregulin (growth factor of the epidermal growth factor family; Das et al. 1995) and ferritin heavy chain in the rat uterus (Zhu et al. 1995). However, most of these markers (uteroglobin, uteroferrin, HB-EGF, calcitonin) are also modulated by estrogen, indicating a dual hormonal regulation of these genes. In addition, their role in implantation is unclear to date.

The list of potential markers of endometrial receptivity is continously growing. However, only two of them (integrin $\alpha_v\beta_3$, LIF) are currently considered as receptivity markers, and only one (integrin $\alpha_v\beta_3$) is currently believed to be associated with infertility in women with endometriosis (Lessey et al. 1994 1995). Several new individual protein bands, recently identified as histones, appear in human endometrial secretion during the receptive stage of the cycle (Beier-Hellwig et al. 1994). Perhaps receptivity is determined by a specific combination (pattern) of various factors rather than by a single receptivity marker (Beier et al. 1994).

Integrins. The integrin expression in the endometrium is characterized by temporal and spatial changes during the menstrual cycle. The integrins $\alpha_v\beta_3$ (the vitronectin receptor), $\alpha_1\beta_1$ (a collagen-laminin receptor) and $\alpha_4\beta_1$ (a fibrinonectin receptor) exhibit increased expression during the luteal phase of the human menstrual cycle. The $\alpha_v\beta_3$ is perhaps a good receptivity marker since it is absent in infertile women with minimal endometriosis even in the presence of normal luteal-phase progesterone levels (Lessey et al. 1994). This observation strongly suggests that the sex steroid hormone effects are modulated by other factors including cytokines (leukemia inhibitory factor [LIF], interleukin 1, colony-stimulating factor 1, etc.) and growth factors (Tabibzadeh and Babaknia 1995).

Leukemia Inhibitory Factor. LIF is a cytokine which is produced by the mouse endometrium just prior to blastocyst implantation (Bhatt et al. 1991). LIF has been suggested to be essential for a successful implantation in mice. LIF-deficient mice (knock-out experiment) show a defect of implantation and an impaired decidualization (Stewart et al. 1992). This finding indicates that LIF is an essential component in the uterine receptivity in mice. In mice uterine LIF expression is upregulated by ovarian estrogens which are high during implantation in rodents. However, it is not known whether LIF is essential for implantation in species which do not require ovarian estrogens for implantation such as guinea pigs and primates. In guinea pigs LIF expression is present in the endometrial luminal epithelium, and endometrial glands and shows cycle-dependent changes. As in mice, it is expressed in the uterus during estrus, i.e., around the time of estradiol surge (Fig. 2).

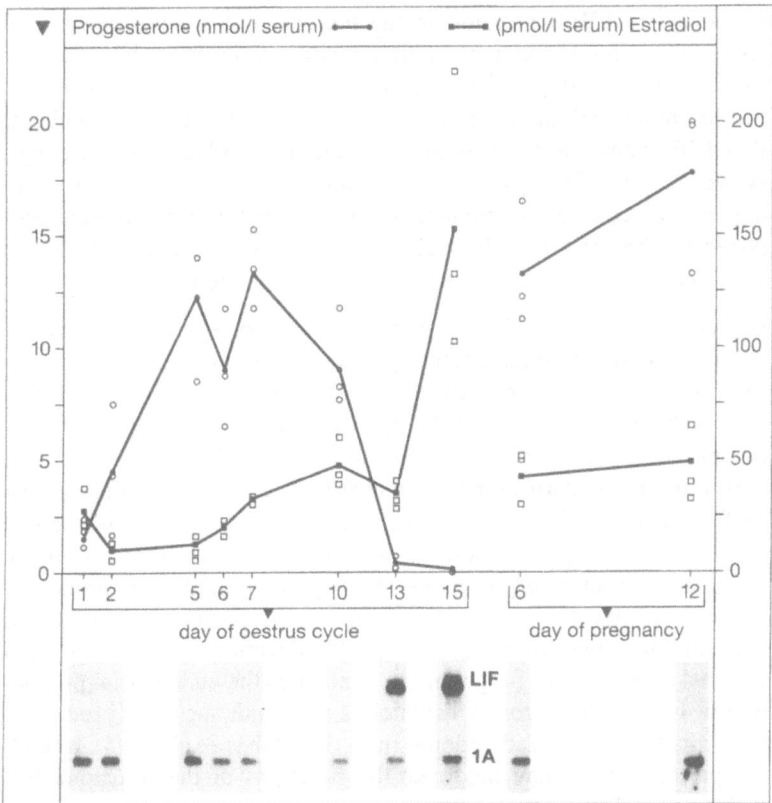

Fig. 2. Expression of LIF mRNA in uterine homogenates during the estrus cycle (*left*) and during pregnancy on day 6 (day of implantation) and 12 in relationship to serum progesterone (*open circles*) and estradiol (*squares*).

Note high LIF expression during estrus (day 15) and the absence of LIF expression during implantation (day 6 p.c.) and early pregnancy on day 12 p.c. Northern blot analysis using specific cDNA probes. The second day of vaginal opening in the fertile cycle was defined as day 1 post coitum (*day 1 p.c.*). Cycle duration in guinea pigs is about 15–16 days. Ovulation (estrus) occurs on day 1 of the cycle; implantation takes place on day 5–6 p.c. In nonpregnant animals uterine LIF expression was measured on days 1, 2, 5, 6, 7, 10, 13, and 15 of the cycle using northern blot analysis and with nonradioactive in situ hybridization ($n=3$/group). Cytochrome c oxidase subunit 1 was used as a reference gene. Blood samples were collected for estradiol and progesterone RIA

However, no LIF expression in the uterine homogenates can be detected either during the implantation window or in the pregnant uterus. In addition, estradiol stimulates uterine LIF expression in ovariectomized animals (Knauthe et al. unpublished data). These data indicate that LIF cannot be used as an implantation marker in guinea pigs. However, these findings do not rule out the possibility that local LIF expression occurs at the implantation site in response to estrogens produced by the blastocyst. In such a situation LIF expression could not have been detected in homogenates of the whole uterus.

Growth Factors. Steroid hormones are known to regulate the activities of many growth factors. Stromal growth factors mediate epithelial effects of steroid hormones. HB-EGF, the stromal mitogenic growth factor which belongs to the EGF family, was suggested to mediate the mitogenic action of progesterone on uterine stromal cells (Zhang et al. 1994). In the rat uterus, progesterone stimulates the production of HB-EGF, which is believed to be involved in the development of stromal sensitivity to decidual stimuli. In rats onapristone was shown to block decidual reaction in response to scratching and inhibited the progesterone-induced HB-EGF expression which indicates that antiprogestins may inhibit implantation by blocking the decidual reaction (Zhang et al. 1994). In baboons, progesterone stimulates the endometrial production of IGF binding protein 1, which is the major secretory product of the primate decidualized endometrium (Fazleabas et al. 1994), a binding protein which may modulate the functions of the somatomedins IGF-1 and IGF-2 in the decidua.

Gap Junctions. Intercellular communication may be important during implantation. In rats, endometrial gap junctions are highly expressed locally at the implantation sites, but are downregulated in other parts of the uterus. Onapristone treatment during the preimplantation phase prevents progesterone-induced downregulation of connexin 26 and connexin 43 in the endometrium in rats (Grümmer et al. 1994). A high expression of connexin 26 and connexin 43 during the preimplantation phase seems to be a suitable biological marker of the nonreceptive endometrium.

The list of potential receptivity markers is continuously increasing. However, a universal marker of endometrial receptivity which would predict a successful implantation is not yet available.

11.2.3.2 Inhibitory Factors

MUC-1. The second concept of endometrial receptivity includes the downregulation of factors which prevent implantation. The properties of mucins, such as MUC-1, indicate that these molecules may serve as anti-adhesion molecules during embryo attachment. The highly glyco-sylated and extended structure of MUC-1 may prevent attachment to the apical surface epithelium under nonreceptive conditions. In mice MUC-1 is highly expressed during the proestrus and estrus but disappears in response to progesterone treatment and during the receptive phase of the cycle (Surveyor et al. 1995). The downregulation of MUC-1 in endometrial epithelial cells of mice is a progesterone-dominated event since estradiol does not restore its expression in the presence of progesterone. Recently it has been shown that the the loss of MUC-1 on the surface epithelium is associated with the acquisition of uterine receptivity in baboons (Hild-Petito S et al. 1996).

Progesterone Receptors. Progesterone is a very potent gene suppressor. Both ER and PR are promptly downregulated in the endometrial epithelium and in many other sex steroid-dependent tissues in response to progesterone. In humans the disappearance of epithelial PR (and ER) in the endometrial epithelium closely correlates with the opening of the implantation window, which indicates that there is a functional loss of both progesterone and estradiol in the receptive surface endometrial epithelium (Lessey at al. 1995).

During pregnancy progesterone induces uterine quiescence by suppressing the expression of a number of proteins including gap junctions (connexin 43), calcium channels, and receptors of uterotonins (Chwalisz and Garfield 1994). Perhaps the downregulation (transrepression) of estrogen-induced factors which prevent implantation by progesterone (such as MUC-1) is the pivotal mechanism of endometrial receptivity. However, progesterone may exhibit many other effects, still undefined, on both the endometrium and blastocysts. In addition, progesterone has immunosuppressant properties and may also control the function (most likely via the cytokine network) of immunocompetent cells, which are quite abundant in the the decidua.

11.3 Progesterone Antagonists

Since the synthesis of the first progesterone antagonist RU-486 by scientists of Roussel Uclaf more than a decade ago (Phillibert et al. 1995) a number antiprogesterone compounds, including onapristone (ZK 98299), lilopristone (ZK 98734; Neef et al. 1984), ORG-31710 and ORG-31806 (Kloosterboer et al. 1994), and CDB-2914 (RTI 3021–012; Cook et al. 1994) have been synthetized and characterized. To date no other compounds have been studied so extensively as RU-486 (mifepristone) and onapristone (ZK 98299). These two compounds show differences in various in vitro and in vivo models with regard to pharmacodynamic and pharmacokinetic properties. Both compounds bind with high affinity to the progesterone (PR) and glucocorticoid receptors (however, the affinity of RU-486 to both receptors is higher than that of onapristone). Both RU-486 and onapristone also bind to the androgen receptor and exhibit practically no binding either to the human or the rat ER. Compared with RU-486, onapristone shows a short half-life in vivo and at the receptor level, the on- and off-rates of onapristone are similar to those of progesterone (Chwalisz et al. 1995). Onapristone has a short half-life of approx. 2–3 h after oral administration in humans (K. Zurth, unpublished data), whereas the half-life of RU-486 is considerably longer and ranges between 24 and 48 h (Heikinheimo 1989).

The molecular mechanisms of action of onapristone (13α-configurated steroid) and RU-486 (13β-configurated steroid) seem to be different. RU-486 promotes dimerization of the PR and its binding to DNA. On the other hand, onapristone (and some other 13α-configurated progesterone antagonists) impair the binding of the PR-complexes to the progesterone responsive element in the promotor of a PR-regulated gene as evidenced by gel retardation assay in T 47 D cells (Klein-Hitpass et al. 1991). This observation has been verified by other groups (Horwitz 1992; Gronemeyer at al. 1992), including our laboratories in COS-1 cells transiently transfected with human PR_B (Chwalisz et al. 1995). RU-486 occupied hPR complexes bind to PREs but are transcriptionally inert and antagonize progesterone action by a conventional competition mechanism. Interestingly, when cellular cAMP levels are raised, RU-486 and some other antagonists which bind to PREs demonstrate strong agonistic activity (Sartorius et al. 1993). In contrast, despite high cAMP levels onapristone is an antagonist in this system. The binding of RU-

486–PR complexes to PREs may explain the occurrence of agonistic activity described in the primate endometrium (Koering et al. 1986). Onapristone (and some other 13α-configurated antiprogestins) may be considered therefore as "pure" progesterone antagonists.

11.4 Effects of Antiprogestins on Endometrial Receptivity

It is meanwhile well known that sequential exposure to estrogen and progesterone are essential for the development of a receptive uterus, and that progesterone is essential for the establishment of pregnancy in all mammals. Therefore progesterone antagonists interfere with all stages of receptivity and early pregnancy. However, their effects may vary in different animal species due to differences in the hormonal regulation of implantation (see above). The effects of antiprogestins on the endometrium are also dose and cycle stage dependent.

11.4.1 Dissociation of Central and Peripheral Effects of Antiprogestins

Experiments with various antiprogestins performed in various animal species, including rats, guinea pigs and nonhuman primates, consistently show that the endometrium is generally more sensitive to antiprogestins than the hypothalamus and/or the pituitary gland. This conclusion is based on comparing antiprogestin doses which are effective in blocking ovulation (central effects) with those inducing endometrial effects including early abortion (rats, guinea pigs) and premature menstruation (monkeys). The differential effects of antiprogestins on ovulation and the endometrium have encouraged us to perform comparative studies in different animal species with different antiprogestins, which are briefly reviewed below. The overall aim of these studies was to establish a treatment regimen of a minidose of antiprogestin that permits continued ovarian (and menstrual) cyclicity but alters gonadal-reproductive tract activity and prevents pregnancy. The ideal antiprogestin for endometrial contraception should exhibit a high degree of endometrial selectivity, i.e., it should be very potent in preventing implantation at

Table 1. Differences in hormonal regulation and implantation process between guinea pigs and rats

	Guinea pigs	Rats/mice
Ovulation	Spontaneous	Spontaneous
Luteal phase	Long	Short
Implantation type	Interstitial	Superficial
Dependency on ovarian steroids	No (partially P)	E_2[a], P
Placentation	Hemo-monochorial	Hemo-trichorial
Luteoplacental shift	Yes	No

[a] Endometrial sensitivity to blastocyst stimulus for decidual transformation is brought about by the action of the luteal-phase estrogen surge.

doses which do not inhibit ovulation or disturb ovarian and menstrual cyclicity.

In rats, guinea pigs, and monkeys all antiprogestins which we have investigated to date show a dissociation between the endometrial and central effects. However, as presented below, the degree of this dissociation varies between compounds and species. The guinea pigs differ from rodents with regard to both hormonal regulation of receptivity and implantation type (Table 1) and may therefore be regarded as a more suitable model for primate implantation than rodents. A comparison of antiovulatory activities of various antiprogestagenic compounds reveals some differences between rats, guinea pigs, and monkeys which point out the limitation of rats and guinea pigs as animal models for endometrial receptivity. A further disadvantage of small laboratory animals is the absence of uterine bleeding. Cynomolgus and bonnet monkeys and baboons show ovarian and menstrual cycles which are very similar to those of women. Therefore in our studies of endometrial effects of antiprogestins emphasis was placed on nonhuman primates.

11.4.2 Effects of Antiprogestins and Antiestrogens on Early Pregnancy in Rats

In rats the endometrium is approximately ten times more sensitive to antiprogestins than the hypophyseo-ovarian axis as demonstrated by comparing the doses of RU-486, onapristone, and other antiprogestins

Table 2. Dissociation of central and endometrial effects of the antiprogestins RU-486 and onapristone in rats: comparison of ED_{50} ($n=6$/group)

Test	RU-486 (ED_{50}) (mg/animal)		Onapristone (ED_{50}) (mg/animal)	
	p.o.	s.c.	p.o.	s.c.
Antiovulatory activity	4.5	7.0	8.8	4.5
Inhibition of receptivity (treatment days 1–4 p.c.)	0.70	n.t.	1.0	n.t.
Early abortion (treatment: days 5–7 p.c.)	1.0	0.81	0.91	0.54

n.t., Not tested.

which inhibit ovulation with those that are effective in preventing implantation or inducing early abortion (Table 2). This dissociation was observed after either oral (p.o.) or subcutaneous treatment (s.c.). Termination of early pregnancy after treatment on days 5–7 post coitum (p.c.), i.e., shortly after nidation had taken place, was clearly due to the endometrial effects. However, the interceptive mechanisms after treatment during the prenidatory stage of pregnancy (days 1–4 p.c.) are more

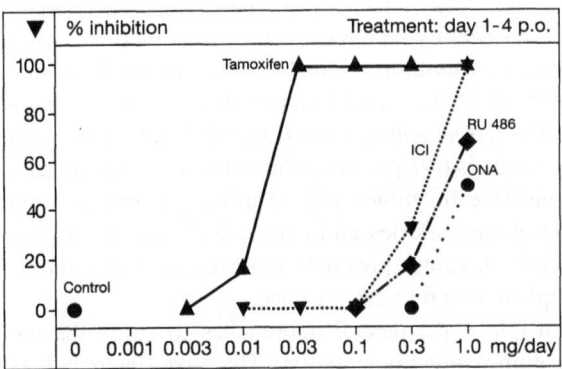

Fig. 3. Critical role of the estrogens in rat implantation. Interceptive effects of the antiprogestins mifepristone (RU-486) and onapristone (*ONA*) and the antiestrogens tamoxifen and ICI-182 780. Oral treatments during the prereceptive phase on days 1–4 p.c. ($n=6–8$/group)

complex and may include disturbances in the transport of the embryo, early embryonic development, endometrial maturation, and its sensitivity to decidualization. An accelerated tubal transport after postcoital administration of RU-486 has been described in rats and mice (Vinijsanun and Martin 1990; Roblero and Croxatto 1991).

The experiments with antiprogestins performed during the prereceptive phase suggest that progesterone is essental for endometrial receptivity in rats. However, in rats and mice the antiestrogens are highly effective interceptive agents, which points to the mandatory role of the perinidatory estrogen. After treatment during the prenidatory phase (on days 1–4 p.c.), the antiestrogens tamoxifen and ICI-182 780 (a pure ER antagonist) are even more effective in preventing implantation than either mifepristone or onapristone (Fig. 3). Whether the interceptive mechanism of antiprogestins administered during the prereceptive phase is solely due to their antiprogestagenic or functional antiestrogenic (antiproliferative) effects remains to be established.

11.4.3 Effects of Antiprogestins on Uterine Receptivity in Guinea Pigs

The guinea pig exhibits a long luteal phase (9–10 days) and an interstitial implantation type which is not dependent on ovarian estrogens (Table 1). Ovariectomy on days 3–5 p.c. does not prevent implantation, suggesting that the embryo is capable of producing progesterone. However, growth retardation and embryo death occur after ovariectomy without progesterone substitution (Deansly 1960, 1971). Implantation takes place on days 6–7 p.c. As in humans, the extravillous trophoblast is highly invasive in guinea pigs. During pregnancy it continuously invades the uterine arteries and causes their dilatation (Nanaev et al. 1995). Therefore, guinea pigs may represent a more suitable model for primate implantation than rats or mice.

We used two experimental approaches to study the antiprogestin effects on guinea pig implantation. The first (interceptive) approach employed a postcoital treatment from day 1–6 of pregnancy. In the second approach the guinea pigs were continuously treated with minidoses of different antiprogestins for two cycles and mated during the second treatment cycle.

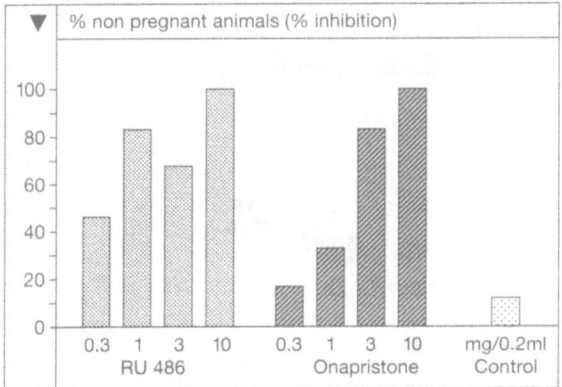

Fig. 4. Interceptive effects of onapristone and mifepristone (RU-486) in guinea pigs. The animals (*n*=5–6) were treated subcutaneously during the prereceptive phase on day 1–6 p.c. Autopsy was performed on day 12 p.c

Interceptive Effects of Antiprogestins. Both mifepristone and onapristone prevented implantation in a dose-dependent manner after postcoital treatment on days 1–6 of pregnancy (Fig. 4), showing a comparable efficacy (day 1 was defined on the basis of leukocytic infiltration in the vaginal smear). We performed serial tubal and uterine flushings to study the antiprogestin effects of onapristone and mifepristone on tubal transports and early embryonic development. In normal early pregnancy the ova could be detected in the fallopian tube until day 4 p.c. The implantation took place between day 6 and 7 p.c., since blastocysts could not be flushed out from the uterus on day 7 p.c (Fig. 5, upper panel). In nonpregnant guinea pigs the tubal transport of ova is slightly accelerated (Fig. 5, lower panel). An accelerated embryo transport was evident on day 4 p.c. after both antiprogestins, and particularly pronounced after RU-486 on day 4 p.c. (Fig. 6).

Interestingly, onapristone caused either an arrest of early embryonic development or a fertilization defect, since only one- or two-cell stages could be recovered from the uterus or the oviducts (Fig. 6).

Synergistic Effects of Antiprogestin with Antiestrogen. Interestingly, both tamoxifen and ICI-182 780 caused interceptive effects in guinea

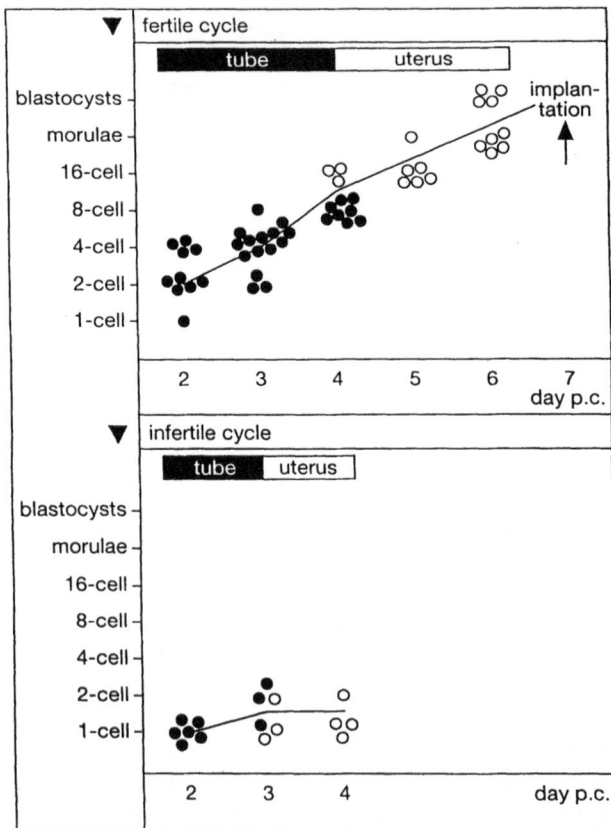

Fig. 5. Tubal ovum transport and developmental stages of fertilized (*above*) and nonfertilized ova (*below*) in normal guinea pigs. Female guinea pigs (Pirbright white; Charles River Wiga, Suthfeld, Germany) were kept in the presence of males and mated. Day 1 of pregnancy was defined by the presence of leukocytes in the vaginal smear. *Lower panel*, results of tubal flushings from the nonfertile cycles

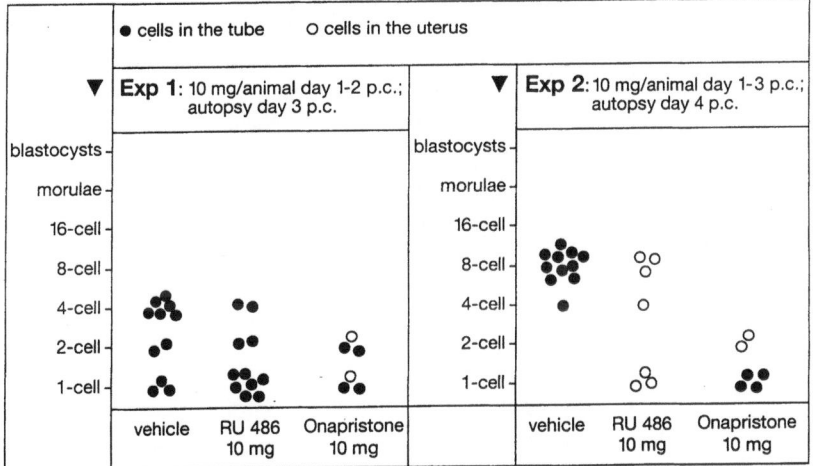

Fig. 6. Effects of onapristone and mifepristone (10 mg/animal s.c.) on tubal transport and early embryonic development after postcoital treatment in guinea pigs. The uterine and tubal flushings were performed on either day 3 (*Exp. 1*) or 4 p.c. (*Exp. 2*) (*n*=6/group). *Black points*, ova recovered from the tube; *open circles*, ova recovered from the uterus. Note the accelerated tubal transport and an developmental arrest after onapristone on day 4 p.c

pigs, although not as pronounced as in rats after postcoital adminitration on days 1–6 p.c. (Fig. 7, upper panel). This observation strongly suggests that estrogens play an important role during the preimplantation phase in guinea pigs as well as in rats. Moreover, a pronounced synergistic effect was found between onapristone and tamoxifen (but not ICI-182 789 at the doses tested) in guinea pigs during the preimplantation phase of pregnancy (Fig. 7, lower panel). It remains to be established whether this synergism was due to endometrial or tubal effects. This observation is intriguing since the guinea pig implantation is believed to be independent of (ovarian) estrogens. Perhaps the estrogen of embryonic origin plays a role during the guinae pig implantation, a phenomenon well known from pig blastocysts (Bazer et al. 1995). This might explain why antiestrogens exert synergistic effects with antiprogestins in guinea pigs. Recently it has ben shown that human blastocysts are also capable of producing estradiol. The preim-

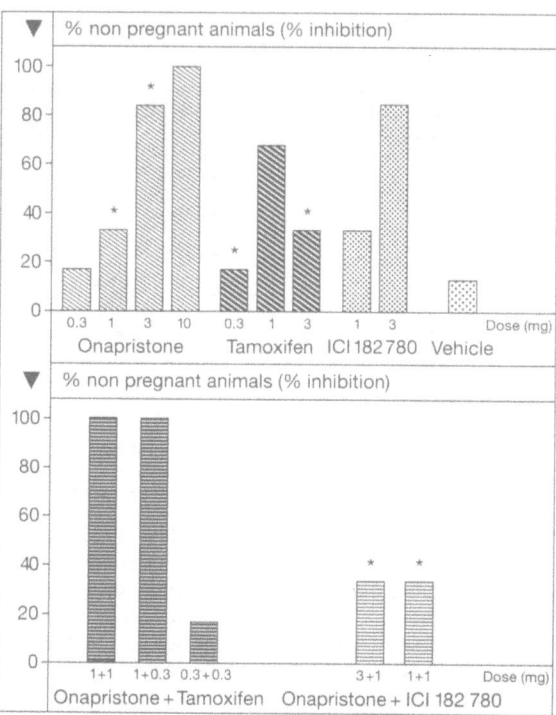

Fig. 7. Synergistic effects of onapristone and tamoxifent in guinea pigs during the preimplantation phase of pregnancy. The guinea pigs (*n*=5–6/group) were treated s.c. with onapristone, tamoxifen and ICI-182 780 alone (*upper panel*) or in combination of onapristone with either tamoxifen or ICI-182l780. Note a pronounced synergistic effect of onapristone with tamoxifen. Data are presented as percent inhibition of pregnancy

plantation human blastocysts at days 5–8 postfertilization, cultured in the presence of testosterone, produce substantial amounts of estradiol and human chorionic gonadotropin (Edgar et al. 1993). Therefore, embryonic estrogens and chorionic gonadotropin could act locally on the uterine stroma in guinea pigs and in primates and in a simlar way in rats and mice to regulate receptivity and the vascular architecture.

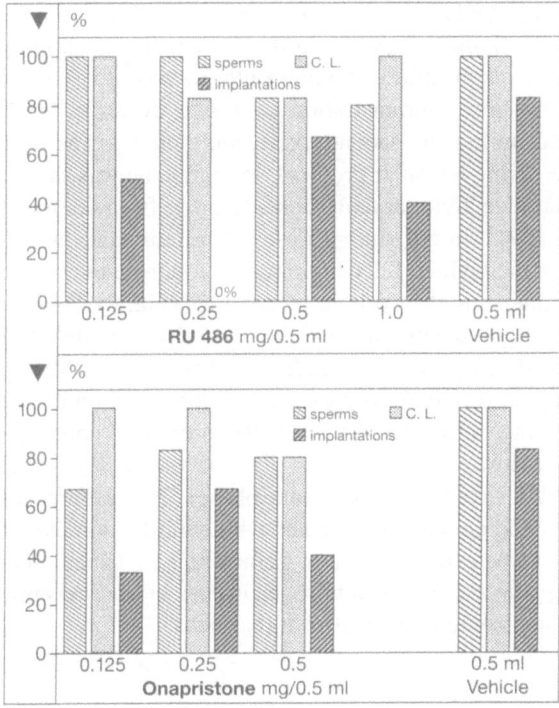

Fig. 8. Inhibition of endometrial receptivity with low-dose antiprogestins mifepristone (RU-486) and onapristone in guinea pigs. Continuous, daily oral administration over two cycles. The guinea pigs were mated during the second cycle, and autopsy was performed on day 12 p.c. For each dose, *first bar,* percentage of animals with the presence of sperm on day 1 after mating; *second bar,* percentage of animals exhibiting fresh corpora lutea (*C.L.*) during autopsy (ovulation marker); *third bar*, percentage of animals with implantation sites. Note the attenuation of fertility after 0.125 mg/mg animal (both onapristone and RU-486), and a complete inhibition of receptivity after 0.25 mg/animal RU-486 in the presence of normal ovulation

Inhibition of Endometrial Receptivity with Continuous Low-Dose Treatment in Guinea Pigs. We tested a number of antiprogestagenic compounds in their ability to inhibit uterine receptivity in guinea pigs by daily low-dose administration over two cycles. The guinea pigs were mated during the second cycle, and autopsy was performed on day 12 p.c. Using a similar protocol, mifepristone was shown to inhibit endometrial receptivity at daily doses ranging from 0.8 to 2.5 mg (Batista et al. 1991). In our studies doses of mifepristone and onapristone could be defined which fully inhibited or attenuated uterine receptivity without influencing the cycle in guinea pigs (Fig. 8). However, in contrast to monkeys, onapristone exhibited a relatively high antiovulatory activity in guinea pigs, which indicates that central effects of antiprogestins vary in different species. In addition, an inhibition of vaginal opening during estrus was observed after prolonged antiprogestin treatment even at low doses (in guinea pigs the vagina remains closed during the cycle except for the estrus phase). The differences between guinea pigs and nonhuman primates with regard to antiovulatory activity limit to some extent the use of guinea pigs as a small animal model in studying the effects of antiprogestins on uterine receptivity, especially in using continuous treatment regimens.

11.4.4 Inhibition of Endometrial Receptivity in Monkeys

In nonpregnant primates the antiprogestin effects are cycle stage and dose dependent. In nonhuman primates and humans administration of mifepristone or lilopristone (ZK 98734) during the follicular phase of the menstrual cycle impairs gonadotropin secretion and, depending on the dose, causes either retardation of the folliculogenesis or blocks ovulation (except for onapristone). When administered during the late luteal phase, high-dose antiprogestin treatment (mifepristone, onapristone, or lilopristone) inhibits the secretory activity of the endometrium and induces premature menstruation, providing the endometrium has been sufficiently exposed to endogenous progesterone.

Dissociation of Endometrial and Central Effects of Antiprogestins in Nonpregnant Monkeys. Studies with various antiprogestins which we performed in nonpregnant cynomolgus and bonnet monkeys demonstrate that central and endometrial effects are dose related, the endometrium being more sensitive than the hypothalamo-hypophyseo-ovarian axis. In cyclic cynomolgus monkeys onapristone, in contrast to RU-486, exhibited very low antiovulatory activity. However, at doses which did not block ovulation, as evidenced by progesterone concentrations in blood serum, onapristone induced a state of prolonged amenorrhea, indirectly indicating an endometrial effect (Williams et al. 1993). Similar effects were observed after RU-486 treatment. However, those doses of RU-486 which blocked ovulation were similar to doses which induced amenorrhea. In addition, both onapristone and mifepristone exhibited antiproliferative effects on the endometrium with a comparable potency in ovariectomized, estradiol-substituted monkeys (Chwalisz et al. 1992). The mechanism of these divergent effects of RU-486 and onapristone on primate ovulation is still unclear. Both the pharmacokinetic properties of onapristone and its different mode of action at the receptor levels might be responsible for these differences.

In bonnet monkeys (Ishwad et al. 1993) onapristone given at very low doses (5, 10 mg/animal, s.c.; $n=3$/group) once-a-week for two consecutive cycles produced endometrial desynchronization without disturbing the ovarian or menstrual cycle after 5 and 10 mg once-a-week. Endometrial biopsy performed around day 20 of the second cycle revealed stromal compaction and impaired growth and development of endometrial glands. Treatment with 20 mg onapristone once-a-week did not inhibit ovulation. However, menstrual bleeding was inhibited, which resulted in the prolongation of the cycle to 66–82 days. Moreover, luteal progesterone levels were reduced in this group.

The Effects of Low-Dose Onapristone on Endometrial Receptivity in Bonnet Monkeys. The differential effects of onapristone on endometrial development and ovulation in bonnet and cynomolgus monkeys have encouraged us to study its effect on fertility. Cyclic bonnet monkeys ($n=5$/group) were treated s.c. with 2.5 and 5 mg onapristone or with the vehicle for four to seven consecutive cycles. Mating was performed during the periovulatory phase of every cycle. All control animals became pregnant within three cycles, whereas only one of nine treated with onapristone became pregnant. Ovulation occurred in 30 of 45 treatment cycles. This study indicates that low-dose onapristone prevents pregnancy without disturbing the menstrual cycle in the majority of cycles after every third day of treatment in bonnet monkeys. Overall, studies with onapristone performed in bonnet monkeys strongly suggest that it should be possible to find a dose and/or a treatment regimen of an antiprogestin which assures antifertile effects in the presence of an undisturbed ovarian and menstrual cycle.

The Effects of Low-Dose Onapristone on Selected Receptivity Markers in Baboon. In this study cyclic baboons (n=3/group) were treated s.c. with either 1 or 3 mg/kg onapristone daily for 9 days, beginning 24 h after the estradiol surge. The endometrium was analyzed on days 10–11 post ovulation. Treatment with low-dose onapristone in baboons during the luteal phase altered the differential regulation of the prereceptive (PR and MUC-1) and receptive (smooth muscle myosin II, SMM II) markers on the surface epithelium without affecting either ovarian function or endometrial morphology. In normal baboons the highest MUC-1 expression on the surface epithelium was observed during the preimplantation phase (i.e., day 8 post ovulation). MUC-1 expression correlated with the presence of PR and ER in this epithelium. On days 10–12 post ovulation the expression of both MUC-1 and PR was markedly reduced as a result of progesterone action. Treatment with onapristone inhibited the downregulation of both MUC-1 and PR in the surface epithelium on day 10 post ovulation (Hildt-Petito et al. 1996). However, onapristone did not exhibit any morphological effects on the endometrium in this study (A. Fazleabas, personal communication).

11.5 General Comments and Clinical Implications

Experimental studies with antiprogestins reviewed above strongly suggest that progesterone plays a pivotal role in endometrial receptivity. Uterine receptivity appears to be a highly sensitive progesterone-dependent event which can be inhibited with low-dose antiprogestin treatment without disturbing the ovarian and menstrual cycle, recognizing the real possibility of endometrial contraception with antiprogestins. Studies with various compounds performed in small laboratory animals and in nonhuman primates indicate that the endometrium is generally more sensitive to antiprogestins than the hypophyseo-ovarian axis.

Therefore, endometrial selectivity depends primarily on the dose and treatment regimen rather than on the specific compound. However, studies performed in nonhuman primates indicate that the degree of dissociation between the central (inhibition of ovulation) and peripheral (endometrial desynchronization, biochemical milieu of the endometrium) effects may vary depending on the compound. In primates onapristone is an example of a highly dissociated compound with low antiovulatory activity. Studies performed in bonnet monkeys (Ishwad et al. 1994; Katkam et al. 1995) and baboons (Hild-Petito 1996) provide therefore ample evidence that it should be possible to define an antiprogestin dose and/or regimen (e.g., the once weekly interval) which would inhibit fertility by altering the biochemical milieu of the endometrium without at the same time influencing normal menstrual and ovarian cyclicity.

Differential effects on ovulation and endometrial morphology and biochemistry were also observed in humans after mifepristone treatment. A daily dose of 1 mg mifepristone disrupted both the morphology and function of the endometrium while preserving steroidogenesis, ovulation, and menstrual cyclicity (Batista et al. 1992). This contrasts with the complete inhibition of ovulation observed with higher mifepristone doses in women (Cameron et al. 1995). In a study in 14 healthy women once-a-week treatment with mifepristone doses as low as 2.5 and 5 mg caused desynchronization of the endometrium in the presence of normal ovulation. However, ovulation was occasionally delayed for 6–13 days (Gemzel-Danielsson 1996). These studies demonstrate that in principle a small daily dose or once-a-week dose of an antiprogestational agent can inhibit both morphological and functional maturation of the human endometrium.

In monkeys the inhibition of endometrial gland development is the major morphological effect of low-dose onapristone treatment (Ishwad et al. 1994; Katkam et al. 1995). Onapristone has been found to have a similar effect on endometrial gland formation in rabbits (Chwalisz et al. 1991). Thus the endometrial epithelium seems to be the primary target of antiprogestin treatment. It remains to be established how growth factors of stromal origin are involved in these effects.

Studies performed in bonnet monkeys and baboons indicate, however, that the morphological effects of low-dose antiprogestins are rather subtle. Thus even discrete endometrial effects of low-dose antiprogestin

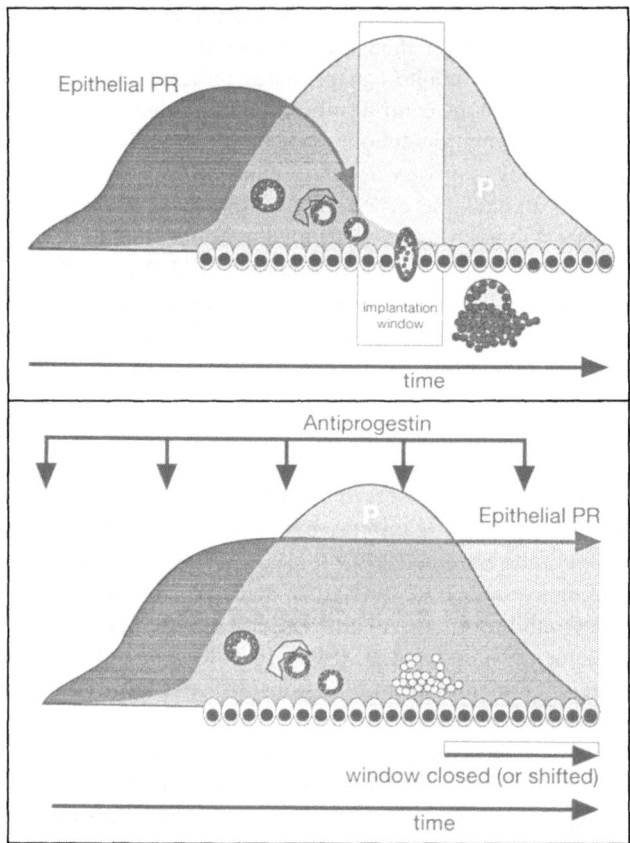

Fig. 9. The effects of antiprogestin treatment on PR expression in the luminal epithelium: Relationship to the implantation window

may result in closing the implantation window (Katkam et al. 1995), either by suppressing endometrial factors that are essential for implantation or by inducing factors such as MUC-1 that prevent implantation (Hild-Petito 1996). Moreover, it is meanwhile evident that the endometrial morphology is not a suitable predictor of a receptive endometrium. A comparison of various morphological parameters of the endometrium in a group of fertile women and infertile subjects during the peri-implantation period revealed almost no differences between these two groups (Saleh et al. 1995). Therefore, assessing the biochemical parameters of endometrial function may be more relevant marker of antiprogestin effects than the classical endometrial morphology. Further work is needed to identify reliable markers of endometrial receptivity (or their pattern).

In primates the establishment of normal endometrial receptivity appears closely associated with the downregulation of epithelial PR. Histological delay, consistent with a luteal-phase defect, is associated with a failure of PR downregulation and a lack of normal markers of receptivity (integrin $\alpha_v\beta_3$; Lessey et al. 1996). Paradoxically, the implantation window, which is highly dependent on progesterone, opens when luminal epithelial PR disappears, i.e., when these cells become functionally insensitive to progesterone. Antiprogestin treatment in general leads to the inhibition of the downregulation of PR (i.e., they increase the endometrial PR concentrations). The upregulation of PR in endometrial epithelium seems to be the most consistent effect of antiprogestins in nonhuman primates (Hild-Petito 1996) and humans (Mäentausta et al. 1993; Cameron et al. 1995, 1996; Gemzell-Danielson et al. 1996). Perhaps the downregulation of epithelial PR is a key event of receptivity, and inhibiting this process is crucial for closing or shifting the implantation window with antiprogestins (Fig. 9).

However, the exact molecular mechanism of action of antiprogestins on endometrial receptivity and the implantation process is still not clear. In particular, further studies are required to investigate the antiprogestin effect on endometrial factors which seem to play an essential role in various stages of implantation.

In addition, the endometrium may not be the only target for antiprogestins during the peri-implantation period. Antiprogestins may also affect other important processes, including the fertilization process, tubal transport, early embryonic development, and embryonic signaling. These potential targets for antiprogestins remain to be investigated.

Overall, the experimental studies, in particular those performed in nonhuman primates, suggest the value of clinical trials in unprotected women to evaluate whether the biochemical and morphological effects of low-dose antiprogestins are consistent with contraception. There is, however, a number of questions concerning efficacy, safety, embryo toxicity, and finally additional health benefits which remain to be answered in future clinical studies. A key concern of long-term antiprogestin use is the possibility of unopposed estrogen action in the endometrium, which might result in endometrial hyperplasia. A desychronous endometrial morphological pattern consistent with estrogenic effects was described after chronic treatment with high-dose RU-486 (25 and 50 mg) of women with endometriosis and leiomyomas (Murphy et al. 1994). On the other hand, the existing short-term studies performed in ovariectomized animals and studies with low-dose onapristone in normal bonnet monkeys suggest that antiprogestins also exhibit an antiproliferative effects on the endometrium, which would argue strongly against the possibility of endometrial stimulation. In addition, numerous political and ethical issues associated with antiprogestins in general may influence their development for fertility control.

Acknowledgments. We are grateful to Mrs. B. Kosub, Mrs. B. Bragulla, Mrs. A. Seipp, Mrs.C. Grund and Mr. Otto for their excellent technical assistance in performing experimantal studies and to Mrs. R. Jäger for the editing.

References

Batista MC, Bristow TL, Mathews J, Stokes WS, Loriaux DL, Nieman LK (1991) Daily administration of the progesterone antagonist RU 486 prevents implantation in the cycling guinea pigs. Am J Obstet Gynecol 165:82–86

Batista MC, Cartledge RN, Zellmer RN, Merino MJ, Axiotis C, Loriaux L, Niemann LK (1992) Delayed endometrial maturation induced by daily administration of the antiprogestin RU 486: a potential new contraceptive strategy. Am J Obstet Gynecol 1992:60–65

Bazer FW, Spencer TE, Ott TL, Ing NH (1995) Regulation of endometrial responsiveness to estrogen and progesterone by pregnancy recognition signals during the preimplantation period. In: Dey SK (ed) Molecular and cellular aspects of preimplantation processes. Serono Symposia USA. Springer, Berlin Heidelberg New York, pp 27–48

Beier HM (1975) Uteroglobin and related biochemical changes in the reproductive tract during early pregnancy in the rabbit. J Reprod Fertil [Suppl] 25:53–69

Beier-Hellwig K, Sterzik K, Bonn B, Hilmes U, Bygdeman M, Gemzell-Danielsson K, Beier HM (1994) Hormone regulation and hormone antagonist effects on protein pattern of human endometrial secretion during receptivity. In Bulletti C, Gurpide E, Flamigni C (eds) The human endometrium. Ann N Y Acad Sci 734:143–157

Beier HM, Hegele-Hartung C, Mootz U, Beier-Hellwig K (1994) Modification of endometrial cell biology using progesterone antagonists to manipulate the implantation window. Hum Reprod 9 [Suppl 1]:98–120

Bergh PA, Navot D (1992) The impact of embryonic development and endometrial maturity on the timing of implantation. Fertil Steril 58:537–542

Bhatt H, Brunet LJ, Stewart CL (1991) Uterine expression of leukemia inhibitory factor coincides with the onset of blastocyct implantation. Proc Natl Acad Sci (USA) 88:11408–11412

Cameron ST, Thong KJ, Baird DT (1995) Effects of daily low-dose mifepristone on the ovarian cycle and on dynamics of follicle growth. Clin Endocrinol 43:407–414

Cameron ST, Critchley HOD, Buckley CH, Chard T, Kelly RW, Baird DT (1996) The effects of post-ovulatory administration of onapristone on the development of a secretory endometrium. Hum Reprod 11:40–49

Chang MC (1950) Development and fate of transferred rabbit ova or blastocyst in relation to the ovulation time of recipients. J Exp Zool 114:197–

Chwalisz K, Hegele-Hartung C, Fritzemeier KH, Beier HM, Elger W (1991) Inhibition of the estradiol-mediated endometrial gland formation by the antigestagen onapristone in rabbits: relationship to uterine estrogen receptors. Endocrinology 129(1):312–322

Chwalisz K, Hsiu JG, Williams RF, Hodgen GD (1992) Evaluation of the antiproliferative actions of the progesterone antagonists mifepristone (RU 486) and onapristone (ZK 98 299) on primate endometrium. Society for Gynecologic Investigation, Scientific Program and Abstracts, 39th Annual Meeting, San Antonio, Texas, March 18–21

Chwalisz K (1993) Role of progesterone in the control of labor. In: Chwalisz K, Garfield RE (eds) Basic mechanisms controlling term and preterm labor. Ernst Schering Research Foundation Workshop 7, Springer, Berlin, Heidelberg, New York. pp 97–163

Chwalisz K, Garfield RE (1994) Antiprogestins in the induction of labor (1994) Ann NY Acad Sci 734:387–413

Chwalisz K, Stöckemann K, Fuhrmann U, Fritzemeier KH, Einspanier A, Garfield RE (1995) Mechanism of action of antiprogestins in the pregnant uterus. In: Henderson D, Philibert D, Roy AK, Teutsch G (eds) Steroid receptors and antihormones. Ann NY Acad Sci 761:202–224

Cook CE, Lee YW, Wani, Fail PA, Petrow (1994) Effects of D-ring substituents on antiprogestational (antagonist) and progestational (agonist) activity of 11β-aryl steroids. Hum Reprod 9 [Suppl 1]:32–40

Cowell, TP (1969) Implantation and development of mouse eggs transferred to the uteri of non-progestational mice. J Reprod Fertiol 19:239–245

Croxatto HB, Salvatierra AM, Croxatto HD, Fuentealba B (1993) Effects of continuous treatment with low-dose mifepristone throughout one menstrual cycle. Hum Reprod:8:201–207

Croxatto, HB, Salvatierra AM, Croxatto HD, Fuentealba B, Zurth C, Beier S (1994) Effects of the antiprogestin onapristone on follicular growth in women. Hum Reprod 9:1442–1447

Das SK, Chakraborty I, Paria BC, Wang XN, Plowman G, Dey SK (1995) Amphiregulin is an implantation-specific and progesterone-regulated gene in the mouse uterus. Mol Endocrinol 9:691–705

Deansley R (1960) Implantation and early pregnancy in ovariectomized guinea pigs. J Reprod Fertil 1:242–248

Deansley R (1971) The differentiation of the decidua at ovo-implantation in the guinea pigs contrasted with the traumatic deciduoma. J Reprod Fertil 26:91–97

Ding YQ, Zhu LJ, Bagchi MK, Bagchi IC (1994) Progesterone stimulates calcitonin gene expression in the uterus during implantation. Endocrinol 135:2265–2274

Edgar DH, James GB, Mills JA (1993) Steroid secretion by early human embryos in culture. Hum Reprod 8:277–278

Edwards RG (1995) Physiological and molecular aspects of human implantation. Hum Reprod 10 [Suppl](2):1–14

Enders AC, Schlafke S (1989) Cytological aspects of trophoblast-uterine interactions in early implantation. Am J Anat 125:1–30

Enders AC (1993) Overview of the morphology of implantation in primates. In: Wolf DP, Stouffer RL, Brenner RM (eds) In vitro fertilization and embryo transfer in primates. Springer, Berlin Heidelberg New York, pp 145-157

Fazleabas AT, Verhage HG (1994) Expression and regulation of insulin-like growth factor binding protein-1 and retinol binding protein in the baboon (Papio anubis) uterus. In: Glasser SR, Mulholland J, Psychoyos A (eds) Endocrinology of embryo-endometrium interactions. Plenum, New York, pp 57–75

Feil PD, Clarke CL, Satyaswaroopp PG (1988) Progestin-mediated changes in progesterone receptor forms in the normal human endometrium. Endocrinology 123:2506–2513

Finn CA, Martin L (1974) The control of implantation. J Reprod Fertil 39:195–206

Fliss AE, Michel FJ, Chen CL, Höfig A, Bazer FW, Chou JY, Simmen RCM (1991) Regulation of the uteroferrin gene promotor in endometrial cells: interaction among estrogen, progesterone, and prolactin. Endocrinol 129:697–704

Gemzell-Danielsson K, Swahn ML, Svalander P, Bygdeman M (1993) Early luteal phase treatment with RU 486 for fertility regulation. Hum Reprod 8:870–873

Gemzell-Danielsson K, Westlund P, Johannisson E, Swahn ML, Bygdeman M, Seppälä (1996) Effect of low weekly doses of mifepristone on ovarian function and endometrial development. Hum Reprod 11:256–264

Ghosh D, Roy A, Sengupta J, Johannnisson E (1993) Morphological characterization of the preeimplantation stage endometrium in rhesus monkeys. Hum Reprod 8:1579–1589

Glasier A, Thong KJ, Dewar M, Mackie M, Baird DT (1992) Mifepristone (RU 486) compared with high-dose estrogen and progestestogen for emergency postcoital contraception. N Engl J Med 327:1041–1044

Gronemeyer H, Benhamou B, Berry M, Bocquel MT, Gofflo D, Garcia T, Lerouge T, Metzger D, Meyer ME, Tora L, Vergezac A, Chambon P (1992) Mechanism of antihormone action. J Steroid Biochem Mol Biol 41:217–221

Grümmer R, Chwalisz K, Mulholland J, Traub O, Winterhager E (1994) Regulation of connexin26 and connexin43 expression in rat endometrium by ovarian steroid hormones. Biol Reprod 51:1109–1116

Hegele-Hartung C, Mootz U, Beier HM (1992) Luteal control of endometrial receptivity and its modification by progesterone antagonists. Endocrinol 131:2446–2460

Heikinheimo O (1989) Pharmacokinetics of the antiprogesterone RU 486 in women during multiple dose administration. J Steroid Biochem 32:21–25

Hild-Petito S, lian J, Carson D (1996) Mucin (Muc-1) expression is differentgially regulated in the uterine luminal and glandular epithelia in the baboon (Papio anubis). Biol Reprod 54:939–947

Hoff JD, Quigley ME, Yen SC (1983) Hormonal dynamics at midcycle: a reevaluation. J Clin Endocrinol Metab 57:792-796

Horwitz KB (1992) The molecular biology of RU 486. Is there a role for antiprogestins in the treatment of breast cancer? Endocr Rev 13 (2):146–163

Horwitz KB, Alexander PS (1993) In situ photolinked nuclear progesterone receptors of human breast cancer cells: subunit molecular weights after transformation and translocation. Endocrinol 113:2195–2201

Ishwad PC, Katkam RR; Hinduja IN, Chwalisz K, Elger W, Puri CP (1993) Treatment with a progesterone antagonist ZK 89 299 delays endometrial development without blocking ovulation in bonnet monkeys. Contraception 48:57–70

Katkam RR, Gopalkrishnan K, Chwalisz K, Schillinger E, Puri CP (1995) Onapristone (ZK 98 299): a potential antiprogestin for endometrial contraception. Am J Obstet Gynecol 173:779–787

Klein-Hitpass L, Cato ACB, Henderson D, Ryffel GU (1991) Two types of antiprogestins identified by their differential action in transcriptionally active extracts from T47D cells. Nucleic Acid Res 19:1227–1234

Kloosterboer HJ, Deckers GH, Schoonen WGEJ (1994) Pharmacology of two new very selective antiprogestagens: ORG 31710 and Org 31806. Hum Reprod 9 [Suppl]1:47–53

Koering MJ, Healy DL, Hodgen GD (1986) Morphologic response of endometrium to a progesterone receptor antagonist, RU 486, in monkeys. Fertil Steril 45:280–228

Lessey BA, Killam AP, Metzger DA, Haney AF, Greene GL, McCarty K (1988) Immunohistochemical analysis of human uterine estrogen and progesterone receptors throughout the menstrual cycle. J Clin Endocrinol Metab 67:334

Lessey BA, Castelbaum AJ, Sawin SW, Buck CA, Schinnar R, Bilker W, Strom BL (1994) Aberrant integrin expression in the endometrium of women with endometriosis. J Clin Endocrin Metab 79:643–649

Lessey BA, Yeh I, Castelbaum AJ, Fritz MA, Ilesanmi AO, Korzeniowski P, Sun J, Chwalisz K (1996). Endometrial progesterone receptors and markers of uterine receptivity in the window of implantation Fertil Steril 65:477–483

Loke YW, King A (1995) Human Implantation. Cell biology and immunology. Cambridge University Press

Mäentausta O, Svalander P, Gemzell-Danielsson K, Bygdeman M, Vihko R (1993) The effects of an antiprogestin, mifepristone and an antiestrogen, tamoxifen, on endometrial 17β-hydroxysteroid dehydrogenase and progestin and estrogen receptors during the luteal phase of the menstrual cycle: an immunohistochemical study. J Clin Endocrinol Metab 77:913–918

McDonnell DP, Goldman ME (1994) RU 486 exerts antiestrogenic activities through a novel progesterone receptor A form-mediated mechanism. J Biol Chem 269:11945–11949

McLaren A (1973) Blastocyst activation. In: Segal SJ, Sheldon J, Crozier R, Corfman PA, Condliffe PG (eds) The regulation of mammalian Reproduction. Thomas, Springfeld, pp 321–334

Murphy AA, Castellano PZ (1994) RU 486: Pharmacology and potential use in the treatment of endometriosis and leiomyomata uteri. Curr Opin Obstet Gynecol 1994:269–278

Nanaev A, Chwalisz K, Frank HG, Kohen G, Hegele-Hartung C, Kaufmann P (1995) Physiological dilatation of uteroplacental arteries in guinea pigs depends on nitric oxide synthase activity of extravillous trophoblast. Cell Tissue Res 282:407–421

Navot D, Scott RT, Droesch KD, Veeck LL, Hung-Ching Liu, Rosenvaks Z (1991) The window of embryo transfer and efficiency of human conception in vitro. Fertil Steril 55:114–118

Neef G, Beier S, Elger W, Henderson D, Wiechert R (1984) New steroids with antiprogestational and antiglucocorticoid activities. Steroids 44:349–372

Padykula HA (1991) Regeneration in primate uterus. The role of stem cells. In: Wynn, RM, Jollie WP (eds) Biology of the uterus. Plenum, New York, pp 279–288

Paria BC, Huet-Hudson YM, Dey SK (1993) Blastocyst's state of activity determines the "window" of implantation in the receptive mouse uterus. Proc Natl Acad Sci USA 90:10159–10162

Phillibert D, Moguilewsky M, Mary M, Lecaque D, Tournemine C, Secchi J, Deraedt R (1985) Pharmacological profile of RU 486 in animals. In: Baulieu EE, Segal SJ (eds) The antiprogestrone steroid RU 486 and human fertility control. Plenum, New York, pp 49–68

Psychoyos A (1986) Uterine receptivity for nidation. Ann NY Acad Sci 476:36–42

Psychoyos A (1973) Endocrine control of egg implantation. In: Green RO (ed) Handbook of physiology, sect 7, vol 2, part 2. American Physiological Society. Washington DC, pp 187–215

Puri CP (1995) Antiprogestins: useful investigative tools and novel contraceptives. Curr Sci 68:407–423

Roblero LS, Croxatto HB (1991) Effect of RU 486 on development and implantation of rat embryos. Mol Reprod Develop 29:342–346

Saleh MI, Warren MA, Li TC, Cooke ID (1995) A light microscopical morphometric study of the luminal epithelium of human endometrium during the peri-implantation period. Hum Reprod 10:1828–1832

Sartorius CA, Tung L, Takimoto GS, Hoerwitz KB (1993) Antagonist-occupied human progesterone receptors bound to DNA are functionally switched to transcriptional agonists by cAMP. J Biol Chem 5:9262–9266

Stewart CL, Kaspar P, Brunet LJ, Bhatt H, Gadi I, Köntgen F, Abbondanzo SJ (1992) Blastocyst implantation depends on maternal expression of leukemia inhibitory factor. Nature 359:76–79

Surveyor GA, Gendlern SJ, Pemberton I, Das SK, Chakraborty I, Julian J, Pimental RA, Wegner CC, Dey SK, Carson DD (1995) Expression and steroid hormonal control of Muc-1 in the mouse uterus. Endocrinol 136:3639–3647

Tabibzadeh S, Babaknia A (1995) The signals and molecular pathways involved in implantation, a symbiotic interaction between blastocyst and endometrium involving adhesion and tissue invation. Mol Hum Reprod 1, Hum Reprod 10:1579–1609

Vegato E, Shabhaz MM, Wen DX, Goldman ME, O'Malley BW, McDonnell DP (1993) Human progesterone receptor A form is a cell- and promoter-specific repressor of human progesterone receptor B function. Molec Endocrinol 7:1244–1255

Vinijsanun A, Martin L (1990) Effects of progesterone antagonists RU 486 and ZK 98 734 on embryo transport, development and implantation in laboratory mice. Reprod Fertil Dev 2:713–727

Williams RF, Chwalisz K, Hodgen GD (1993) Anti-progestins: dissociation of antiovulatory and anti-proliferative actions. Society for Gynecologic Investigation. Scientific Program and Abstracts, 40th Annual Meeting, March 31-April 3 (abstract S59)

Zhang Z, Funk C, Glasser SR, Mullholand J (1994) Progesterone regulation of heparin-binding epidermal growth factor-like growth factor gene expression during sensitization and decidualization in the rat uterus: Effects of the antiprogestin, ZK 98 299. Endocrinol 135:1256–1263

Zhu Li-Ji, Bagchi MK, Bagchi IC (1995) Ferritin heavy chain is a progesterone-inducible marker in the uterus during pregnancy. Endocrinol 136:4106–4115

12 Clinical Strategies for the Achievement of Endometrial Contraception with Progesterone Antagonists

H.B Croxatto, B. Fuentealba, A.M. Salvatierra, and R. Massai

12.1 Possible Modes of Action of Antiprogestins on the Endometrium

Since the first antiprogestin, RU-38486 (mifepristone), was reported to the scientific community in 1982 (Philibert et al. 1982), many others have been synthesized, but very few of them, including mifepristone (Roussel Uclaf), ZK-98299 (onapristone), ZK-98734 (lilopristone), ZK-98993 (Schering AG), ORG-31710, and ORG-31806 (Organon

Oss) have been tested in primates to assess effects on the reproductive system in general and the endometrium in particular.

At various times throughout the menstrual cycle progesterone is involved in the regulation of a number of processes which take place at each level of the reproductive axis from brain to genital tract. Progesterone intervenes in their control not only at the elevated serum levels of the luteal phase but also at the slightly rising levels around the onset of the gonadotropin surge and even at the very low and stable levels of the follicular phase. It is therefore expected that antiprogestins affect endometrial development and function through a direct action on this tissue, as well as indirectly from the consequences of blockade of progesterone action on the ovary, pituitary, or hypothalamus. An example of this is the variable effect of a high dose of mifepristone given in the midluteal phase. At times it causes immediate endometrial bleeding followed by a second bleeding at the normal time of corpus luteum demise. At other times it causes immediate luteolysis with total shedding of the endometrium, and no second bleeding is observed (Schaison et al. 1985; Shoupe et al. 1987).

Considering the complexity of the spectrum of progesterone actions it is predictable that variables such as the time of the menstrual cycle, dose level, mode of administration, and particular antiprogestin given affect the response of the endometrium. Therefore results obtained with a given regimen should not be extrapolated or generalized without great caution.

Ideally one should distinguish direct from indirect effects of antiprogestins to interpret the endometrial response. Those attributable to their direct action on endometrial cells should be defined under experimental conditions in which all indirect effects are excluded. This may be attained easily in vitro, but also in vivo if the endometrium is the most sensitive tissue to the action of an antiprogestin, and the dose used is below the threshold for the upper levels of the axis. When the treatment with antiprogestin decreases steroid production, replacement therapy with estradiol and progesterone should be used to ensure that none of the effects observed on the endometrium can be attributed to deficient production of these hormones, caused by the antiprogestin actions elsewhere in the body. Theoretically the effects of antiprogestins on the endometrium can be mediated via progesterone receptor blockade as well as glucocorticoid receptor blockade. Although specific effects of glucocorticoid hormones on the human endometrium have not been considered important in the past, they cannot be excluded a priori. Given the fact that antiprogestins are also endowed with antiglucocorticoid activity, this should be kept in mind when interpreting endometrial effects of antiprogestins However, at low doses such as 1 mg/day, mifepristone is very unlikely to compete significantly with cortisol for its receptor.

Concerning the direct effects of antiprogestins on the endometrium, some apparent agonistic, estrogenic and antiestrogenic effects have been observed in some particular experimental conditions. Examples of such effects are: (a) mifepristone induces secretory changes in the endometrium of estrogen-primed postmenopausal women (Gravanis et al. 1985), (b) mifepristone increases estrogen receptor levels in the endometrium in cycling women (Berthois et al. 1991) and in ovariectomized estrogen-supplemented monkeys (Haluska et al. 1990; Neulen et al. 1990; Slayden et al. 1993; Brenner and Slayden 1994), and (c) mifepristone and onapristone block estradiol-induced endometrial proliferation in ovariectomized monkeys (Wolf et al. 1989; Chwalisz et al. 1992; Slayden et al. 1993). The intracellular mechanisms involved in these effects still await elucidation and may be related to the ability of the antiprogestin-receptor complex to bind DNA and/or the differential expression of progesterone receptor (PR) isoforms A and B in the target cells (See Chap. 1, this volume).

In contrast to onapristone, RU-486 allows PR binding to DNA (Klein-Hitpass 1993), and through a novel mechanism involving cAMP-regulated proteins (Horwitz et al. 1995) it can present agonistic effects under some conditions (Beck et al. 1993). On the other hand, the binding of the antiprogestin to isoform PR-A appears to be involved in the antiproliferative effect seen in some targets cells through its ability to alter the transcriptional activity of estrogen receptors (McDonnell and Goldman 1994). The relative expression of the PR isoforms seems to be differentially regulated in progesterone target cells (Feil et al. 1988; Brandon et al. 1993) and may be critical for the cellular response to progesterone or antiprogestins.

The current body of knowledge is insufficient to anticipate the clinical implications of the apparent agonistic, estrogenic, and antiestrogenic effects of antiprogestins on the endometrium. The balance of such effects is critical since they antagonize each other, and this has not been assessed in real life situations. The fact that increased estrogen receptor levels in the endometrium, caused by antiprogestins in ovariectomized estrogen-supplemented monkeys, are associated with decreased proliferative activity, tells us that the complexity of this area still escapes our understanding. The bottom line is that not all the effects of antiprogestins on the endometrium may be attributed only to blockade of progesterone action in this target tissue.

12.2 Observed Effects on Endometrial Development and Function

Most of studies concerning the effects of antiprogestins on the menstrual cycle in women have been carried out with mifepristone, and alterations in endometrial development have been a constant finding, with this and with other antiprogestins.

A single dose of mifepristone, ranging from 5 to 200 mg, has been given to women between days 2 and 6 after the surge in luteinizing hormone (LH). Three days after treatment the effects observed by morphometric analysis include inhibited glandular secretory activity, accelerated degenerative changes, and increased stromal but not glandular mitosis (Li et al. 1988). Another study reported increasing retardation of endometrial development from 12 to 84 h after a single dose of 200 mg administered on LH+2. The main differences with the control tissues were observed in the glandular elements. A lesser number of vacuolated cells, observed as early as 12 h after drug intake, smaller glandular diameter, evident on LH+4 and, persisting pseudoestratification and increased number of mitosis on LH+6 were indicative of retarded or blunted response to progesterone (Swahn et al. 1990).

Additional assessment of the effects of this treatment on endometrial development was carried out near the time implantation is believed to start, namely on days LH+6 to LH+8. Immuno- and lectin-cytochemistry showed increased staining of progesterone receptors in the glandular epithelium and decreased staining of secretory components, respectively. Both of these findings indicate that the secretory transformation, which normally occurs in response to progesterone, was inhibited (Gemzell-Danielsson et al. 1994). More recently the endometrial effects of 200 mg mifepristone or 400 mg onapristone given on LH+2 were compared (Cameron et al. 1995). With both treatments retarded secretory development was observed in the morphological assessment on days LH+4 or LH+6. In addition, both treatments decreased the immunostaining of the progesterone-dependent enzyme 15-hydroxyprostaglandin dehydrogenase and increased that of the cell proliferation marker Ki67, both in the glandular epithelium.

Retarded endometrial secretory transformation was also observed when 10 mg mifepristone was administered daily for 4 days from ovulation onwards (Berthois et al. 1991) or on days 5 and 8 after the LH surge (Greene et al. 1992).

A differential threshold for mifepristone effects on pituitary, ovarian, and endometrial function has been found after continuous administration of 10, 5, or 1 mg/day for 30 days (Croxatto et al. 1993). Of these three levels the endometrium seems to be the most sensitive target for the action of the antiprogestin. With the dose of 1 mg/day no consistent central or ovarian effects were observed, but endometrial histology was disturbed in all five cases (inactive, proliferative, or asynchronous secretory; Croxatto et al. 1993). With the same dose of mifepristone, 1 mg/day given for one cycle, endometrial samples taken 7–9 days after the LH peak, showed a histological dating lagging 3 or 4 days behind the chronological dating in six out of nine biopsies (Batista et al. 1992). No hyperplastic endometrial development was observed in these studies.

The effects of onapristone and lilopristone on endometrial development have been assessed in bonnet monkeys. Onapristone, 5–10 mg given s.c. at weekly intervals during two cycles, induced atrophic changes both in the glands and in the stroma while the pattern of estradiol and progesterone levels was suggestive of normal ovulatory cycles (Ishwad et al. 1993). On the other hand, lilopristone, 25 mg given s.c. at weekly intervals, suppressed gonadotropin and ovarian steroid secretion, and therefore direct effects on the endometrium could not be assessed (Puri et al. 1992).

It is clear that administration of antiprogestins, in a wide range of doses, alters endometrial development, but the question remaining is whether these alterations would preclude successful implantation in the majority of women.

Several substances produced in the endometrium have been proposed as molecular markers of endometrial receptivity, and are expected to reflect more specifically than morphology the potential of antiprogestins for interfering with implantation. One of these is the $\alpha_v\beta_3$ vitronectin receptor, an integrin with a role in cell-cell adhesion that may be involved in endometrial-trophoblast association (Lessey et al. 1992). This molecule is present in human trophoblast and appears also in the epithelial cells of human endometrium on cycle days 19–20 and remains for a period of 4 days (Tabibzadeh 1992; Lessey 1994; see Lessey, this volume).

The determination of the protein pattern of the human uterine fluid has been proposed as another tool for diagnosing normality or alteration of endometrial secretory activity and, presumably, endometrial receptivity. Electrophoretic analysis of secreted proteins shows differences throughout the phases of the cycle. At the beginning and at the end of the cycle, days 1–5 and 25–28 respectively, there is a pattern of quiescense. The number and intensity of the bands increases during the period of proliferation, days 6–14, reaching their maximum during the secretory phase, days 15–24 (Beier-Hellwig et al. 1989 1994; see also Beier, this volume).

Other endometrial markers, proposed as being essential for endometrial receptivity, which are downregulated by antiprogestins, are an endometrial secretory glycan (Graham et al. 1991) and a metalloproteinase inhibitor (see Aplin, this volume and Bischof, this volume).

Key questions at the moment are whether lower doses of antiprogestins can produce subtle alterations detected only at the molecular level, without the more profound changes expressed in altered endometrial morphology, and whether they are sufficient to impair endometrial receptivity.

12.3 Clinical Strategies

The alterations induced by mifepristone on endometrial development are the basis for the concept of endometrial contraception. It is widely accepted that there is a limited time period during which the human endometrium is receptive for successful implantation, and clinical observations support this concept (Navot et al. 1991). Therefore the delay in endometrial development caused by antiprogestins could result in failure of implantation. Different strategies to achieve endometrial contraception have been designed and tested in monkeys and the human: (a) a single high dose given in the early luteal phase, (b) intermittent

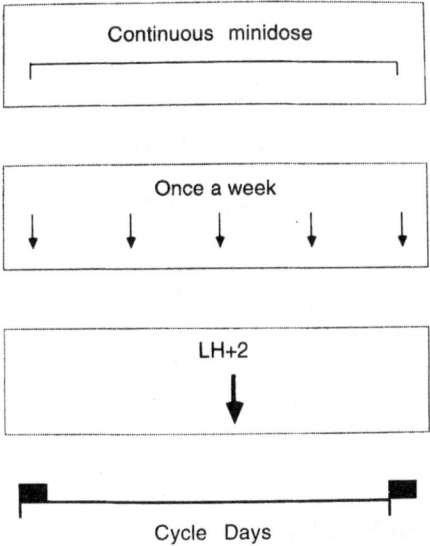

Fig. 1. Schematic representation of treatment schedules proposed to achieve endometrial contraception. These schedules differ both in the time distribution of the total dose per cycle (daily, once a week, once per cycle) and in the amount of drug given each time. See text for details. *LH*, luteinizing hormone

administration during the menstrual cycle, or (c) continuous minidose administration (Fig. 1).

12.3.1 Single High-Dose Administration in the Early Luteal Phase

A single dose of 200 mg mifepristone on LH+2 was sufficient to alter endometrial development (Swahn et al. 1990; Cameron et al. 1995). When the contraceptive efficacy of this regimen was tested in 21 unprotected women, with a total of 157 ovulatory treated cycles, for up to 12 months, only one clinical pregnancy occurred (Gemzell-Danielsson et al. 1993). The same approach was tested in 17 mated rhesus monkeys. After giving mifepristone, 2 or 10 mg/kg body weight, s.c., 3 days after the estradiol peak, no pregnancy was detected in a total of 33 cycles. The low dose did not change any event of the cycle, but the dose of 10 mg unexpectedly produced a threefold prolongation of the luteal phase (Ghosh and Sengupta 1993).

12.3.2 Intermittent Administration During the Menstrual Cycle

Onapristone, 2.5 mg s.c. every third day for 17 consecutive cycles was given to four bonnet monkeys. Another animal received 5 mg every third day for 21 cycles. Depending on the pharmacokinetics, these intermittent injections in oil may in fact act as a continuous low-dose treatment. None of these monkeys conceived, but the five control animals became pregnant within the first three cycles. Endometrial growth and development was retarded in all treated animals (Katkam et al. 1995).

12.3.3 Continuous Minidose Administration

The effects of a continuous low-dose treatment with mifepristone on the menstrual cycle were assessed in women by giving 10, 5 or 1 mg/day for 30 days (Croxatto et al. 1993). The doses of 10 and 5 mg/day, but not that of 1 mg/day, inhibited ovulation consistently. All doses disturbed endometrial maturation. The constancy of this effect, even at the dose of

Table 1. Effect of continuous mifepristone (1 mg/day) over a 5-month period on ovarian function

Type of cycle[a]	Patients[b] (n)
Monophasic	
Follicular rupture (–); rise in progesterone levels (–)	12
Biphasic anovulatory	
Follicular rupture (–); rise in progesterone levels (+)	2
Ovulatory	
Follicular rupture (+); rise in progesterone levels (+)	16

[a]Assessed by serial echographic imaging to detect follicular rupture and by serial plasma progesterone determinations.
[b]Only the first, third, and fifth months of treatment were assessed in each of ten treated women.

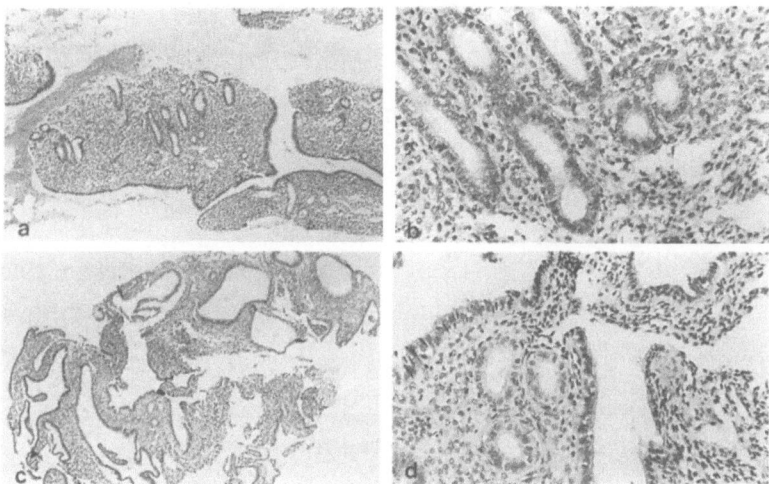

Fig. 2a–d. Light micrographs of biopsies taken on day 22 (**a,b**) and on day 148 (**c,d**) of a continuous treatment with mifepristone 1 mg/day. Endometrial samples taken from to a woman who presented monophasic cycles and amenorrhea throughout the 5 months of treatment. **a** On day 22 of treatment: note that most glands are straight and with narrow lumen. Stroma is compact, ×35. **b** Glandular epithelium with cubic or cylindric cells and these, with cytoplasmic vacuoles, ×170. **c** On day 148 of treatment: note the dilated glands, few straight glands and compact stroma, ×35. **d** At higher magnification the epithelium of the dilated glands is pseudostratified with cytoplasmic vacuoles, or cubic. Straight glands with cubic epithelium and scanty secretion in the lumen, ×170

1 mg/day, indicates that the endometrium is more sensitive to mifepristone than upper levels of the reproductive axis. Therefore the results of this study suggested the possibility of altering endometrial development without affecting ovarian function.

The long-term effects of this treatment were tested in a two-center study in which a daily dose of 1 mg/day was given continuously for 5 months (Croxatto et al., unpublished). Histological assessment of endometrial biopsies taken during treatment confirmed the effectiveness of this dose for altering endometrial development (Figs. 2, 3). The protein pattern of the uterine fluid during treatment (Croxatto et al., unpublished) and the distribution of estradiol and progesterone receptors as-

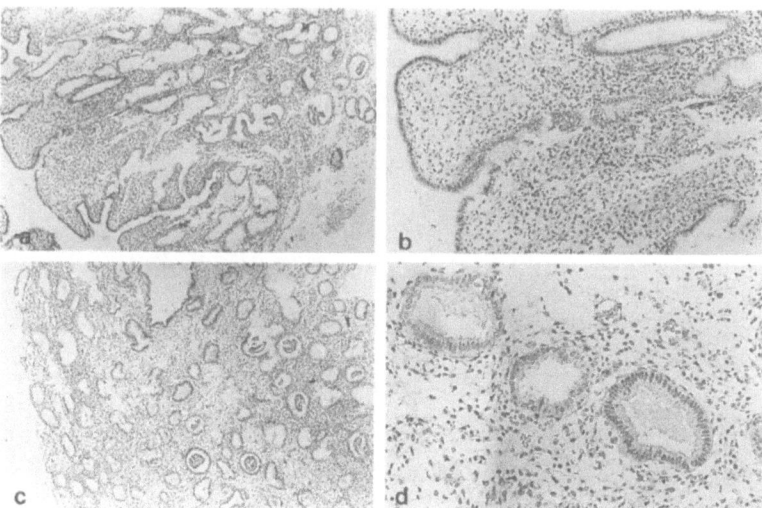

Fig. 3a–d. Light micrographs of biopsies taken on day 23 (**a, b**) and on day 144 (**c, d**) of a continuous treatment with mifepristone 1 mg/day. Endometrial samples taken from a woman who presented ovulatory cycles and regular bleeding pattern throughout the 5 months of treatment. **a** On day 23 of treatment: intense stromal edema close to the surface and secretory glands with cytoplasmic vacuoles or luminal secretion, ×35. **b** Blood vessels with thin walls close to the surface but arteriolar development in deeper areas, ×86. **c,d** On day 144 of treatment (**c,** ×35; **d,** ×170). Note the delayed development of glands in relation with the stroma, similar to that observed during the first month of treatment

sessed by immunocytochemistry confirmed the delay in endometrial development and suggested that this may be even longer than that estimated by the histological assessment. Ovulation was suppressed in nearly 50% of the cycles, indicating that a dose of 1 mg/day is still too high for dissociating ovarian and endometrial effects in the majority of women (Table 1).

This treatment did not interfere with bleeding cyclicity in those women who had ovulatory cycles, while amenorrhea or prolonged inter-bleeding periods were observed in association with anovulation. The occurrence of prolonged periods of amenorrhea, in which the endometrium is constantly exposed to unopposed estrogen action, is believed to be associated with increased risk of endometrial hyperplasia and neoplastic disease, and it is generally considered an undesirable condition from a medical point of view. The induction of such condition by continuous administration of minidoses of antiprogestins gives rise to the same concerns, although the previously mentioned apparent agonistic and antiestrogenic activities of some antiprogestins could make a significant difference, yet to be explored. Nonetheless, such concern had led to the search for ways in which to circumvent the condition of unopposed estrogen and amenorrhea. Such attempts are described in the following section.

12.4 Other Applications

12.4.1 Antiprogestin-Progestin Regimen

A different approach, in which several effects of the antiprogestin on the menstrual cycle are involved, including those on the endometrium, is the sequential regimen (Fig. 4). In this scheme the antiprogestin is given in the first half of the cycle to impede maturation of the leading follicle, and therefore ovulation and a progestin is given for the remaining of the cycle to induce secretory transformation of the endometrium and with-

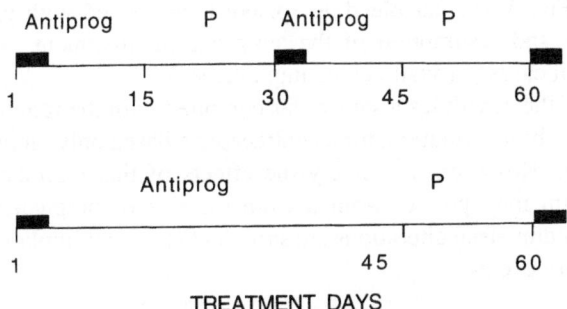

Fig. 4. Schematic representation of an antiprogestin-progestin sequential regimen. Two modalities are depicted. *Above*, antiprogestin (*Antiprog*) is given during the first half of the cycle and the progestin (*P*) in the second half. *Below*, antiprogestin is given for 45 days and the progestin during the succeeding 2 weeks, so that menses occurs only six times per year

Table 2. Effect of a sequential regimen of mifepristone-medroxyprogesterone acetate[a] on endometrial morphology

Endometrium[b]	Patients (n)
Secretory initial	2
Secretory day 16–18	3
Glandular-stromal asynchrony	2
Mixed types of glands	3
Normal	0

[a]Mifepristone 5 mg/day was given from day 1 to day 15 and medroxyprogesterone acetate (MPA) 10 mg/day was given from day 16 to day 28 for three consecutive periods. The first mifepristone pill was taken on the first day of the first cycle and on the day after the last MPA pill in subsequent cycles.
[b]The endometrial biopsy was taken during the third treatment cycle, 6–9 days after initiating MPA treatment (LH+0 to LH+6).

drawal bleeding. The effects of this treatment on ovarian function have been tested administering mifepristone in combination with medroxyprogesterone acetate or norethindrone (Kekkonen et al. 1990, 1993, 1995). A more recent study assessing endometrial development (Croxatto et al., unpublished) found secretory changes induced by the progestin, but endometrial development was impaired (Table 2). As shown in Fig. 5, regular bleeding episodes, associated with progestin withdrawal and resumption of the antiprogestin treatment, were observed in all cases (Croxatto et al., unpublished).

None of the schedules tested so far complied with the required high efficacy to inhibit ovulation, for a contraceptive based only on ovulation suppression. However, it is likely the effects of this regimen on the endometrium may protect women from the risk of pregnancy if the observed endometrial alterations are sufficient to inhibit implantation in the ovulatory cycles.

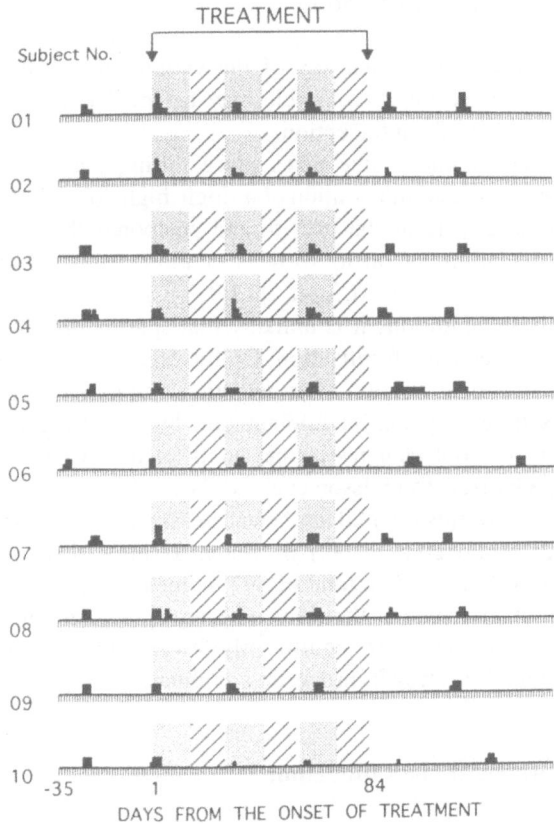

Fig. 5. Bleeding pattern during antiprogestin–progestin sequential treatment. Mifepristone 5 mg/day was given from day 1 to day 15 (*shaded area*) followed by medroxyprogesterone acetate 10 mg/day on days 16–28 (*hatched area*) for 84 days. High case at the bottom of each time line indicates bleeding and low case indicates spotting. Note that withdrawal bleeding was somewhat less predictable at the end of the third course of treatment (subjects 05, 06, 09, and 10), when medroxyprogesterone acetate withdrawal was not followed by mifepristone because of study design

12.4.2 Postcoital Contraception

Another approach, in which any of the various effects that antiprogestins have on the menstrual cycle may be involved, is their use in
emergency postcoital contraception.

If unprotected intercourse takes place during the middle or late
follicular phase, the administration of a single high dose of mifepristone
at this time arrests follicular growth and postpones the gonadotropin
surge and ovulation for up to 10 days or more, with the consequent
prolongation of the cycle (Liu et al. 1987; Croxatto and Salvatierra
1988). In these conditions it is unlikely that spermatozoa will survive
long enough to achieve fertilization. On the other hand, if unprotected
intercourse occurs at or soon after ovulation, mifepristone administration at this time may inhibit implantation by impairing endometrial
development without changes in the length of the cycle, as has been
reported by Gemzell-Danielsson et al. (1994).

The efficacy of this method has been assessed in two studies (Glasier
et al. 1992; Webb et al. 1992) in which a single dose of 600 mg
mifepristone was given to a total of 597 women within 72 h of unprotected intercourse. None of the women became pregnant with this treatment, and side effects were significantly fewer than with those of the
standard high dose estrogen-progestin combination.

12.4.3 Expected Menses Induction

The administration of antiprogestin at the time of expected menses,
regardless of whether or not implantation has occurred, is another mo-
dality of potential contraception in which endometrial functioning is
involved. Since the integrity of the endometrium depends on the action
of progesterone, it seems likely that by giving an antiprogestin, monthly,
before menses, endometrial bleeding with complete shedding of this
tissue may occur.

Administration of mifepristone 100 mg/day for 4 days in the late
luteal phase for three successive cycles to nonpregnant women induced
bleeding 30–48 h after the ingestion of the first dose, without disrupting
the menstrual rhythm or the hormonal profile (Croxatto et al. 1987).
When simulated early pregnancy was achieved, by giving exogenous

human chorionic gonadotropin (hCG), the administration of mifepristone, 100 mg/day from on days 12–15 after the LH surge, induced bleeding despite the high circulating estradiol and progesterone levels subsequent to hCG treatment (Croxatto et al. 1985).

Several studies have tested the efficacy of this approach (Ulmann 1987; van Santen and Haspels 1987; Lähteenmäki et al. 1988; Dubois et al. 1988; Couzinet et al. 1990). Mifepristone was given monthly as a single dose of 600 or 400 mg 1 day before the expected menses, or 100 mg for 4 consecutive days in the late luteal phase to women who had experienced unprotected intercourse during the midcycle. Pregnancy continued after treatment in 17%–19% of the subjects who had detectable levels of hCG. This failure rate is similar to that of mifepristone when used after missed menses to interrupt pregnancy without prostaglandins (Baulieu 1989; Van Look and von Hertzen 1995).

12.5 Conclusions

The concept of endometrial contraception is closely associated with the ability of antiprogestins to interfere with progesterone action on the endometrium. The contraceptive potential of antiprogestins based on this concept is only beginning to be explored. Several modalities in terms of mode of use and mode of action appear feasible, but in fact only one compound, mifepristone, has been tested in phase II trials in the modalities of single administration in the early or late luteal-phase administration or expected menses induction, and emergency contraception.

At low doses, mifepristone compares favorably with existing oral contraceptives in terms of subjective side effects. In spite of this advantage antiprogestins are unlikely to replace existing hormonal contraceptives but will expand the options of users.

Acknowledgments. Previously unreported work on the sequential regimen was supported by the Contraceptive Research and Development Program (CONRAD), and on continuous minidose was supported by the WHO Special Program of Research, Development and Research Training in Human Reproduction (project WHO/HRP 92017).

References

Batista MC, Cartledge TP, Zellmer AW, Merino MJ, Axiotis C, Loriaux L, Nieman LK (1992) Delayed endometrial maturation induced by daily administration of the antiprogestin RU 486: a potential new contraceptive strategy. Am J Obstet Gynecol 167:60–65

Baulieu EE (1989) Contragestion and other clinical applications of RU486, an antiprogesterone at the receptor. Science 245:1351–1357

Beck CA, Weigel NL, Moyer ML, Nordeen SK, Edwards DP (1993) The progesterone antagonist RU486 acquires agonist activity upon stimulation of cAMP signaling pathways. Proc Natl Acad Sci USA 90:4441–4445

Beier-Hellwig K, Sterzik K, Bonn B, Beier HM (1989) Contribution to the physiology and pathology of endometrial receptivity: the determination of protein patterns in human uterine secretions. Hum Reprod 4:115–120

Beier-Hellwig K, Sterzik K, Bonn B, Hilmes U, Bygdeman M, Gemzell-Danielsson K, Beier HM (1994) Hormone regulation and hormone antagonist effect on protein patterns of human endometrial secretion during receptivity. Ann N Y Acad Sci 734:143–156

Berthois Y, Salat-Baroux J, Cornet D, De Brux J, Kopp F, Martin PM (1991) A multiparametric analysis of endometrial estrogen and progesterone receptors after the postovulatory administration of mifepristone. Fertil Steril 55:547–554

Brandon DB, Bethea CL, Strawn EY, Novy MJ, Burry KA, Harrington BS, Erickson TE, Warner C, Keenan EJ, Clinton GM (1993) Progesterone receptor messenger ribonucleic acid and protein are overexpressed in human uterine leiomyomas. Am J Obstet Gynecol 169:78–85

Brenner RM, Slayden OVD (1994) Oestrogen action in the endometrium and oviduct of rhesus monkeys during RU486 treatment. Hum Reprod 9 [Suppl 1]:82–97

Cameron ST, Critchley HOD, Buckley CH, Kelly RW, Baird DT (1995) Effects of post-ovulatory administration of two antiprogestins (mifepristone and onapristone) on the differentiation of a secretory endometrium. J Reprod Fertil (Abstr Ser) 16:22

Chwalisz K, Hsiu JG, Williams RF, Hodgen GD (1992) Evaluation of the antiproliferative actions of the progesterone antagonists mifepristone (RU486) and onapristone (ZK98299) on primate endometrium. 39th annual meeting of the Society for Gynecologic Investigation, p 317, abstract no 417

Couzinet B, Le Strat N, Silvestre L, Schaison G (1990) Late luteal administration of the antiprogesterone RU486 in normal women: effects on the menstrual cycle events and fertility control in a long-term study. Fertil Steril 54:1039–1044

Croxatto HB, Salvatierra AM (1988) Effects of RU486 on the menstrual cycle. In: Puri CP, van Look PFA (eds) Hormone antagonists for fertility regulation. Indian Society for the Study of Reproduction and Fertility, India, p 141–153

Croxatto HB, Spitz IM, Salvatierra AM, Bardin CW (1985) The demonstration of the antiprogestin effects of RU486 when administered to human during hCG-induced pseudopregnancy. In: Baulieu EE, Segal SJ (eds) The antiprogestin steroids RU486 and human fertility control. Plenum, New York, p 263–269

Croxatto HB, Salvatierra AM, Romero C, Spitz IM (1987) Late luteal phase administration of RU486 for three successive cycles does not disrupt bleeding patterns or ovulation. J Clin Endocrinol Metab 65:1272–1277

Croxatto HB, Salvatierra AM, Croxatto HD, Fuentealba B (1993) Effects of continuous treatment with low dose mifepristone throughout one menstrual cycle. Hum Reprod 8:201–207

Dubois C, Ulmann A and Baulieu EE (1988) Contragestion with late luteal administration of RU486 (Mifepristone). Fertil Steril 50: 593–596

Feil PD, Clarke CL, Satyaswaroop PG (1988) Progestin-mediated changes in progesterone receptor forms in the normal human endometrium. Endocrinology 123:2506–2513

Gemzell-Danielsson K, Swahn ML, Svalander P, Bygdeman M (1993) Early luteal phase treatment with mifepristone (RU486) for fertility regulation. Hum Reprod 8:870–873

Gemzell-Danielsson K, Svalander P, Swahn ML, Johannisson E and Bygdeman M (1994) Effects of a single post-ovulatory dose of RU486 on endometrial maturation in the implantation phase. Hum Reprod 9:2398–2404

Ghosh D, Sengupta J (1993) Anti-nidatory effect of a single, early post-ovulatory administration of mifepristone (RU486) in the rhesus monkey. Hum Reprod 8:552–558

Glasier A, Thong KJ, Dewar M, Mackie M, Baird DT (1992) Mifepristone (RU486) compared with high-dose estrogen and progestogen for emergency postcoital contraception. N Engl J Med 327:1041–1044

Graham RA, Li T-C, Seif MW, Aplin JD, Cooke ID (1991) The effects of the antiprogesterone RU486 (mifepristone) on an endometrial secretory glycan: an immunocytochemical study. Fertil Steril 55:1132–1136

Gravanis A, Schaison G, George M, de Brux J, Satyaswaroop PG, Baulieu EE, Robel P (1985) Endometrial and pituitary responses to the steroidal antiprogestin RU 486 in postmenopausal women. J Clin Endocrinol Metab 60:156–163

Greene KE, Kettel LM, Yen SS (1992) Interruption of endometrial maturation without hormonal changes by an antiprogesterone during the first half of luteal phase of the menstrual cycle: a contraceptive potential. Fertil Steril 58:338–343

Haluska GJ, West NB, Novy MJ, Brenner RM (1990) Uterine estrogen receptors are increased by RU486 in late pregnant rhesus macaques but not after
spontaneous labor. J Clin Endocrinol Metab 70:181–186
Horwitz KB, Tung L, Takimoto GS (1995) Novel mechanisms of antiprogestin
action. J Steroid Biochem Mol Biol 53:9–17
Ishwad PC, Katkam RR, Hinduja IN, Chwalisz K, Elger W, Puri CP (1993)·
Treatment with a progesterone antagonist ZK 98.299 delays endometrial
development without blocking ovulation in bonnet monkeys. Contraception
48:57–70
Katkam RR, Gopalkrishnan K, Chwalisz K, Schillinger E, Puri CP (1995)
Onapristone (ZK 98.299): a potential antiprogestin for endometrial contra-
ception. Am J Obstet Gynecol 173:779–787
Kekkonen R, Alfthan H, Haukkamaa M, Heikinheimo O, Luukkainen T,
Lähteenmäki P (1990) Interference with ovulation by sequential treatment
with the antiprogesterone RU486 and synthetic progestin. Fertil Steril
53:747–750
Kekkonen R, Lähteenmäki P, Luukkainen T, Tuominen J (1993) Sequential
regimen of the antiprogesterone RU486 and synthetic progestin for contraception. Fertil Steril 60:610–615
Kekkonen R, Croxatto HB, Lähteenmäki, Salvatierra AM, Tuominen J (1995)
Effects of intermittent antiprogestin RU486 combined with cyclic medroxyprogesterone acetate on folliculogenesis and ovulation. Hum Reprod
10:287–292
Klein-Hitpass L, Cato A, Henderson D, Ryffel G (1993) Two types of antiprogestins identified by their differential action in transcriptionally active extracts for T47D cells. Nucleic Acids Res 19:1227–1234
Lähteenmäki P, Rapeli T, Kääriäinen M, Alfthan H, Ylikorkala O (1988) Late
postcoital treatment against pregnancy with antiprogesterone RU 486. Fertil
Steril 50:36–38
Lessey BA (1994) The use of integrins for the assessment of uterine receptivity. Fertil Steril 61:812–814
Lessey BA, Damjanovich L, Coutifaris C, Castelbaum A, Albeda SM, Buck
CA (1992) Integrin adhesion molecules in the human endometrium. Correlation with the normal and abnormal menstrual cycle. J Clin Invest
90:188–195
Li TC, Dockery P, Thomas P, Rogers AW, Lenton EA, Cooke ID (1988) The
effects of progesterone receptor blockade in the luteal phase of normal fertile women. Fertil Steril 50:732–742
Liu JH, Garzo G, Morris S, Stuenkel C, Ulmann A, Yen SSC (1987) Disruption of follicular maturation and delay of ovulation after administration of
the antiprogesterone RU486. J Clin Endocrinol Metab 65:1135–1140

McDonnell DP, Goldman ME (1994) RU486 exerts antiestrogenic activities through a novel progesterone receptor A form-mediated mechanism. J Biol Chem 269:11945–11949

Navot D, Scott RT, Droesch K, Veeck LL, Liu H-C, Rosenwaks Z (1991) The window of embryo transfer and the efficiency of human conception in vitro. Fertil Steril 55:114–118

Neulen J, Williams RF, Hodgen GD (1990) RU 486 (mifepristone): induction of dose dependent elevations of estradiol receptor in endometrium from ovariectomized monkeys. J Clin Endocrinol Metab 71:1074–1075

Philibert D, Deraedt R, Tournemine C, Mary I, Teutsch G (1982) RU38486 – a potent antiprogesterone. Proceedings of the 6th international congress of hormone steroids, Jerusalem, abstract no 204

Puri CP, Katkam RR, Vadigoppula AD, Gopalakrishnan K, Elger WA, Billimoria FR, Patil RK (1992) Contraceptive potential of an antiprogestin ZK 98.734: reversal of ZK 98.734-induced blockade of folliculogenesis with FSH and LH and their differential effects in bonnet monkeys. Indian J Exp Biol 30:987–995

Schaison G, George M, Lestrat N, Reinberg A, Baulieu EE (1985) Efects of the antiprogesterone steroid RU486 during midluteal phase in normal women. J Clin Endocrinol Metab 61:484–489

Shoupe D, Mishell DR Jr, Lähteenmäki P, Heikinheimo O, Birgerson L, Madkour H, Spitz IM (1987) Effects of the antiprogesterone RU486 in normal women. I. Single-dose administration in the midluteal phase. Am J Obstet Gynecol 157:1415–1420

Slayden OD, Hirst JJ, Brenner RM (1993) Estrogen action in the reproductive tract of rhesus monkeys during antiprogestin treatment. Endocrinology 132:1845–1856

Swahn ML, Bygdeman M, Cekan S, Xing S, Masironi B, Johannisson E (1990) The effect of RU486 administered during the early luteal phase on bleeding pattern, hormonal parameters and endometrium. Hum Reprod 5:402–408

Tabibzadeh S (1992) Patterns of expression of integrin molecules in human endometrium throughout the menstrual cycle. Hum Reprod 7:876–882

Ulmann A (1987) Uses of RU486 for contragestion: an update. Contraception 36 [Suppl]:27–31

Van Look PFA, von Hertzen H (1995) Clinical uses of antiprogestins. Hum Reprod Update 1:19–34

van Santen ME, Haspels AA (1987) Interception IV: failure of mifepristone (RU486) as a monthly contragestive, lunarette. Contraception 35:433–438

Webb AMC, Russell J, Elstein M (1992) Comparison of Yuzpe regimen, danazol, and mifepristone (RU486) in oral postcoital contraception. Br Med J 305:927–931

Wolf JP, Hsiu JG, Anderson TL, Ulmann A, Baulieu EE, Hodgen GD (1989) Noncompetitive antiestrogenic effect of RU486 in blocking the estrogen-stimulated luteinizing hormone surge and the proliferative action of estradiol on endometrium in castrate monkeys. Fertil Steril 52:1055–1060

Subject Index

Ernst Schering Research Foundation Workshop

Editors: Günter Stock
Ursula-F. Habenicht

This series will be available on request from
Ernst Schering Research Foundation, 13342 Berlin, Germany